Athlete First
A History of the Paralympic Movement

Athlete First
A History of the Paralympic Movement

Steve Bailey
Winchester College, UK

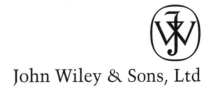

John Wiley & Sons, Ltd

Copyright © 2008   John Wiley & Sons Ltd, The Atrium, Southern Gate, Chichester,
West Sussex PO19 8SQ, England

Telephone (+44) 1243 779777

Email (for orders and customer service enquiries): cs-books@wiley.co.uk
Visit our Home www.wiley.com

Other Wiley Editorial Offices

John Wiley & Sons Inc., 111 River Street, Hoboken, NJ 07030, USA

Jossey-Bass, 989 Market Street, San Francisco, CA 94103-1741, USA

Wiley-VCH Verlag GmbH, Boschstr. 12, D-69469 Weinheim, Germany

John Wiley & Sons Australia Ltd, 33 Park Road, Milton, Queensland 4064, Australia

John Wiley & Sons (Asia) Pte Ltd, 2 Clementi Loop #02-01, Jin Xing Distripark, Singapore 129809

John Wiley & Sons Canada Ltd, 6045 Freemont Blvd, Mississauga, Ontario, L5R 4J3

Wiley also publishes its books in a variety of electronic formats. Some content that appears
in print may not be available in electronic books.

Library of Congress Cataloging-in-Publication Data

Bailey, Steve.
    Athlete first : a history of the paralympic movement / Steve Bailey.
       p. cm.
    ISBN 978-0-470-05824-4
    1. Special Olympics—History.   2. Paralympics—History.   3. Sports for people with disabilities.
    4. Athletes with disabilities.   I. Title.
    GV722.5.S64B35 2007
    796.087′4—dc22

                                                                        2007024559

British Library Cataloguing in Publication Data

A catalogue record for this book is available from the British Library

ISBN: 978-0-470-05824-4

Typeset in 10/12 Times by Integra Software Services Pvt Ltd. Pondicherry, India
Printed and bound in Great Britain by Antony Rowe Ltd, Chippenham, Wiltshire.
This book is printed on acid-free paper responsibly manufactured from sustainable forestry
in which at least two trees are planted for each one used for paper production.

To Paula,
Tim, Will and Rosie

Contents

Figures and Boxes

FIGURES

BOXES

Foreword

Sir Philip Craven

President of the International Paralympic Committee

The International Paralympic Committee (IPC) is one of the largest and most dynamic sport organizations in the world; with a constituency that comprises the vast majority of athletes with a disability. The IPC's democratic structure has ensured the centrality of the athlete since its inception in 1989.

This is the first published history of the Paralympic Movement, presenting a detailed examination from the early enthusiasms of different groups and individuals to the creation of the International Paralympic Committee, and the IPC's first fifteen years of operation. Although there has been a growing body of work in a number of areas of sport science, sport for athletes with a disability has not so far received comparable attention from historians. This study goes some way towards bridging that gap.

Bringing this rigorous study of the Paralympic Movement to fruition has been the undertaking of Dr Steve Bailey, a respected historian and author. The enormous volume of material that Dr Bailey has worked with has been provided willingly by the IPC, as well as additional resources being put at his disposal by the International Olympic Committee. The author has provided the perspective of an outside observer, and the synthesis and interpretations are entirely those of the author. But many others have given their time and support to advise on points of accuracy and fill in gaps where the written record is incomplete.

This project has arisen out of the relationship between the International Paralympic Committee, the International Olympic Committee and the International Council of Sport Science and Physical Education, and it is this strength of cooperation that will continue to promote the objectives of bringing sporting opportunities to all athletes with a disability.

Foreword

Prof. Dr Gudrun Doll-Tepper

President of the International Council of Sport Science and Physical Education

What started as a formal meeting between the then President of the International Olympic Committee (IOC), Juan Antonio Samaranch and myself in 1997 about the lack of a documented history of the Paralympic Movement, developed into an international collaborative project, bringing together three of the world's major sports bodies. The International Council of Sport Science and Physical Education (ICSSPE) proposed a project to the IOC that would see, for the first time, an in-depth collation of the activities, challenges and achievements that have made the Paralympic Movement what it is today.

Athlete First: A History of the Paralympic Movement is the result of this project. Dr. Steve Bailey, a scholar recognised by the International Olympic Committee, has compiled not only the most extensive history of the Paralympic Movement, but also an honest and thought provoking account of the development of the IPC from the first Stoke Mandeville Games in 1948 and the aspirations of Sir Ludwig Guttmann, through to the first Paralympic Summer Games in 1960, the formation of the IPC in 1989 and the Paralympic Games in 2004 in Athens. Personalities who have enabled the Paralympic Movement to grow are seen close-up, as they worked to establish this very special movement.

Athlete First is also filled with stimulating stories and drama, which is to be expected when such a huge collection of individuals comes together to progress an ideal. What is most inspirational is how divergence is overcome and the collective commitment of individuals keeps the IPC working toward their vision 'to enable Paralympic athletes to achieve sporting excellence and inspire and excite the world'. The extensive work that the IPC does in development of sporting opportunities at the grass-roots is also testament to how complex and engaging the organisation is. It is certainly not before time that the whole world can get to know this through reading *Athlete First*.

The book has received the full backing of the International Paralympic Committee, where the author was given unrestricted access to all minutes of meetings and archives of the International Paralympic Committee, as well as being welcomed as an accredited scholar at the International Olympic Committee's research centre in Lausanne, for which I would like to express my sincere gratitude to both organisations.

I commend this book to you and would like to declare my honour at having been involved in such a valuable and inspiring project. Steve has done a magnificent job and I offer him my whole-hearted thanks at taking on such an all-consuming task.

International Council of Sport Science and Physical Education (ICSSPE)

2008 marks the 50th Anniversary of the International Council of Sport Science (ICSSPE). Since 1958, ICSSPE has been connecting professionals in all disciplines of sport science and physical education. As a result of its initiatives, ICSSPE is recognised as a Formal Associate of UNESCO. It has held this status since 1997, not only for its past history of major contributions, but also for its ongoing ability to contribute effectively to UNESCO's ongoing objectives. As a further testament to the importance and relevance of its goals, ICSSPE is also a recognised organisation of the International Olympic Committee (IOC) and cooperates with the World Health Organization.

ICSSPE provides its members with a wide range of benefits, as part of its network encouraging international cooperation in all areas of sport science and physical education, and actively promotes the practical application of innovative research in these fields.

In 1995, the International Paralympic Committee (IPC) joined ICSSPE, and since then, the two organisations have collaborated successfully on a number of activities, for example, with publications like ICSSPE's May 2002 *Bulletin* no.35 focusing primarily on 'The Paralympic Movement and the 2007 *Perspectives* no. 7 addressing 'Sport for Persons with a Disability'.

Another one of these activities is ICSSPE's major Sports Science Congress, which has taken place immediately prior to the summer games in its host country since the 1972 Olympic Games in Munich, Germany. In 2004, ICSSPE, the IPC, FIMS (International Federation of Sports Medicine), and the IOC agreed to form a partnership to have the top four international sport organisations working together to support and organise this regular congress, the International Convention on Science, Education and Medicine in Sport (ICSEMIS) 2008.

ICSSPE looks forward to another healthy 50 years in active cooperation with its members like the IPC, and to continue to be at the forefront of social change through the use of sport and physical activity.

For more information, please visit us at www.icsspe.org.

Preface

My purpose has been to trace and interpret the phenomenon that has become the Paralympic Movement; how it came into being, and how it has served the needs and ambitions of athletes with a disability from its beginnings in the middle of the 20th century. The later period of study has necessarily focused on the development of the International Paralympic Committee, now providing the biggest global sporting phenomenon for athletes with a disability. Recognising that an organisation such as the International Paralympic Committee is far more than the sum of its administrative parts, I have sought to include much personal and anecdotal information through interviews and correspondence, as well as the study of thousands of documents. Often in the growth of the Paralympic Movement, differing views have promoted quarrels; sometimes people working together may appear to have been obstinate or even self-promoting. But my interpretation of the many forms of evidence I have seen and heard is that the development and advancement of ideas has been made possible by the interaction of highly dedicated individuals passionately expressing their vision of the future for athletes with a disability. Much of the time this has meant that they have challenged established barriers to access and societal structures. It was Oscar Wilde who welcomed this sort of conflict as encouraging growth: 'Disobedience, in the eyes of anyone who has read history, is man's original virtue. It is through disobedience and rebellion that progress has been made.'

Although it has been possible to record many examples of the tireless work of a number of individuals and international organisations, I need to apologise for the inevitable omissions. We can only show a sample of the type of dedication that has been evident in the growth of the Paralympic Movement.

One overriding point is that my research has had to draw on thousands of pages of documentary evidence, and that I have inevitably had to interpret both meaning and value to this study with relatively little opportunity to recreate the precise historical context in which these records were made. The errors and omissions are mine, as are the interpretations. I have had the benefit of many hours of sage advice from people involved with all aspects of the Paralympic Movement. But this is still not the same as experiencing the meetings and the events first-hand. The International Paralympic Committee agreed to give me access to more recent documents only with a written agreement on the specific use of the material and the right of a factual review of the manuscript. I have been pleased to provide this, and this work has been improved as a result of the written comments subsequently provided by Phil Craven, Clare Wolfensohn, Leen Coudenys and Jean Stone. The opinions reflected in this book remain my own, as do the mistakes.

My thanks go to a number of people who have helped me make sense of the mass of documentation and opinion. In particular I would like to recognise the help offered by the following people: Christophe Maillet, Tamie Devine, Amandeep Chima, Susanne Reiff, Siân Ölschläger, Leen Coudenys, Nanami King, Horst Strohkendl, Tip Thiboutot, Phil Craven, Bob Steadward, Clare Wolfensohn and Jean Stone. Celia Carden at John Wiley & Sons, Ltd. has been a great supporter; I am grateful to Celia for her patience and advice in the final stages. Gudrun Doll-Tepper has remained a strong motivator, and it was her initial encouragement that got this project underway. I am grateful to Juan-Antonio Samaranch, who intervened personally to ensure that I had unfettered access in Lausanne to the IOC correspondence files and the normally closed minutes of IOC meetings. Without the extensive advice and scrutiny of draft chapters by Hans Lindström, Carl Wang and Bernard Atha, this text could not have been brought to life. Finally I must record my gratitude to Joan Scruton, who was willing to receive me with a cup of tea at her home on many occasions over a period of two years. Joan permitted me to record hours of interviews and to study a number of unpublished manuscripts that were in her possession. She was able to recount her many years of involvement with the Paralympic Movement with total accuracy: a fact later borne out by my scrutiny of the minutes of hundreds of meetings – I know which process I enjoyed more.

Throughout this study the many prestigious titles and honours of the people referred to have been omitted, not out of disrespect for the individuals concerned, but because this history has tried to deal with the people, and not the positions they have represented. Also, all spellings have been anglicised for the benefit of consistency.

This research project and subsequent publication has only been possible with the tolerance and support of my family: I am grateful to Paula, Tim, Will and Rosie for their patience and encouragement.

Steve Bailey
Winchester
2007

Abbreviations

ACOG	Atlanta Olympic Organising Committee
ANOC	Association of National Olympic Committees
APOC	Atlanta Paralympic Organising Committee
ATHOC	Athens Organising Committee
CAID	Commission for Inclusion of Athletes with a Disability
CFSOD	Canadian Federation of Sports Organisations for the Disabled
CISS	Comité International des Sports des Sourds / International Committee for Deaf Sports
COJO	Comité d'Organisation des Jeux Olympiques (French)
COOB	Comite Organizador Olimpico Barcelona
COPTA	Organising Committee for the Paralympics in Tignes Albertville
CP-ISRA	Cerebral Palsy – International Sports and Recreation Association
ECISOD	European Committee of the International Sports Organisation for the Disabled
EUROCOM	European Regional Committee of IPC
EUROPC	European Paralympic Committee
FESPIC	Far East and South Pacific Games for the Disabled
GAISF	General Association of International Sports Federations
IBSA	International Blind Sport Association
ICC	International Coordinating Committee of World Sports Organisations for the Disabled
ICSSPE	International Council of Sport Science and Physical Education
IF	international federation
IFAPA	International Federation for Adapted Physical Activity
IFSOD	International Federation of Sports Organisations for the Disabled
INAIL	Istituto Nazionale per l'Assicurazione contro Infortuni sul Lavoro
INAS-FID	International Sports Organization for Athletes with an Intellectual Disability
INAS-FMH	International Association for Sport for Persons with Mental Handicap
IOC	International Olympic Committee
IOSD	International organisations of sport for people with a disability
ISMGF	International Stoke Mandeville Games Federation
ISMWSF	International Stoke Mandeville Wheelchair Sports Federation
ISOD	International Sports Organisation for the Disabled
IWBF	International Wheelchair Basketball Association
LAOOC	Los Angeles Olympic Organising Committee
LPOC	Lillehammer Paralympic Organising Committee
NAPOC	Nagano Paralympic Organising Committee
NBA	National Basketball Association
NGOs	Non-governmental organisations
NWAA	National Wheelchair Athletic Association

NWBA	National Wheelchair Basketball Association
ONCE	Organisatión Nacional de Ciegos Españoles
SANROC	South African Non-Racial Olympic Committee
SCEC	Sports Council Executive Committee
SLOC	Salt Lake Organising Committee
SPOC	Seoul Paralympic Organising Committee or Sydney Paralympics Organising Committee
USOC	United States Olympic Committee
WCWB	World Council for the Welfare of the Blind
WVF	World Veterans' Federation

CHAPTER 1

A Showcase of Ability

It's all about discovery. My discovery is that Swimming opened the door to everything: first it gave me freedom, then a place in society (Béatrice Hess, France, IPC Brochure 2004)

INTRODUCTION: NO EXCUSES, NO LIMITS

For anyone who has witnessed the determination of athletes striving to push themselves beyond their own limits it is quite easy to understand how competitive sport can play such a key part in the life of an individual with a disability. There are more opportunities for accomplishment of personal goals through sport than in many other aspects of life, and sport certainly can change the way other people see us. For some persons with a disability competitive sport provides a vehicle for levelling out some of the inequalities that are faced day-to-day. But for everyone it is thrilling, fun and satisfying.

This book attempts to examine the route through which the Paralympic Movement has advanced. On its way to the present day we will see personal crusades, conflict and consensus. But the overriding message is one of heartfelt enthusiasm to make a difference. This study should allow us to understand something of the early sacrifices and successes of a small group of people, but it will also trace the emergence of a highly complex worldwide organisation, the International Paralympic Committee. In this sense it is both an institutional history and a weaving together of several biographies. The sketching of the personalities is vitally important to our understanding of the emergence of the modern phenomenon.

The Paralympic Movement effectively began with the recreational and rehabilitative use of sport for persons with a disability, turning gradually into a broad-based pyramid of competitive sport that has ultimately led to the elite level of the Paralympic Games. The philosophy of the Paralympic Movement is one of self-realisation through competitive sport. The expression of personal determination and the exploration of one's own boundaries are there for those brave enough to commit themselves.

The Paralympic Movement has developed over the last fifty years to become the pinnacle of achievement for athletes with a disability. Ludwig Guttmann, a German neurosurgeon who had established the Stoke Mandeville Spinal Injuries Unit in Aylesbury in 1944, used sport as part of a process of rehabilitation for patients with spinal injuries. As his employment of competitive physical activity became more sophisticated, he also saw the benefits of drawing people with similar injuries together: sport enabling individuals to meet and strive for 'normal' goals. As the first Stoke Mandeville Games coincided with the opening day of the Olympic Games being held in London in 1948, the parallel with the Olympic Games was drawn. Today the Paralympic Movement is recognised as a global

Athlete First: A History of the Paralympic Movement Steve Bailey
© 2008 John Wiley & Sons, Ltd

sporting phenomenon: a wonderful celebration of competitive physical activity that fuels dreams, encouraging many to participation and to excellence.

THE INTERNATIONAL PARALYMPIC COMMITTEE

The International Paralympic Committee was formed in 1989 out of the earlier cooperation of several international organisations looking to stabilise and extend the world of elite sport for persons with a disability. These organisations have had their own colourful and distinct histories, and their full genesis is beyond the scope of this study. However it is essential to understand how these organisations have moved towards a vision of international elite sport for individuals with disabilities. The International Paralympic Committee now organises the Paralympic Winter and Summer Games, as well as acting as the international federation for 12 sports – in which it also coordinates the World and Regional Championships. The successes of the IPC have allowed the organisation to target activities in developing countries, and to focus specifically on improving the participation levels of women with disabilities, and of those athletes with severe disabilities. 'Through sport, its ideals and activities the IPC seeks the continuous global promotion of the values of the Paralympic Movement, with a vision of inspiration and empowerment' (IPC 2004).

In the period after the end of the Second World War Ludwig Guttmann was involved in the institutionalisation of organisations serving the needs of persons with a disability other than those with spinal injuries, although he held a fiercely personal grip on organisations he had brought into being. Guttmann was instrumental in the promotion of sporting competition for athletes with disabilities, establishing the International Stoke Mandeville Games organisation. Work was being done in some European nations to provide for people who were blind and for amputees, but Guttmann was keen to hold off their entry into the Stoke Mandeville movement. He was later to be more broadly inclusive of people with other disabilities through the International Sports Organisation for the Disabled (ISOD).

As international federations strengthened partisanship towards the needs of their own population, they also built restrictions to access by others. In turn, this had a slowing effect on progress towards the wider acceptance on the world stage of elite sport for athletes with a disability. Major international non-governmental organisations (NGOs) have tended to encourage interest groups to get together and speak with one voice so as to ensure consistent and fair representation and support, as well as enabling these agencies to serve complete constituencies more effectively. This has been true of United Nations agencies and the International Olympic Committee (IOC). The Olympic Movement has always insisted on being able to respond to one lobby rather than receiving numerous different petitions for assistance or attention from groups with overlapping interests. Just as the IOC has sought to encourage a single umbrella organisation to represent sports science, it has also been instrumental in prompting confederacy among disability sports organisations. In 1982 an International Coordinating Committee of World Sports Organisations for the Disabled (ICC) was established, with the intention of 'speaking with one voice' with regard to sport for persons with a disability. This committee undertook the management of what became the Paralympic Games: international multi-disability world championships organised in conjunction with the timing and location of the Olympic Games cycle. Although the time was right for cooperation between the separate disability organisations, it was particularly the call of the International Olympic Committee for unity from within the organisations serving athletes with a disability that consolidated the actions that led to the foundation of the International Paralympic Committee. This was no impulsive act: national organisations wished to create a sport-specific organisation rather than a disability-specific one. The national organisations also drove the movement towards a democratic structure. The International Paralympic Committee is the most prominent evidence of success in drawing the early development of elite disability sport into a fully coordinated world organisation.

Certain issues regularly became focal points as the international organisations were establishing themselves and as the movement progressed towards a single international body for athletes with disability: among them whether representation should be based on disability, sport or country; and whether classification of athletes for competition should be medical/anatomical or functional. These issues emerged in the historical context of the development of sport for those with disabilities. It is inevitable in preparing a history of the Paralympic Movement that the emphasis will change as we move through time: new problems arise and new horizons permit fresh setting of targets. The early pioneers brought their own specialisations to the attention of a larger audience, inevitably inviting a smaller section of the population into the limelight for a time – until ideas broadened and others worked to help bring the same benefits to their particular population. In this respect sport for people in wheelchairs was in the public eye earlier than some other sporting opportunities for persons with other disabilies.

The reasons for prominence of one particular group are not always easy to pinpoint. Sometimes it can result from the particular drive and commitment of an appropriately poised individual; sometimes the regional or national political environment can suit the emergence of a dominant influence. Conspiracy theories have pointed to Eurocentric attitudes of colonialism being historically at the root of all successful international sporting organisations: 'arrogantly teaching the world how to play'. Certainly some chance is likely to contribute to the circumstances being right for initiatives to become wholly supported in society – particularly where more marginalised populations have been concerned. It is essential to explore the background to these localised energies so as to understand better the emerging picture of the Paralympic Movement. Inevitably there are difficulties in ascribing meaning and determining the prime movers in a diverse subject such as this, and it is best to emphasise that no particular merit is intentionally being bestowed on individual participants in the process. Adaptation and emulation are the means of progress, and international sport for persons with a disability has benefited from the nebulous identities of groups with different needs. By definition the pursuit of sporting excellence within particular populations will always require some reassessment of established concepts relating to elite sport and international competition.

Funding and research recognition will inevitably affect the progress and development of highly specialised areas of sports science. The impact of the Paralympic Movement has been far-reaching in its effects on attitudes towards all those persons with a disability. Governments have addressed aspects of educational reform, accessibility and prejudice against disability in recent decades. Seeing elite athletes on a world stage promotes an inclusive stance towards all members of society, helping to bring down barriers.

Today, the International Paralympic Committee is the principal force for the Paralympic Movement, identifying as its vision: 'To enable paralympic athletes to achieve sporting excellence and inspire and excite the world'. The IPC seeks to enable athletes with a disability to be involved with decisions about their own future, to maintain a sports-centred organisation and to provide the appropriate opportunities for the development of all athletes – from early stages through to elite levels. To capture the essence of these aims the International Paralympic Committee introduced a new Paralympic Motto: 'Spirit in Motion' (IPC 2003).

QUALIFICATION, ELIGIBILITY AND CLASSIFICATION

It has been natural for organisations to define eligibility so as to provide for 'fair' competition. Classification in sport for those with disability has a similar basis to the early distinctions made between the amateur and the professional athlete in Olympic sport in the early 20th century: participants wished to compete against those with similar opportunities and against those with similar limitations, so that competition itself was meaningful – a victory or defeat had significance. In the creation of structures and definitions for classification in disability sport, as identified by Ludwig Guttmann just after the Second World War, there was also the inevitable development of barriers to access. Qualification meant distinction and also exclusion. Guttmann logically encouraged competitive sports events among former patients of spinal units. Others followed Guttmann's model and took the institutionalised system of sporting participation back to their own countries and units after spending time at Stoke Mandeville. Using disability categories to specify who could and who could not compete necessarily excluded certain athletes who did not fit into a particular classification. The motive of clarity also brought a greater difficulty in moving towards integration within sports movements, although segregation was a by-product and was not usually intentional.

THE 'MEDICAL MODEL OF DISABILITY' VERSUS THE 'SOCIAL MODEL OF DISABILITY'

Before embarking on an examination of how the Paralympic Movement has emerged to become the world phenomenon that it is today, it is important to understand the nature of disability in society.

From centuries past it had been common to treat persons with a disability in terms of those requiring medical cure, rehabilitation or segregation from the rest of 'normal' society. This legacy has been called the 'medical model' of disability, and it was commonly sustained until only a few years ago. This model (also sometimes called the 'individual model') relies on a designation of a person in terms of negative classification – disability prevents a person from functioning within society. The inability of people to participate fully in society is seen in terms of their disability. The humanity of individuals becomes subordinated to their disability.

More appropriate to us today is the 'social model' of disability: individuals' impairment becomes a disability when the organisation of society prevents them from participating fully. This could be in relation to access, mobility, communication or other barriers. So, in the social model of disability, a distinction is made between 'impairment' and 'disability'. Impairment is considered to be a long-term limitation of body function, structure or physical appearance that has usually been caused by illness, injury or a congenital condition. Disability is defined as the loss of opportunity to function equally with others because of impediments put in their way either by the environment or by the way society is structured. The World Health Organization's Action Plan for Disabilities and Rehabilitation 2006–2011 defines 'disability' as: 'the outcome or result of a complex relationship between an individual's health condition and personal factors, and of the external factors that represent the circumstances in which the individual lives'. Effectively, society causes the disablement of those individuals who are impaired in some way. Inflexibility in organisational policies can be a barrier to enabling normal functioning of persons with a disability in society, as can cultural representations that patronise or dehumanise. In the social model disability is necessarily a political concept.

DISABLING BARRIERS AND THE ROLE OF COMPETITIVE SPORT

There can be no doubt that sport has the power to bind people together, make them feel as though they belong and create 'community'. The many positive benefits sport has to offer all individuals are even more meaningful to persons with a disability. Motivation and socialisation are obvious rewards to add to health maintenance. For many people sport has provided levels of freedom that have not been normally experienced by them, due to barriers, ignorance and prejudice. Sport can offer a means of navigating past the barriers that have limited participation in other facets of their lives. For many people sport has given new goals and targets that have lifted them out of a sometimes unwelcoming environment. The high profile of the Paralympic Movement has served to force communities to address questions of accessibility and inclusion for persons with a disability. In more recent years this could mean that a career path has opened up through sport, but for most individuals sport has helped physical and mental well being.

As changes in policy and legislation have come into effect, society has become more accepting of persons with a disability, but this has not been enough. Compliance with what is required does not in itself lead to changes in attitude. The difference is made by active provision of opportunities, inclusion of all individuals in communities as citizens.

Language Defines and Restricts

Concrete change in use of language has been encouraged in the past decade, bringing people's attention to removing seldom-considered negative connotations. Language and ascribed meaning are relentlessly evolving. Value systems also continuously change, causing a need for redefinition of what is meant by particular words and phrases. A phrase from the past becomes a hackneyed cliché with familiarity and overuse. The worst prejudices and misunderstandings in society have frequently been exacerbated by particular use of language, perpetuating myths that have affected the treatment of marginalised groups. Resolute campaigning in many quarters in more recent years has led to a change in the way language is used to refer to persons with a disability. Labels can generalise and stigmatise so that differences become problematic. Certainly labels can dehumanise. Stigma can imply threat, inferiority, or that the 'different' individual does not deserve the same levels of courtesy and consideration as other people. As Goffman (1963) explained, stigma could act to be socially discrediting and to exclude individuals from acceptance in society. Stereotypes are reinforced through language that confines definition of persons in terms of their disability, rather than recognising the humanity of individuals in their own right. Apprehension and misunderstanding have blighted the progress of persons with a disability.

The currently preferred principle is to use positive, 'people-first' language when referring to individuals with disabilities. It is more appropriate to refer to the person first and to the impairment afterwards – if it is relevant to do so at all. So terms such as 'crippled', 'afflicted', 'suffering from', 'wheelchair-bound' and 'handicapped' are considered negative, and are to be discouraged. A wheelchair provides the mobility that can be enabling, rather than 'binding'. Putting people first means recognising the value of people as individuals, rather than patronisingly defining them in terms of their disability. 'Disabled people', therefore, are referred to as 'persons with a disability'. Political correctness in language can have its own problems, however. The purpose of being politically correct is reportedly to reduce the chance of offending others. Politically correct language can still apply labels and it can ignore individuality. But it can signal an intent that is positive – effectiveness is in the understanding or in the actions rather than in the language. Respect can be conveyed through sensitivity. Appropriate and thoughtful use of language may avoid labelling altogether.

Not everyone agrees that the preoccupation with political correctness in language is a good thing: overdoing people-first language can be unacceptable to the very populations believed to benefit. In a reaction against the oversensitivity that had arisen, the US National Blind Federation passed a resolution in 1993 declaring that politically correct language 'does the exact opposite of what it purports to do since it is overly defensive, implies shame instead of true equality, and portrays the blind as touchy and belligerent' (Jernigan 1993). Some extensions to politically correct language can overreach their purpose and become condescending in their use: terms such as 'challenged' and 'differently able' might fall into this category. While society has made some effort to correct the wrongs of the past, it is essential to remember that individuals often see their disability as a crucially identifying feature of their persona. While the fact that individuals have a disability that causes some limitation of function is part of who they are, it should not affect society's attitudes towards them as individuals in the community.

READING AND WRITING A HISTORY OF THE PARALYMPIC MOVEMENT

In the discussions that follow it has been essential to make use of contemporary sources: principally documents and publications. Extensive support has been forthcoming from people who were involved in the events themselves, to corroborate the documentary evidence and to provide the necessary 'colour' that makes the Paralympic Movement what it is: a thriving and energetic celebration of sport for persons with a disability. In reflecting the evidence as accurately as possible, some outdated terminology used by the participants of the day has been retained, although this necessarily means that more recent sensitivities in language already discussed might be affronted. No offence is intended, only a wish to keep the language of the discussions accurate to the historical context in which they took place. It should become apparent to the reader that the central participants in the Paralympic Movement are much less constrained by the language used to describe their disability or social situation than are people who are trying to enter the debate from an external viewpoint. As this study heads towards analysis of the very recent past one might observe that the language being quoted from meetings, interviews and written evidence is often of a nature that would be judged not to be politically correct at all. Those involved do not tiptoe around their subject – they act with passion so as to affect change.

Paralympic Terminology

The employment of the term 'Paralympics' has been in dispute off and on for many years. It is interesting to look at the different ways that individuals and organisations have employed the term, and how they have explained its origins and meaning. The earliest users of the term for the quadrennial games tended to perceive 'para' as a prefix that was associated with paraplegia, combined with 'Olympic' – the association with the Olympic ideals in sporting distinction. As time progressed, the International Coordinating Committee moved towards a derivation that was coupled to the idea of 'para' as 'being attached to' or 'parallel to'– so accordingly the Paralympics were defined in terms of the broadened participation of disability groups in a sporting celebration timed to closely precede or follow the Olympic Games. The wish to aspire to the highest sporting accomplishments, as epitomised by the celebration of the Olympic Games, has always been present in the identity of the Paralympic Movement.

In 1949 Ludwig Guttmann declared that he hoped the International Stoke Mandeville Games would be the 'disabled person's equivalent of the Olympic Games' (Guttmann 1949b); he seems to have been adamant that the use of the word 'Olympic' must be maintained, even in the face of pressure from the International Olympic Committee to protect what it saw as its own copyright. Jens Bromann (former President of the International Blind Sport Association and former Vice President of IPC) comments: 'Guttmann told the IOC that as long as he was living he would call these games "Olympic" and he would never give up that term because sport for the disabled was as ideal as the spirit of the Olympic Games for the able-bodied' (Jennings 1996). Roger Bannister, neurosurgeon and inspiration to many athletes for his achievements on the track, presented the prizes at the 1955 Stoke Mandeville Games and announced that he considered the recipients 'wonderful record holders in their own "Paraplegic Olympics"'.

A recent, more intricate, explanation was published by the International Paralympic Committee: 'The word "Paralympic" derives from a combination of three sources: the Latin adjective "par" ("similar" or "the same"), the Greek preposition "para" ("next to" or "alongside"), and the word "Olympics" (the Paralympic Games being held parallel to the Olympic Games)' (Reinecke and Reiff 2002). While this may be a suitable explanation now, it has been demonstrated that nothing so precise was intended at the outset.

Organisers of the Tokyo 1964 Paralympic Games were among those to try to clarify the meaning of the title. Although Ludwig Guttmann referred to the 1964 13th International Stoke Mandeville Games as the 'Tokyo Games for the Paralysed' in his welcome address at the Opening Ceremony, throughout his official reports he called the event the Paralympic Games. This was the same in most official reports of Tokyo – the term used was 'Paralympics'. The Japanese press also used the term 'Paralympics' to report the events at the time. For various reasons, usually connected with the legal rights to usage of Olympic-related terminology, the name used for the four-yearly international games has been varied until more recently: World Wheelchair Games, World Winter Games, International Games for the Disabled, Olympiad for the Physically Disabled, Torontolympiad, Olympics for the Disabled and finally the Paralympic Games. Since 1988, when the Games were held in Seoul, Korea, the Paralympic Games has been accepted as the official name.

ORIGINS OF ORGANISATIONS OF SPORT FOR PERSONS WITH A DISABILITY

Any attempt to understand the development of the Paralympic Movement will be aided by a look at the various organisations that emerged in the 20th century serving specific populations of persons with a disability. They each came into existence in differing ways, often riding the enthusiasm of particular individuals. But they provided an essential stability for those individuals who wished to express themselves through competitive sport, and eventually these organisations gave the platform for efforts to bring the different disability groups together. In an effort to provide greater fluency in preparations for quadrennial multi-disability games, discussions between international organisations led to the creation of the International Coordinating Committee of Sports for the Disabled (ICC), on 22nd March 1982. The President, Vice President and Secretary General from four international federations began meetings that would have much wider impact. The organisations involved were: Cerebral Palsy – International Sports and Recreation Association (CP-ISRA), the International Blind Sport Association (IBSA), the International Stoke Mandeville Games Federation (ISMGF) and the International Sports Organisation for the Disabled (ISOD). In 1986 these four organisations were joined in their efforts by the International Committee for Deaf Sports (CISS) and the International Sports Association for Persons with Mental Handicap (INAS-FMH). Understanding the beginnings of the different international organisations serving sport for persons with a disability will aid any detailed exploration of the Paralympic Movement, because they represent the constituents of the Movement itself. Below is a brief introduction to the very diverse origins of the international federations.

Comité International des Sports des Sourds / International Committee for Deaf Sports

The oldest of the international federations for sport for individuals with a disability is the Comité International des Sports des Sourds / International Committee for Deaf Sports (CISS). This organisation, at first called the International Committee of Silent Sports, was set up just before the end of the inaugural World Games for the Deaf, held in Paris in 1924 on 16th August. The preferred name for the CISS Games is now the Deaflympics. The prime movers were Antoine Dresse (Belgium) and Eugène Reuben-Alcais (France). The latter had encouraged the six existing national federations for the deaf (Belgium, Czechoslovakia, France, Great Britain, the Netherlands and Poland) to send competitors to the First International Silent Games. Some athletes from other countries without a national organisation also competed (from Hungary, Italy and Romania). At a meeting in the Café de la Porte Dorée, adjacent to the Bois de Vincennes, Paris, 13 representatives from these nine countries met and sketched out the formation of an international organisation. The constitution was formally adopted at the first Congress, in Brussels, on 31st October 1926. The Summer Silent Games has operated on a four-year cycle since 1924, apart from a ten-year gap from 1939, with Winter World Games for the Deaf starting in 1949. As the only federation representing people who are deaf, the International Olympic Committee recognised the CISS in 1951. The particular independence that the CISS has had since its very early beginnings has strengthened its ability to represent its members. At the same time the isolation that has come with total self-sufficiency, and its singular population, has tended to make it more difficult to persuade the members of CISS to embrace the potential benefits of bringing all disability sports organisations together. The fact is that the International Committee for Deaf Sports has not really needed to hang on the coat-tails of any other global body for survival. CISS became a member of the International Coordinating Committee in 1986, and was a founder member of the International Paralympic Committee. But its early misgivings were confirmed: that there was little to gain from maintaining its involvement. The elected officials of CISS felt that valuable resources were being squandered attending meetings that had little relevance to their ability to represent athletes who are deaf. In 1995, at the Congress held in Helsinki before the Winter Silent Games in Yllas, Finland, the membership of CISS voted to withdraw from the International Paralympic Committee.

International Stoke Mandeville Games Federation

The International Stoke Mandeville Games Federation (ISMGF) arose from the annual festivals of sport held at Stoke Mandeville Hospital, Aylesbury, UK. Originally the games were organised by the Paraplegic Sports Endowment Fund, which later became the British Paraplegic Sports Society and is now the British Wheelchair Sports Foundation. The participants at these annual gatherings were mainly from the spinal injuries units or other rehabilitation centres around the United Kingdom. The tendency of the Stoke Mandeville Committee to be Eurocentric was historically related to its origins in England, and by the expansion mostly into Europe via medical exchange contact. When an International Stoke Mandeville Games Committee was set up at the Meeting of Managers and Trainers in 1959, it was not surprising that the five members should include Great Britain and the Netherlands holding permanent positions. The Netherlands was suggested as a permanent member 'as the country which, with Great Britain, first put the Games on an international basis' (Scruton 1998); the country in which the next games were to be held (if not at Stoke Mandeville) would also be a member. In 1959, Italy was included as the host country for the 1960 Games, with France and Belgium constituting the five.' It might help to add another sentence explaining the basis on which the final two were chosen. Membership of the Committee was initially intended to change regularly. The country in which the next games were to be held (if not at Stoke Mandeville) would be a member, with France and Belgium constituting the five. Delegates on the first Committee were: Dr L. Guttmann, President (Great Britain), Dr A. Maglio, Treasurer (Italy), Dr A. Tricot (Belgium), Mr M. Boubee (France) and Capt. H. Tjebbes (Netherlands). Joan Scruton was appointed Honorary Secretary. Only two years later the membership was extended to include representatives from the USA and Austria: Mr R. Simon (Austria) and Mr B. Lipton (USA). Then in 1964 the full Committee was enlarged to include: Dr A. Lococo

(Argentina), Dr G. Bedbrook (Australia), Mr W. Weiss (Germany), Mr Y. Kasai (Japan) and Mr G. Pentland-Smith (Rhodesia). The fundamental pattern of events was agreed in 1960: that the Games would be held annually for three years at Stoke Mandeville, then the Games should have 'Olympic Status' in the fourth year, and efforts should be made to hold them in the city or country in which the Olympic Games were taking place. The International Stoke Mandeville Games were the starting point for the phenomenon we see as the ultimate event today. Although participation in the Games was restricted to people with spinal cord lesions, the Games would eventually give rise to the most spectacular multi-disability sports celebration – the Paralympic Games.

At a meeting in Heidelberg in 1972 it was agreed to change the name to the International Stoke Mandeville Games Federation. ISMGF changed its name again to the International Stoke Mandeville Wheelchair Sports Federation (ISMWSF) in 1990. A merger later amalgamated the International Stoke Mandeville Wheelchair Sports Federation and the International Sports Organisation for the Disabled from 1st January 2004, becoming the International Wheelchair and Amputee Sports Federation (IWAS).

International Sports Organisation for the Disabled

The International Sports Organisation for the Disabled (ISOD) was established in 1964, serving amputees and 'les Autres'. A large number of persons with a disability did not qualify for participation under the aegis of one of the organisations established so far, and discussion took place in 1977 to find a way of providing for this disenfranchised group of athletes. Representatives of ISOD from France, United Kingdom and Spain met in February to consider systems of classification that would bring another group into ISOD – 'les Autres'. This term serves to identify people with other conditions that had not been represented within the other federations, including people with locomotor disabilities such as dwarfism, muscular dystrophy, osteogenesis imperfecta (brittle bones), Guillain's Syndrome and arthrogryposis, some types of cerebral palsy, spinal cord conditions such as polio, and multiple sclerosis. When the interested parties considered the formation of ISOD it was with an umbrella function in mind, a multi-disability sports organisation to cater for the sporting needs of people other than those with spinal lesions.

The organisation followed from meetings of the World Veterans' Federation at its Paris headquarters that began in 1960. Eleven countries attended the 1961 gathering, at which an International Working Group was set up, and elections took place for membership of an Executive Board and Medical Committee. They agreed a constitution that would receive significant modification over the next few years. The President of the Working Group was also Secretary General of the World Veterans' Federation, Curtis Campaigne, with Guttmann and Van Rijn (Netherlands) elected as Vice Presidents. Guttmann welcomed the development of ISOD as a logical extension of the British Sports Association for the Disabled (BSAD), founded on his initiative in February 1961. Joan Scruton says that Guttmann saw a need to embrace other disability organisations into his original vision of Paralympic Games as sporting celebrations for people with spinal lesions, and required a corporate structure that could administer this (Scruton 2000). The inaugural meeting of the International Sports Organisation for the Disabled was in 1964 in Paris. Norman Acton took over from Campaigne as President (he was the new Secretary General of the World Veterans' Federation as well). Vice Presidents elected were Guttmann and J Westerhoff (Netherlands). Countries recognised as founder members were Austria, Belgium, Finland, France, Germany, Italy, Luxembourg, the Netherlands, Norway, Poland, Switzerland and the United Kingdom. Later, the World Veterans' Federation could no longer offer the same level of involvement in ISOD, and in 1966 Norman Acton resigned from the Presidency. The Secretary General was also from the WVF, Mr E. Joubert, and he also tendered his resignation. Although some financial support had been pledged from the WVF, the International Sports Organisation for the Disabled had to suddenly draw itself up to its full height and use the strength of its member nations to stand confidently, after eight years of being propped up. A new Executive Committee was elected, with Guttmann as President.

In 1967 ISOD appointed a sub-committee to prepare rules for sports for amputees, and to assemble a report on the range of sports opportunities for athletes who were blind. Involvement with the International Cerebral Palsy Society (ICPS) began unsteadily, but meetings in 1976 and 1977 brought medical experts from ISOD and the ICPS together to establish classifications under which competitors with cerebral palsy could take part in multi-disciplinary events.

As disability-specific sports organisations such as IBSA and CP-ISRA were begun in the 1970s, (with INAS-FMH being formed in 1985), the International Sports Organisation for the Disabled began to lose its significance as a coordinating body for athletes outside the ISMGF framework. In 1978 Ludwig Guttmann, still President of ISOD, put together a paper with Joan Scruton on the concept of the ISOD becoming the equivalent of the International Olympic Committee. It would 'become the coordinating committee of sport for all disabled'. Guttmann saw confusion within different countries being the barrier to progress in the late 1970s, with several organisations acting separately. The paper suggested that ISOD could 'assume the role of an overall umbrella organisation, coordinating the work of the individual international organisations'. But the establishment of the International Coordinating Committee in 1979 did not lead to this logical transition for ISOD. Its work continued, and eventually it became prudent to establish a merger between ISOD and ISMWSF.

Cerebral Palsy – International Sports and Recreation Association

Cerebral Palsy – International Sports and Recreation Association (CP-ISRA) was created in 1978. Until this time all sporting activities for people with cerebral palsy were coordinated through the Sports and Leisure Group of the International Cerebral Palsy Society, which had been founded in 1968. The first Cerebral Palsy World Games were held in Denmark in 1982, and athletes with cerebral palsy first took part in the Paralympic Games in Arnhem, the Netherlands, in 1980. Recreational Seminars have been a feature of the CP-ISRA, beginning in Portugal in 1983. The 1994 General Assembly of CP-ISRA adopted the following mission statement. The aim of CP-ISRA is: 'To promote the development of sporting and recreational activities, both competitive and non-competitive, for people with cerebral palsy and allied conditions'. Under the banner of 'allied conditions' CP-ISRA has given emphasis to individuals with neurological impairment, including people who have been affected by strokes and traumatic brain injury. CP-ISRA 'strives to be an athlete-centred organisation, involving athletes and ex-athletes in discussion and formulation of decision-making at all levels'. In relation to the Paralympic Games, CP-ISRA takes responsibility for the level of participation of athletes with cerebral palsy 'based on fair classification and appropriate sports'. Functional classification has been employed throughout CP-ISRA's existence. Its own Sports Rules Manual is used to determine eligibility criteria, and to consider minimum disability. The different sports have to be considered separately because the criteria will vary for each.

Cerebral palsy can be described as a brain lesion that is non-progressive. It causes varying impairment of coordination, muscle tone and strength. Characteristics include: difficulty in maintaining posture and in controlling some movement; central motor disturbance that can lead to deficiency in perceptual areas; some hearing, speech and visual deficits; and epilepsy. 'Eligible participants must have a diagnosis of cerebral palsy or other non-progressive brain damage with locomotor dysfunction, either congenital or acquired. If an abnormality can only be detected by a detailed neurological examination of the athlete and there is no obvious impairment of function, the person is not eligible for CP-ISRA competitions'. CP-ISRA has been very actively involved, with the International Paralympic Committee, in examining ways of best providing appropriate elite sport opportunities for people with severe disabilities.

International Association for Sport for Persons with Mental Handicap

The International Association for Sport for Persons with Mental Handicap (INAS-FMH) was established in 1986 to further sport for people with intellectual disability. As society has altered its use of related language, this organisation became the International Association for Sport for Persons with Intellectual Disability (INAS-FID) in 1999. The terms used to describe individuals with intellectual disability have changed steadily through the 20th century. Some language used in past years could now be considered derogatory. Another complication is that language is culturally dependent – some countries employ a term to describe what is now called intellectual disability that, when transliterated into another language, equates to a word that has become insulting. Some other terms that have been used to describe individuals with intellectual disability in the 20th century include: mentally defective, mentally deficient, mentally handicapped, mentally retarded, learning disabled.

The federation takes 'normalisation' as a main principle in its activities. This starts from the premise that people with intellectual disabilities are equal members of society, and as such they possess the same rights and obligations as everyone else. There are particular needs that individuals have as a result of their disability, just as some other individuals are blind or are elderly and have specific needs. These rights extend into the realm of opportunities to participate and to compete in sports. INAS-FID is democratic in structure, arranged on a basis of national representation. Ignorance and prejudice within the broader community is seen to be its greatest barrier to progress. A tendency for families and carers to have low expectations of athletes with intellectual disability has also been a restriction to people gaining the greatest benefits from their involvement. But more recently the difficulty of effectively classifying eligibility has caused significant problems in the relationship between INAS-FID and the International Paralympic Committee.

International Special Olympics, Inc.

Another organisation that has catered for individuals with intellectual disability is International Special Olympics, Inc., which was founded in 1968 as a result of the very personal commitment of Eunice Kennedy Shriver. Special Olympics Inc. was established with the stated mission to 'provide physical fitness, sports training, and athletic competition for mentally retarded individuals'. This organisation, largely funded from its inception by the Joseph P. Kennedy, Jr Foundation, is a very wide-ranging organisation providing competitive athletic programs for persons with intellectual disability. Having held a day camp for children with intellectual difficulties in 1963, Shriver was inspired to extend these events to other cities in the United States over the next five years. Bringing together the Chicago Park District and the Kennedy Foundation, Shriver nurtured the First International Special Olympic Games in Soldier Field, Chicago, in July 1968. Special Olympics remains some distance from the Paralympic Movement, serving mostly North America and wishing mainly not to associate itself directly with the development of the International Paralympic Committee. The International Olympic Committee, as we will see, tried to bring Special Olympics and INAS-FID together so that they could 'speak with one voice'.

International Blind Sports Association

The International Blind Sports Association (IBSA) was established in 1980 serving blind and visually impaired sportspersons. There is a very long history of athletic endeavour being an integral part of the education and recreation of blind people; many residential schools and colleges had established extensive competitive programmes in the first half of the 20th century, and some athletic associations were formed to help coordinate the expanding competitive schedule. The World Council for the Welfare of the Blind (WCWB) recognised the value of sports and competition to all blind people, and passed a resolution at its 1979 General Assembly encouraging the formation of an international sports federation conspicuously catering for the distinctive requirements of blind athletes. The resolution was crafted by Helmut Pielasch (German Democratic Republic) and a small group of other delegates from around the world. IBSA endorsed renewed objectives in 2001.

CONCLUSION

> Broadly speaking, the aims of sport embody the same principles for the disabled as they do for the able-bodied; in addition however, sport is of immense therapeutic value and plays an essential part in the physical, psychological and social rehabilitation of the disabled. Sport helps the disabled person to restore contact with the world around him; in other words, to facilitate and accelerate his social re-integration or integration. (Ludwig Guttmann 1976)

There have been many obstacles to overcome in providing opportunities for persons with a disability to participate in elite competitive sporting environments. This book is intended to guide us through some of the great efforts made by individuals and organisations. More than 50 years ago, efforts were made to employ sport systematically for rehabilitation. These efforts lead us to look more closely at the early coordination of competitive opportunities for individuals with a disability – usually organised on disability-specific lines. This could be said to mark the start of a Paralympic Movement. This book aims to explore the mechanisms by which the Paralympic Movement developed, leading to the foundation of the International Paralympic Committee, and to trace the formidable work of this body to the present day.

Attitudes are all-important however, and it is noticeable immediately that barriers have been constructed in the minds of the general public and in the minds of some athletes themselves. The literature of post-Second World War sport for people with a disability shows a clear misunderstanding on the part of the public: that all early provision for athletes with a disability had therapeutics as its primary aim, rather than elite athletic performance and competition. The misconception associated the efforts of those participating in competitions nationally or internationally with rehabilitation, rather than acknowledging the highly trained, elite sportspersons as athletes in their own right. People did not think of these competitions in the same terms as their understanding of the Olympic Games or world championships in different sports. It is inevitable that this negativity would slow down any progress in attracting sponsorship or governmental support for the furtherance of sport for disabled persons. The extent of negativity existing within the community of persons with disability was ironic, and also a factor in slowing the initial development of the Paralympic Movement. There was certainly some reluctance for a global encouragement and promotion of sport for all people with a disability. While reading this account we should bear in mind the contemporary shifts in attitudes both of the participants and of society more broadly to sporting opportunities for persons with a disability.

CHAPTER 2

An Air of Hopelessness

INTRODUCTION

'One of the most devastating calamities in human life', is how Ludwig Guttmann described severe injury or disease of the spinal cord (1973). This description can equally be applied to many other debilitating causes that so radically affect the mobility and functioning of individuals in society. Although attitudes have changed significantly through the last century, it is only relatively recently that it has been possible to consider that sport might play a part in providing opportunities for people with disabilities to be placed in the spotlight of elite athletic endeavour.

The 19th century was a time of new developments in scientific discovery, particularly in medicine. Responses towards people with ailments or injuries that prevented them from normal participation in society tended to be clinical: prevent further deterioration where possible and withdraw the individual from the midst of the community to be 'cared for' separately. To some extent the emergence of remedial and therapeutic gymnastics improved the situation, as rehabilitation became more scientifically focused, but the overriding preoccupation was with anthropometrical testing and measurement. Hygiene was also a major focus: there was an urgency to examine ways to improve health and living conditions as countries came to realise and accept the inherent problems associated with industrialisation. Governments of the newly industrialised nations were becoming used to measuring the efficiency of the populace in terms of productivity. This was reflected in governmental support for initiatives that might serve to keep people working. Technology permitted the measurement to become more accurate, and data was collected in great quantities. Physical efficiency generally drove research directions. Competing systems of gymnastics probably hindered progress as the nineteenth century ended; squabbling between proponents of different methods did little for the sharing of new ideas. Hygiene, posture and 'correct' physical development featured in the systems of gymnastics encouraged in schools around the world in the early 20th century. Influence from various quarters diverted the specific attention of different countries: in England, for example, physical training for physical efficiency was promoted in government elementary schools, while the leadership qualities of team games were preferred in the public schools. The Office International d'Hygiène Publique (OIHP) was established by the Treaty of Rome in 1907, as a result of a recommendation at the 11th International Sanitary Conference in Paris, 1903. Very little of the work of this office was concerned with individuals with disabilities, and the Health Committee of the League of Nations, which superseded the OIHP, was similar in its concerns.

Athlete First: A History of the Paralympic Movement   Steve Bailey
© 2008 John Wiley & Sons, Ltd

Sports medicine remained a distant specialisation as the first years of the 20th century opened, with Germany providing the catalyst for the establishment for the first federation. At the first congress of sports physicians, held at Oberhof/Thüringen in September 1912, the Deutsches Reichskomitee zur wissenschaftlichen Erforschung der Leibesübungen (German State Committee for Scientific Investigation of Physical Exercise) was formed. In 1924 this group was renamed the Deutscher Ärtzebund zur Förderung des Leibesübungen (German Federation of Physicians for the Promotion of Physical Exercise). Arthur Mallwitz and August Bier began the first lecture series on sports medicine in Berlin in 1919. In 1927 the German sports physicians arranged a conference at which delegates from 12 countries discussed the sharing of research and future cooperation. Arising from this first gathering was the agreement to form a world body: the first official meeting of the Association Internationale Medico-Sportive (International Association for Sports Medicine), later to become the Fédération Internationale de Médecine Sportive (FIMS) was held in St Moritz, Switzerland during the Olympic Winter Games of 1928. The subject of sport for individuals with disabilities does not emerge for many years in the context of FIMS; there is no recognition of relevance until the middle of the 20th century.

Much of the earliest documentary information on the use of sport for people with disabilities relates to spinal injury, and as such it does not represent other forms of disability, but tracing this particular path is still fruitful. It illustrates patterns of development and obstacles that have required attention. Historically the emergence of sporting activity as a benefit to individuals with spinal injury has received greater public exposure due to a number of factors. In history an air of hopelessness has hung over many descriptions of disabling conditions: an ancient Egyptian medical treatise, dating from about 3000 BC, suggests that lesion of the spinal cord following dislocation or fracture of the spine is 'an ailment not to be treated'. Galen, Hippocrates and Paulen of Aegina all wrote of treatment of spinal injuries, particularly detailing mechanisms for reducing dislocation. Hippocrates (460–377 BC) described his 'extension bench' for aiding spinal deformities through traction. The 19th century saw a consensus of medical opinion against surgery for spinal injury, even with the new possibilities offered up by discoveries and developments by Pasteur, Lister and others.

There is good evidence that sport and physical activity were part of the treatment of individuals with disabilities early in the 20th century. R. Tait McKenzie, highly influential in the fields of medical gymnastics as well as competitive sport, wrote extensively of their use in his 1909 book: *Exercise in Education and Medicine*. Much of the physical activity and sport was extracted from its usual setting to serve the needs of measurement or diagnosis, but it was rarely experienced by the participants in the context that would have lent it so much of the psychosocial benefits recognised later. McKenzie describes a range of activities that were taken in a fully competitive context at the Overbrook School for the Blind in Pennsylvania, including a form of baseball, football, gymnastics and track and field athletics. McKenzie's account includes an appraisal of the limitations of provision possible for individuals with intellectual disabilities; the language of description is particularly startling: classification of children as idiots, imbeciles or morons according to Henry Goddard's system of testing.

Guttmann describes the body of knowledge and publications up to the First World War: 'The literature of that time in every country, though containing many excellent publications on problems of pathology and physiology, reveals a profoundly defeatist attitude of the medical profession towards these unfortunate sufferers, when dealing with the problem of prognosis and rehabilitation'. Mortality rates among those who received spinal injuries in the First World War were similar for both British and American casualties: approximately 80% did not survive. The view that very little could be done for the spinally injured continued to be held between the wars, and Guttmann describes those who survived their injuries as those who 'dragged out their lives as useless and hopeless cripples, unemployable and unwanted ... with no incentive or encouragement to return to a useful life' (Guttmann 1973b). Very soon after the Stoke Mandeville Spinal Unit was established in 1944, Ludwig Guttmann set out on his mission to change established views about the return of individuals with spinal injuries to a more positive existence.

> It was quite revolutionary to teach and impress on the authorities of medical and social services, in particular the Ministries of Labour and Housing Authorities, that the mere fact that a person was a paraplegic did not justify care in one of the institutions for incurables, but that in spite of permanent and severe physical handicap, rehabilitation to a useful life and employment was possible. With this object in view, regular work and sport were introduced from the beginning as essential parts of the clinical treatment of these patients which, in due course, proved so very successful for their physical, psychological and social rehabilitation.

FROM REHABILITATION TO SPORT: LUDWIG GUTTMANN'S LEGACY

Unquestionably Ludwig Guttmann had the most profound effect on the early progress of sport for people with a disability. As a respected and experienced Jewish neurologist who escaped the increasingly oppressive Germany of 1939, Guttmann took up the position of Research Fellow at the Nuffield Department of Neurosurgery at the Radcliffe Infirmary, Oxford. This post had been secured through the efforts of the British Society for the Advancement of Science and Learning. In Oxford, however, Guttmann felt less than fulfilled; he was desperately waiting to do more than just the research to which he had been assigned. This reduced responsibility was a major change from his previous work as Medical Director of a large hospital in Breslau, as a full professor of neurology and an inspirational teacher.

Guttmann's experience in Germany had included being the first neurosurgeon to work in a psychiatric hospital. His own research interests centred on the physiological responses of the sweat glands, work he continued right through to the end of his life. In Germany his research had also included electrical stimulation of nerves for diagnosis and curative purposes. While in Oxford during the war Guttmann worked on peripheral nerve regeneration, which was also to prove central to his later career. Although constrained in his direct contribution to medical services at the time, Guttmann was asked in 1941 by Brigadier George Riddoch of the London Hospital, to write and submit two major reviews to the Peripheral Nerve Committee of the Research Council. The subjects were to be: 'surgical aspects of spinal injuries' and 'rehabilitation after injuries to the nervous system'. Riddoch had been appointed Neurological Consultant to the British Army and the Ministries of Health and Pensions. Guttmann, a firm believer in fate, regularly asserted that these reviews commissioned by Riddoch were to enable his progress towards his destiny. Riddoch met with Guttmann in 1943 to invite him to put his somewhat provocative ideas into practice in a new spinal injuries unit that was to be established. Guttmann jumped at the opportunity; he was invited to look at sites at Barnsley Hall, Basingstoke, and Stoke Mandeville, Aylesbury. Stoke Mandeville was a better match for his vision of what was needed.

At the heart of Guttmann's success was to be his dogged attitude towards the need for purposeful movement and activity on the part of the spinally injured, for both physical and mental rehabilitation, beginning at the earliest possible opportunity. He puzzled some of those with whom he had worked in Oxford and elsewhere because of his passion for the work he was about to undertake. Hopelessness and pity were the most common emotions associated with these patients, yet Guttmann had a vision that had so far not been pursued in hospitals. Guttmann clearly understood the current thinking relating to people with spinal injuries, but he was determined that his ideas could reverse the pessimism:

> The victims of war, road, industrial and sporting accidents did not establish a social problem in the past, as their life expectancy was very short, two to three years at the utmost as a rule. Complications such as sepsis from ascending infection of the bladder into the kidneys, and pressure sores, were

considered inevitable. Therefore, any attempt to restore such a person to his or her former social activities seemed to be out of the question, and the view generally held was the sooner they died the better for all concerned. (Goodman 1986)

Guttmann had seen and heard all of the negative attitudes towards paraplegia, but he felt that it was essential to develop a systematic and scientific approach to this branch of medicine – it was just as worthy of conscientious and optimistic treatment as any other area. Some inroads in treatment of paraplegia were evident in the work of Donald Munro, neurosurgeon at the Boston City Hospital in the USA, but his writings seemed not to reach a large or appreciative audience. Munro was writing between the mid-1930s and the early 1950s, and his work certainly broke new ground in its emphasis on returning spinally injured patients to productive and valued working lives. He sought total rehabilitation and self-supporting status for patients who had often been regarded as long-term burdens on medical resources. It is difficult to guess at the communication or exchange of information and ideas between Guttmann and Munro, but Guttmann would certainly have cast his net widely to appreciate the work of any practitioner in fields related to his own. We can assume that the two enthusiasts communicated. Munro had certainly published articles in areas essential to Guttmann's work. Other early respected neurosurgeons in the United States were Harvey Cushing and Charles Harrison Frazier.

Much earlier in his life Guttmann had been deeply affected by attitudes towards disabling injuries. While working as an 18-year-old orderly in the Accident Hospital for Coalminers (Knappschaftslazarett) in Königshütte, Upper Silesia, a coalminer was brought in with severe spinal injury. Guttmann never forgot being told by a doctor that 'this man would be dead in six weeks at the latest. I, incredulous, asked the reason for this sad prognosis. "Just watch him and you will see and learn," was his laconic reply' (Goodman 1986). The tall young miner steadily proved the doctor correct in just five weeks. This acceptance of inevitability by those medical professionals in Königshütte indelibly marked itself in the young Guttmann's mind forever. He acknowledged later that spinal injuries remained 'one of the most depressing and neglected in medicine and society' (Guttmann 1954).

The new unit at Stoke Mandeville was to stand prominently for Ludwig Guttmann's particular outlook: each of the other spinal units in the UK was attached to other departments on the premise that the patients should remain together. But this limited the specific care that they could receive. There was not, as yet, a concept of specialised nursing care for the spinally injured. Guttmann saw a long-term focus of care into a complete specialised area of medicine. 'The basic principle of this new philosophy was to provide a comprehensive paraplegia and tetraplegia service to rescue these men, women and children from the human scrapheap and return most of them, in a permanent, profound disability – by clinical measures and psychological readjustment – to a life worth living, as useful and respected citizens in the community' (Goodman 1986). It was Guttmann's intention to move away from the idea that units with patients with spinal injuries became 'merely an accumulation of doomed individuals' (Guttmann 1954).

The Stoke Mandeville Spinal Injuries Unit opened on 1st February 1944, as optimism was emergent in the outlook towards the war. The new spinal unit, located in Ward X, was of necessity housed in prefabricated buildings that were uninspiring for their physical appearance and provision of appropriate facilities – but this was wartime. It was for the new Director to emphasise that the task before the men and women drawn together as staff was crucial and worthwhile. This was quite a feat given the existing attitude of despair and dilution of resources. The staff consisted of two nurses and eight Army orderlies. Guttmann's determination and doggedness ensured that his principles were prominent from the start. In particular he was insistent that all patients must be turned every two hours, day and night, so as to minimise the chances of pressure sores, already identified as one of the two most serious complications facing paraplegics. Joan Scruton recalled that Guttmann used to appear on the ward unannounced at any time to check that patients had been turned and that bedpans had been emptied, and that he also took to measuring and recording the size of patients' bedsores so as to monitor their reduction and disappearance. Urinary tract infection was the other major hazard to threaten the paraplegic. Infection rising to the kidneys could prove fatal. As voluntary urination was often not evident in the earliest stages of the spinally injured it was necessary to enable urine to be voided either by catheterisation or by surgical intervention (suprapubic cystotomy). Guttmann was insistent that aseptic catheterisation should always be preferable to opening the abdomen to install a collecting receptacle. In the later days of the war antibiotics were scarce and infection was all too often catastrophic.

Another feature of Ludwig Guttmann's philosophy was to oppose almost every call for surgery on the spinal cord. Stoke Mandeville probably saw fewer operations of this sort than all other spinal units. Guttmann's experience in Germany led him to refer to surgical intervention as 'irresponsible meddling'.

Guttmann had assessed the physiotherapy department of Stoke Mandeville Hospital before the spinal unit opened. He thought the facilities unsuitable and was dismayed because it portrayed the traditional massage-based approach. Guttmann wanted 'purposeful, dynamic physical management'. Apart from the facilities and equipment, the attitude of the physiotherapists had to be overcome – what value was there in dedicating time and effort to the hopeless? The physiotherapists who became involved with the Spinal Injuries Unit soon saw that the rewards were countless. Miss Elvira Hobson said of the early days of the unit: 'all those things we tried out for the first time but with a good deal of anxiety ... because there was no pattern of treatment for the physiotherapist to follow ... A new dynamic approach was envisaged' (Goodman 1986). It is no surprise that the discipline of physiotherapy would later find Guttmann's work essential to its own professional development, just as the doctors and staff of the Spinal Unit learned much about the patients and their injuries from the caring determination of the physiotherapists. Guttmann's ability to cement a team together was again being proven. In character he was pushy, loud and insistent but no one could question his motivation or his example of pure hard work. His leadership style might owe more to bullying than diplomacy but the cult of personality often behind this type of person was completely overshadowed by Guttmann's fervent desire to give the spinally injured a more positive future. Where did Guttmann get his own motivation and philosophy? His student days had been filled with high levels of competitiveness, fencing being his particular passion. As a student he had been a devout member of one of the University fraternities that held duelling to be the way of maintaining honour, and his own duelling scars were displayed with pride. From Guttmann's student days he was drawn to the example of the motivated and dominant professors as role models. He idolised the strong-willed and confident leadership of those under whom he trained, and he would lead in exactly this way as he established working practices at Stoke Mandeville. His stubborn streak fitted in perfectly with the need to reject earlier approaches to management and care in his chosen speciality.

The workshop was an essential extension to the ward at Stoke Mandeville. Traditional occupational therapy was mixed with innovative developments as Guttmann and those he encouraged to be inventive explored ideas. Rehabilitation for spinally injured patients in the past had been crude and relatively lacking in structure – there were some restrictions due to war austerity, but the outlook was also possibly affected by the inherent attitudes of hopelessness towards the population. Woodwork, shoe repair, engraving, typing and draughtsmanship gave occupation and encouragement. Bill Parker, the instructor, also constructed a 'sweat box' for Guttmann to continue his research. Movement was always central to Guttmann's idea that patients could help their own recovery. Motivation and morale were higher for seeing a patient take his first steps after injury – always when possible to be taken in the middle of the ward rather than in the physiotherapy department. This was to help build up the sense of camaraderie and duty to others in recovery, as well as to emphasise the wish to 'normalise' the recovery process. Support from others in similar circumstances would be more of a driving force than those family members who retained the more traditional outlook of forlorn hope. Relatives could be more hindrance than help. Susan Masham (1968) (later Lady Masham), in the 21st Anniversary issue of *The Cord*, expressed the difference that Stoke Mandeville's special outlook could make: 'A spinal unit could be a depressing place, but not Stoke, which was a place of hope and progress – full of interesting people and activities'.

The Cord was founded in 1947 by Captain P. F. Stewart and five other patients as a journal 'to promote the best interests of all those suffering from spinal troubles and to employ the influence and machinery of the British Legion in all Pension matters and such problems of Housing and Employment; to spread abroad all information of particular interest to paraplegics; and to foster in civilian life that spirit of comradeship that has grown up in the services and in hospital'. In time *The Cord* became both the voice of patients and former patients of Stoke Mandeville, and a means of lobbying and spreading the word.

The National Health Service took over control of Stoke Mandeville in 1951, by which time it had 160 beds – an increase that reflected the acceptance of spinal injuries requiring specialist treatment, and an increase in civilian paraplegics being admitted. Stoke Mandeville then became a National Spinal Injuries Centre, with patients coming from all over the country. Some patients from other nations were admitted as private patients. It had become normal by this time for medical experts from all over the world to spend time observing and working with Guttmann at Stoke before taking their experiences back to help shape procedures at home.

THE STOKE MANDEVILLE SPIRIT GOES INTERNATIONAL

The first competitive team sport developed at Stoke Mandeville was wheelchair polo, emerging in the autumn of 1944. The players were soon taking on local teams of able-bodied men, earning the nickname 'the professionals' for their expertise and for their almost invincible record. Other sporting activities employed at Stoke Mandeville in the early years were badminton, netball, athletics (Indian club-swinging, javelin, shot-put), rope climbing, table tennis, snooker, darts and archery. Archery in particular was enthusiastically pursued, lending itself most suitably to the performance capabilities of paraplegic athletes. At the 1951 Festival of Britain, sportsmen and sportswomen who were paraplegics gave demonstrations in basketball and archery.

In July 1948 Ludwig Guttmann encouraged the first annual 'sports day' for patients and former patients of Stoke Mandeville Hospital. In this first competition, eight ex-servicemen from the Star and Garter Home in Richmond competed against six ex-servicemen and two ex-servicewomen from Stoke Mandeville at archery. Ludwig Guttmann wrote that 'it was a good omen' that the foundation of the Stoke Mandeville Games 'should coincide with the Opening Ceremony of the London Olympic Games' (Guttmann 1949b). Although Guttmann implied that the matching date was more chance than design, he was never one to miss an opportunity, and there is little doubt that he arranged for the first Stoke Mandeville Games to usurp some of the symbolism of the Olympic Games. His vision of the future was clearly evident in 1948. As the second Stoke Mandeville Games drew to a close, Guttmann addressed the gathering and spoke of the day when the event would be 'truly international', and when it would become 'the disabled men and women's equivalent of the Olympic Games'. Writing some six years later Guttmann admitted that he didn't carry everyone along with him in his beliefs: 'Many people had difficulty in sharing my optimism, but events confirmed my confidence in the determination of the paraplegic sportsmen to make this new sports movement a success'.

At the first Stoke Mandeville Games the competition was limited to archery, but by 1949 netball and 'dartchery' – an adaptation of archery making use of an enlarged darts target and the scoring system from the game of darts – had been added. This significant national competition moved on to an international footing in 1952 when a team from the Netherlands travelled to take part. In the 'First International

Inter-Spinal Unit Sports Festival', as the official programme described these first International Stoke Mandeville Games, the sports events were: 'Archery, Wheel-Chair Netball, Throwing the Javelin, Table Tennis, Snooker and a Demonstration of Club Swinging'. From these early beginnings the attraction of participation from teams worldwide was ever increasing. The connections between Stoke Mandeville and the Netherlands go back to a study visit by medical and administrative staff from the Dutch Army to Stoke Mandeville towards the end of the Second World War. Dr van Gogh headed up a rehabilitation centre for ex-servicemen with a disability at Aardenburg, near Doorn. It was a team from this centre that then travelled to Aylesbury to compete, on 26th July 1952, in the first international games for the paralysed – the beginnings of the International Stoke Mandeville Games.

It is generally accepted that progress towards a more inclusive global phenomenon is related to the 1960 Rome Games: 'Actually, the first International Stoke Mandeville Games ever held in the Olympic year in connection with the Olympic Games took place in Rome in 1960, when 400 paralysed sports-men and women representing 23 countries were accommodated in the Olympic Stadium'(Guttmann 1973).

The regular sports day at Stoke Mandeville soon became recognised as the opportunity for elite paraplegic athletes, and on 8th August 1953 representatives from Australia, Canada, Finland, France, Great Britain, Israel, South Africa and the Netherlands took part in what was becoming known as the International Stoke Mandeville Games. Recognition for the sterling work being done through the fledgling international sports organisation was recognised by the World Veterans Federation. In November 1953, at its fourth annual assembly in The Hague, it passed a resolution to assist the Stoke Mandeville Games on a regular basis through a special fund established to help with the purchase of equipment and with some transport costs. These athletes came from spinal units, sports clubs associated with spinal units and other such centres nationally and internationally. But it was not until 1958 that countries were required to organise their entries into national teams. This promoted further organisation within countries; for example, in the United Kingdom the 1958 National Stoke Mandeville Games were held in June so as to aid selection of the national team for the International Stoke Mandeville Games to be held in July.

Wheelchair basketball was introduced to the International Stoke Mandeville Games in 1955, by which time there was a recognised need to improve the competitive structure of wheelchair netball. Just as James Naismith had invented basketball within the environment of the YMCA training school in Springfield, Massachusetts, in 1891, so the game of netball was adapted from basketball within the teacher-training environment of Dartford College in England towards the end of the 19th century (Bailey and Vamplew 1999). Both games began with a player possessing the ball having to remain stationary, and with each 'goal' counting as one point, before basketball players found that they could effectively advance the ball by rolling it or throwing it ahead and running after it – dribbling was then refined (Peterson 1990). It was a Canadian team, however, the Wheelchair Wonders from Quebec, that first represented the North American continent at the International Stoke Mandeville Games, partici-pating in the second Games in 1953 – they competed in the wheelchair netball. Basketball replaced netball on the sports programme of Stoke Mandeville in 1955, when the Pan Am Jets defeated two teams from UK spinal units and one team from the Netherlands. The exchange was seminal. Basketball eventually replaced netball as the wheelchair team sport of preference, but not without resistance from a number of European proponents. Also, the autocratic and domineering control of Guttmann meant that not everything was smooth in international relations: the Pan Am Jets maintained a total hold on the championship at Stoke for successive years, but Guttmann instructed that the Jets should be disqualified from the 1957 International Stoke Mandeville Games for 'rough play'.

There were other complications that were the result of sporting events being developed through units predominantly for veterans' hospitals: the games administrators were principally physicians who held a view of the participants as patients, whereas the sport itself was the focus of the athletes. Thus the restrictive medical model of the earliest administrators led to an authoritarian, paternalistic – and possibly patronising – approach. A fundamentally different outlook was in the minds of the founders of the National Wheelchair Basketball Association (NWBA) in the United States, principally Tim Nugent, in 1949. The structure of the NWBA was democratic, insisting that players must hold the key positions on the Executive Committee. As an educator, Nugent placed the control of the sport in the hands of those with most to gain from its successful administration – the players (Strohkendl 1996).

WHEELCHAIR BASKETBALL DEVELOPS IN THE UNITED STATES

Wheelchair basketball was becoming firmly established as a competitive sport in the United States at the same time that Guttmann was beginning to make headway with the development of his methods at Stoke Mandeville Hospital in England. The influence of the vigorous young men who found themselves in the Veterans' Hospitals in the United States at the end of the Second World War was crucial (Strohkendl 1996). The New England Clippers wheelchair basketball team was formed at Cushing Veterans' Administration Hospital, Framingham, by a number of veterans who had sustained disabling spinal injuries. Stan Labanowich and Armand 'Tip' Thiboutot have recorded the details of a match between the New England Clippers and the Boston Celtics professional basketball team, held at Boston Garden on 6th December 1946 (NWBA Newsletter, 1995). The result was a resounding defeat for the able-bodied Celtics (18 to 2). Thiboutot described his personal reaction on hearing of this event:

> I was a 10 year old and without a disability in 1947, shooting baskets on an outdoor court in Fall River, Massachusetts. A friend ran up and shouted to me that he had just heard a news report on the radio indicating that 'a bunch of guys in wheelchairs had easily defeated the Celtics'. I manifested both astonishment and gullibility, the latter attributed to the fact that I immediately concluded that the veterans in wheelchairs had handily defeated the Celtics, who had played on their feet!' (Thiboutot to Bailey 2003)

The efficient administration of the Paralyzed Veterans of America led to the organisation of wheelchair basketball tournaments and exhibition matches all across the United States from 1946. An astonishing 15 561 spectators witnessed a demonstration game of basketball at Madison Square Garden, New York, on 10th March 1948 between the Clippers and a team from the Halloran Hospital in New York. The Flying Wheels team from Long Beach, California even toured the country by plane.

MEETINGS OF EXPERTS

A sign of the need for common approaches to the now flourishing international sports competitive world for those with disabilities is the meeting convened by the World Veterans' Federation in the early summer of 1957. Delegates of several countries met in Paris for what was called a 'Meeting of Experts on Sports for the Disabled'. The main content of the agenda was to accept standardisation for sports regulations, and to aid in the organisation of competitions both nationally and internationally. In the past the Stoke Mandeville Committee had made modifications for participants in its events, but there could be variation as competitors travelled elsewhere. The international sporting regulations for 'able-bodied' sports were to be applied as closely as possible, but adaptations were to be standardised through regular communication between technical experts. In this process it is understandable that the Stoke Mandeville Committee would loom large in its involvement, and this was seen as obvious and necessary. But here was a subtle transition to permit the sporting events for persons with a disability to belong to the international sporting community – the participants – rather than to Stoke Mandeville out of respect for the 'senior partner'. The first technical meeting, called Managers' and Trainers' Meetings, followed the 1957 Stoke Mandeville Games, when an elected tribunal was established for appeals; it was also agreed that Stoke Mandeville should continue to take the lead in centralising rules, and that referees should be drawn from the country in which the competition was taking place. The regular communication established through these meetings would enable the much more demanding coordination of the International Stoke Mandeville Games in Rome in 1960 to change the movement phenomenally.

As the International Stoke Mandeville Games brought together larger numbers of competitors and coaches, the Games also provided opportunities for medical experts to discuss their research and techniques. Ludwig Guttmann started organising scientific meetings in conjunction with the International Stoke Mandeville Games in 1952, continuing when the Games were first held outside the United Kingdom, in Rome in 1960. The 1961 meeting at Stoke led to the founding of the International Medical Society of Paraplegia, with Guttmann as President. The United Nations Educational, Scientific and Cultural Organization (UNESCO) provided support for a major conference in Helsinki in August 1959, organised by Martti Karvonen and Aarni Koskela from the Institute of Health in Finland. The broad theme of the conference was 'Sport, Work and Culture', but the presentations were divided into sections that had not frequently been on the agenda of the predomi-nantly medico-scientific conferences of the past: Sport and International Understanding, Sport and Work, Sports in Africa and Asia, Sport and Culture, the Road to the Future. Among the papers were some diverse themes: industrialisation and sport; sport and military training; gymnastics in intervals at the place of work; the significance of sport for the disabled; sport and the prevention of accidents at work; sport, physical activities and social adaptation; sport and cultural activity; sport and aesthetic education; sport and ethical education; sport and music; sport and dramatic performance; and a charter for sportsmanship. This was a welcome involvement of the United Nations agency in sport and physical education, and its influence was to help bring people together to share research and good practice through the International Council of Sport Science and Physical Education (Bailey 1996).

CONCLUSION

Superpower rivalry had established itself during this important period: the Berlin Blockade and subsequent airlift stressed the absolute polarisation of the political ideologies of East and West. Germany was divided and the Iron Curtain was in place. War in Korea was in the near future. Yet this was the world that was nurturing the gentle growth of sport for people with spinal injuries. It was natural for the medical specialists to consult each other on their latest practices; Ludwig Guttmann was magnetic in his ability to draw experts to examine the breakthrough at Stoke Mandeville Spinal Injuries Unit. Sport as rehabilitation for spinal paralysis was going to be carried far and wide – the setting was ideal for the spread of such innovations. Some people with other disabilities were well provided for separately, but isolation characterised their endeavour.

The centre of attention for the Paralympic Movement at this time was certainly European, promoted by the patriarchal weight of Ludwig Guttmann. His influence was emphatically positive, driving forward to open new avenues for people with spinal injuries. Later there would be unease at the reliance on such a singular personality, and his unwillingness to accommodate diversion from his goals – even if that route would benefit other disabled populations.

From here the story moves to the launch of the public spectacle that would be the Paralympic Games of the future: beginning with Rome in 1960. The annual celebration of the Stoke Mandeville Games was interspersed with a Paralympic Games in the Olympic year.

CHAPTER 3

The Era of Development: 1960 to 1980

INTRODUCTION

> Sport should become a driving force so that handicapped persons will seek or establish contact with the world that surrounds them and, consequently, obtain recognition as equals and respected citizens (Ludwig Guttmann)

The growth of the Paralympic Movement during the twenty years from 1960 could be described as significant but isolated – some might suggest that any growth during this time was intermittent and patchy. While some countries were developing a positive attitude towards people with disabilities within the community, others were continuing to act in a medieval way: to hide the 'problem' away and certainly not to encourage any public opportunities for display! There was a feeling that some changes for the better were happening in isolation; organisations proceeded with initiatives, but did not always look to see how they could cooperate more widely. The influence of Ludwig Guttmann was at its height, with the ensuing growth and reliance on the International Stoke Mandeville Games as the peak of competition for people with spinal injuries. The establishment of the International Sports Organisation for the Disabled (ISOD) was to extend provision to the needs of amputee and blind athletes. Eventually ISOD and the International Stoke Mandeville Games Federation (ISMGF) would cooperate to organise Paralympic Games catering for a wider range of disabilities, including athletes with cerebral palsy competing in 1980.

Rome in 1960, the first Games took place outside the United Kingdom so as to immediately connect with the location and timing of the Olympic Games. The Paralympic Movement had begun in earnest at this point. From Rome onwards there was a gradual expansion of sports events and of countries involved in the International Stoke Mandeville Games, and eventually other disability groups had the opportunity to take part. The pattern was set for annual International Stoke Mandeville Games in Aylesbury three years out of four; in the Olympic Years they were held in conjunction with the Olympic Games. The first steps were very encouraging, with the Rome and Tokyo Games using the same facilities as the Olympic Games. But the next five Olympic Years (1968, 1972, 1976, 1980 and 1984) did not continue this meaningful pattern, and some possible associated benefit was lost to the Paralympic Movement. Although the sports gatherings of the International Stoke Mandeville Games were not by any means the 'whole story', it was this phenomenon that gave rise to the eventual interlocking of the Paralympic Games with the celebration of the Olympiad. Several disability sports groups were continuing to build vital followings for annual and biennial Games, but we follow the International Stoke Mandeville Games in particular because of the framework they provided for the future.

This period saw a transformation in the aspirations of athletes with a disability. The targets were altered beyond belief – the medical model would still restrict progress, but now athletes could visualise their efforts leading them on to a rostrum at what was to become the Paralympic Games. The prestige accruing from the improved acceptance of their labours would help them as individuals and as role models. On the way through the next years they would begin to see the advancement of a pattern of athletic competitions: national and regional games leading to world championships and the Paralympic Games. The unforeseen consequences of the success of athletes were probably greater for a person with a disability than anyone else: 'Prestige enhances symbolic identification as an elite athlete and perhaps instrumental recognition in the form of economic inducements' (Brandmeyer and McBee 1986). Although financial rewards would still be many years away, for some they would be approaching.

All this took place within the context of social unrest around the world, from anti-war campaigning to superpower rivalry between socialist and capitalist blocs. But attitudes towards individual freedom were also being redefined. These found their expression in the movements of young people wanting to throw off the restrictions of previous generations, and they found dynamic expression in the civil rights movement in the United States. All this was to serve, eventually, to provide a background and a vocabulary for people with disabilities to vigorously demand an involvement in decision making about their own position in society. Governments and international bodies began to accept that they would need to divert attention and funding, to help rectify the circumstances of a section of society that had consistently not received appropriate support. This was not a pathetic call for handouts, but a cry for opportunities, for fairness, for access to what the community had put out of reach. At least, it was the beginning of a recognition that society itself must be responsible for setting right the myths and stigma that had attached themselves to people with disabilities.

THE EARLY YEARS: 1960–1970

First Paralympic Games, Rome, 1960

'Dr Guttmann, you are the De Coubertin of the Paralysed!' His Holiness Pope John XXIII exclaimed these words, as a crowd of several hundred enthusiastic wheelchair athletes greeted him in the Vatican City. The first International Stoke Mandeville Games to take place in the Olympic year in direct and intentional relation to the Olympic Games took place in Rome in 1960. The Opening Ceremony, held in the spectacular Acqua Acetosa Stadium, offered Ludwig Guttmann the perfect opportunity to declare how extensive his vision was: Guttmann spoke of dreams coming true, of history being made – not just in sporting terms but in terms of humanity. The Rome Games were being made possible through the support of Centro Parapligici INAIL (Istituto Nazionale per l'Assicurazione contro Infortuni sul Lavoro), the Italian national insurance organisation for injured workers, located in Ostia. INAIL offered to provide funding for the accommodation of all team members during their stay in Rome (Scruton 1960).

Ludwig Guttmann had begun discussions with Antonio Maglio, Director of the Spinal Centre at INAIL in mid-1957, about bringing the International Stoke Mandeville Games to Rome. They went together to the World Veterans' Federation in Paris and canvassed support, as well as looking at how INAIL itself could act as the local organiser. The World Veterans' Federation (WVF) had, until 1957, provided financial support to the Stoke Mandeville Games; the WVF recognised this competition as a fundamental tonic in the rebuilding of lives through the realisation of dreams. The time came when the World Veterans' Federation had to adopt a more globally identifiable outlook, and parallel organisations were becoming more prominent. Other groups, serving different disability populations, were asking for legitimate attention. But this was also the right time for the expansion of the International Stoke Mandeville Games; it would establish the Paralympic Games as a permanent four-yearly celebration of elite sport for athletes with a disability, alongside and in conjunction with the Olympic Games. Annual Stoke Mandeville Games would still be held in Aylesbury. When the International Olympic Committee voted to award the Fearnley Cup to the International Stoke Mandeville Games in 1956, there had been great satisfaction among the key personalities in Aylesbury. This recognition was made for actions in keeping with the true spirit of Olympism, and endorsed the strides made by the Stoke Mandeville Games in providing athletic opportunities. Ludwig Guttmann accepted the award from Sir Arthur Fearnley himself, at a ceremony in London in 1957. As he received the Cup, Guttmann spoke of 'another cherished dream and looked forward to the day when disabled athletes would be allowed to compete in the Olympic Games' (Scruton 1998).

There was massive enthusiasm for the proposal to hold the 9th International Stoke Mandeville Games in Rome immediately following the Olympic Games, but there was also some reticence and nervousness at the enormity of the proposed project. To have the desired impact, the 1960 Rome Games for the Disabled would have to compare well with the Olympic Games that would immediately precede it, ending just six days earlier.

The world was witnessing increasing tensions between the West and the Eastern Bloc. The space race had heated up, and early in the summer of 1960 the American pilot, Gary Powers, was shot down in Soviet air space in his U-2 spy plane. This led to a wave of expulsions of numerous private citizens from the USSR, and in return the United States returned some Soviet diplomats to their country. November 1960 brought John F. Kennedy Jr to the highest office in the United States – an inspirational and charismatic leader who would not survive long. The apprehension being experienced in world politics did pervade the Olympic Games itself, and there was suspicion and ideological propaganda surrounding the activities of the athletes. But this was still not something that affected the community of athletes with spinal injury gathering for their own Olympiad.

The 23 participating countries in the Rome Paralympics offered up more than 400 competitors, all with spinal cord injuries. The results show that competitions took place in archery, athletics (javelin, precision javelin, shot, club throwing), wheelchair basketball, dartchery, fencing, snooker, swimming, table tennis and pentathlon. The pentathlon had been introduced to the Stoke Mandeville Games in 1957 with a combination of events comprising archery, swimming, javelin, shot and club throwing. The Italian fencers struck not only gold, but took nine medals altogether. Franco Rossi stood out as a particularly dynamic and worthy example of the peak of elite sport. Wheelchair basketball was very popular with the spectators, especially supporting the United States team in their victories over Israel and the Netherlands.

In Rome there was a gathering of learned specialists sharing their expertise, and a great opportunity for medical staff accompanying competitors to share ideas and best practice. The time of the Rome Games also saw the foundation of International Medical Society of Paraplegia – scientific meetings had first taken place at Stoke Mandeville Hospital in 1955, but Guttmann suggested the formation of a society following the meetings at the Rome Games and it formally saw life in 1961. As expected, Guttmann took on the Presidency.

Even with the obvious success of this international sporting event, there were still times that the small-scale administration of the Rome Games, with their reliance on personal knowledge and flair, reminded participants that this was essentially a localised gathering trying to stretch out and offer its benefits to a much wider clientele. In contrast, the Olympic Games were beginning to be used for unprecedented political purposes. The Rome Olympic Games had seen a very delicate stage management in the athletes' domestic arrangements to encourage the greatest distance between the teams supposedly divided by the Cold War. As expected, when the competitions began, political ideology took second place. But future Olympic Games would be used as a world political stage more and more.

Guttmann expressed modest satisfaction with the way the Rome Paralympics had gone:

> It can now be concluded that the first experiment to hold the Stoke Mandeville Games as an entity in another country, as an international sports festival comparable with the Olympic Games and other international sports events for the able-bodied has been highly successful. It justifies the hope that this achievement will be a stimulus to continue the same pattern.

Unfortunately the main sporting venue had to be changed to the Tre Fontane Stadium, further away than planned. Everyone appreciated the competitive facilities, but transport logistics became the nightmare of the five days. The Closing Ceremony, on 25th September, was both a joyful and a sad occasion: so many people had been made to feel part of what was to become the pinnacle of sporting opportunity for individuals with disabilities. The bond of sharing in this experience made it harder for participants to leave and go home. The Rome Games had taken the Paralympic Movement to the true starting line for its future. From this point onwards the struggles to bring people and organisations together would seem like a natural progression: even if not a smooth route at times. Ludwig Guttmann stressed the importance of this moment in his speech in the Palazetto dello Sport: 'The vast majority of competitors and escorts have fully understood the meaning of the Rome Games as a new pattern of re-integration of the paralysed into society, as well as the world of sport'. Of course the Paralympic Movement was to be greater than even Guttmann's dream, and yet it would take many years of toil and setbacks to get there.

Commonwealth Paraplegic Games, Perth, Western Australia, 1962

After the euphoria of the Rome Games, work continued on building the future of sport for individuals with disabilities. The initiative of George Bedbrook, Director of the Spinal Unit in Perth, Western Australia, led to the first Commonwealth Paraplegic Games. The arrangements again relied on a very small number of people who were professionals in other areas, but gave their time and energy to stage this major international event. The Games, based mostly at the Royal Agricultural Showground, opened with nine countries attending and with crowds in their thousands present for much of the competition.

This was an important new phase in the expansion of the Paralympic Movement because it was the beginning of a break away from the locus of Stoke Mandeville having the controlling influence. Regional games would follow, and a widening of outlook would also permit initiatives for multi-disability games to be organised – either nationally or internationally.

'The World United in One': Tokyo 1964

As late autumn decorated the Japanese countryside with traditional chrysanthemum blossom, competitors gathered to celebrate the International Stoke Mandeville Games in 1964.

> The aim of the 'Stoke Mandeville Games' is to unite paralysed men and women from all parts of the world in an international sports movement, and your spirit of true sportsmanship today will give hope and inspiration to thousands of paralysed people. No greater contribution can be made to society by the paralysed than to help, through the medium of sport, to further friendship and understanding amongst nations.

So declared the preface to the official report of the Games, held in Tokyo between 8th and 12th November 1964. As His Imperial Highness The Crown Prince of Japan greeted the athletes and spectators at the Opening Ceremony, he drew a parallel between the International Stoke Mandeville Games and the 18th Olympic Games that had just ended by employing the same motto: 'The World United in One'. Ludwig Guttmann had devised an appropriately evocative emblem for the International Stoke Mandeville Games – three interlocking wheels – and a motto to go with the symbols – Friendship, Unity and Sportsmanship. The similarity to the Olympic five interlocking rings would be a hot issue in the future.

Following the great success of the Games in Rome in 1960, the International Stoke Mandeville Games Committee was filled with self-assurance about the experience gained in organisational and administrative matters. In Guttmann's view the 'Rome Games were undoubtedly an important mile-stone in the development of our sports movement' (Guttmann 1964). The International Games really could be exported to any country, believed the Committee, and their ambition and confidence was proven in the Tokyo Games. In his official report, Guttmann identified three key features of outstanding consequence arising from the Tokyo Games: medical significance; the Games as a demonstration of international cooperation and goodwill; and the educational value of the Games. It was impressive to see that the old concept of paraplegia – that of forlorn hope – had been so obviously replaced with energetic striving and worthwhile application of effort.

A Mrs Watanabe had attended a Congress in Rome at the time of the International Stoke Mandeville Games. She spent time watching the events and met Ludwig Guttmann, expressing great interest in the Games being held in Japan. When Mrs Watanabe returned to Tokyo, she seemed to enthuse people in a number of quarters to explore further. A team from Japan then competed in the International Stoke Mandeville Games in 1962.

> It was Dr Nakamura from Beppu who in 1962 brought the very first small team of Japanese Paraplegics to England to take part in the International Games, which on the team's return, aroused increasing interest in the rehabilitation of traumatic paraplegics in Japan. In the Olympic year of 1964, these were held immediately after the Olympic Games in the magnificent Olympic Stadium of Tokyo, under the leadership of Mr Kasai and his committee more than 100,000 people watched the excellent sportive performances of the 350 paraplegic athletes representing 23 countries (Guttmann 1973)

The Chairman of the Japanese Organising Committee of the 1964 International Stoke Mandeville Games was Yoshisuke Kasai, who had led a group of eight officials and two competitors to those 1962 Games in Aylesbury. Kasai attended the International Stoke Mandeville Games Committee meeting at the time of the 12th Games, and consulted widely with the organisers on practical matters that he would face over the next two years. The response of governmental and prefectural bodies to the need for assistance in setting up facilities and infrastructure in Japan was enormous. Fundraising for the Japanese national games and the International Stoke Mandeville Games had an amazingly broad reach: subsidies from national and regional government, Lions Clubs International and the Japanese Junior Chamber of Commerce, but then direct appeals and unsolicited donations produced results from pharmaceutical companies, automobile manufacturers' associations, and even the Professional Baseball Association. The media in Japan took a keen interest in the planning. Kasai commented that almost every day the radio, television or newspapers would call for people to support 'the less fabulous but very humane paralympic in the shadow of the Olympic Games' (Kasai 1964). The success of the financial support was to ensure that the Tokyo Games were fully funded from these sources, with some surplus being of benefit to sport in Japan for people with disabilities beyond the Games themselves. Kasai and his team of administrative staff had only three days to marshal the volunteers to prepare the Olympic Village for the International Stoke Mandeville Games – the Organising Committee of the 13th Olympic Games handed the Village over on the 5th November. In his understated way, Yoshisuke Kasai commented that he would have liked a little more time 'for rearranging the living quarters for use by the disabled competitors'. He was also concerned that volunteers might not have received enough orientation in order to permit the competitors to fend for themselves as they were used to. He felt that they might have been over helpful towards the participants 'which might have offended the spirit of independence on the part of the paraplegics'.

Stoke Mandeville had undertaken to make arrangements for aeroplanes to be chartered from KLM and Air France to transport the Scandinavian, Israeli, Irish, Maltese, British and some other European teams. They could join the flights in London, Paris, Amsterdam or Hamburg. 'Necessity is the mother of invention' goes the maxim, and when the Dutch national airline produced a narrow wheelchair for use in the cramped aisle space on the aircraft, the Air France technicians rushed to have one made up overnight for use on their Boeing 707B. From the moment of their arrival in Tokyo competitors and officials could see the signs posted around the city for the 'International Paralympic Games' that had recently replaced the Olympic signs a few days before.

The Opening Ceremony was a colourful and moving experience, with hundreds of doves symbolising peace being released to flutter and swirl around the stadium before disappearing into the bright Tokyo sky. A Japanese athlete took the oath; undertaking on behalf of all competitors that the Games would proceed according to the ideals of the Stoke Mandeville spirit – 'Friendship, Unity and Sportsmanship'. The Imperial Family took unprecedented interest in the activities and the phenomenon of the International Stoke Mandeville Games, visiting on several occasions and hosting an elaborate reception. Her Imperial Highness Princess Michiko told Joan Scruton that the young Prince had even thought to help ensure good weather for the period of the Games by making the traditional paper doll 'to invoke good luck'. This might have worked in harmony with Ludwig Guttmann's constant claim that he had 'special arrangements' over the weather for the Stoke Mandeville Games, wherever they might be held.

Daphne Legge-Willis could claim to have been one of the most unfortunate competitors in the Tokyo Games, although her story had a happy ending. Negotiating the transfer from the toilet to her wheelchair in her accommodation, she had the misfortune to fall badly and break her ankle. With her right leg duly set in a plaster cast she still went on three days later to take the silver medal in the Columbia Round of the archery competition. The programme of events held in Tokyo included: archery, athletics, dartchery, wheelchair basketball, fencing, weightlifting, table tennis, snooker, swimming, wheelchair dash, wheelchair relay, wheelchair slalom and pentathlon. Particularly popular with spectators were the wheelchair slalom, relay and the sprints. The relay and the 'dash' were appearing for the first time in the International Games.

While some countries were fledgling members of the international sporting movement for people with disabilities, the US team of 66 athletes had been selected according to their qualifying performances at the National Wheelchair Games in New York in June 1964, and approached competition in Tokyo with a seriousness that had come to be a trademark of the progress made in North America. It was necessary to impose a limit on participation in certain combinations of multiple events, as the time taken to complete the table tennis competition, in particular, was prohibitive. But it was the case in Tokyo, as elsewhere, that competitors arrived with very little experience in some of the events they wished to enter. There was also a noteworthy amount of exchange in technical matters relating to equipment during the Games – sometimes directly, such as in the form of the loan of a wheelchair by the Americans, enabling athletes from the Philippines to participate in the wheelchair relays. Competitors also went home with ideas of lowering handrails, strengthening axles, changing from solid to pneumatic tyres and so on. The technical limitations of different countries would remain a dividing factor for a while still: just as the first wheelchair basketball competitions between teams from the USA and Great Britain in 1955 had seen the Pan Am Jets using lightweight chairs and their British counterparts having to work with converted armchairs.

Officiating was sometimes made more complicated by the invitation to use officials from the Olympic Games that had just finished, although they had little or no experience in the adaptations needed for sport for athletes with a disability. Before the swimming competitions could begin in Tokyo, the Swimming Technical Advisor, W. Elson, had to communicate the vagaries of the adapted regulations to the thoroughly enthusiastic Japanese Olympic judges, but through an interpreter who had great difficulties with the technical distinctions. Elson had to resort to drawing pictures, using gestures, and even stretching out on a table in the briefing room to explain – when this was not enough he transferred the meeting to the swimming pool and demonstrated from the water himself. As the Olympic swimming venue was being converted into an ice-skating rink by this time, swimming competitions had to take place in the nine lane, 50 metre Tokyo Metropolitan Pool.

As well as numerous social events during the Games, the competitors, escorts and officials were taken on an excursion to the serene mountain resort of Hakone, and with a police escort throughout, they felt very special indeed. At one point hundreds of children lined the streets welcoming them with traditional flag waving and cheering. The scientific meeting of the International Medical Society of Paraplegia took place in Tokyo, with the further sharing of beneficial technical and medical research findings. Some specific concerns of the particular situation of individuals with paraplegia in Japan were explored in discussion.

The Closing Ceremony was held in the indoor gymnasium in front of some 8000 Japanese spectators. A very typical finish to the International Stoke Mandeville Games was the singing of 'Auld Lang Syne', following which competitors and officials launched their array of different hats to the crowds of spectators around the gymnasium as gifts and souvenirs.

As has been described, it was in Tokyo that the use of the label Paralympic Games became cemented among all the participants. This was confirmed in the common usage of the title in reports and publications of almost all the Tokyo events. Franco Rossi, the fencing champion from the Rome Games, competed again in Tokyo. He described the progress from Rome to Tokyo as a 'miracle': 'It had been possible to make paralytics compete on the same fields and in the same spirit as the Olympic athletes. Thus the Paralympic Games had been born and had become a reality.' The manager of the French Team at the International Stoke Mandeville Games, Philippe Berthe, entitled his official report '18th Olympic Games, 2nd Paralympic Games' (Berthe 1964). He certainly did not tread delicately around the sensitive area of Olympic terminology: 'After the first paralympic games in Rome in 1960, where we began to organise our olympiades (sic), I feel it impossible to compare these two great sports occasions with the exception, perhaps, of certain events in which handicapped and able-bodied people would compete [together]'. Berthe writes of his conviction that the Tokyo Paralympics broke down barriers between participants and spectators: 'we felt some kind of depersonalisation, of all the thousands melting into one spirit, we quite forgot that these competitors were handicapped. We achieved the finest victory there can be; yes, our games were the true brothers of the Olympic Games.'

Progress in public acceptance of disability and official provision for special care and rehabilitation was immense in Japan as a result of the Games in Tokyo. While the competitors and officials who had travelled to Tokyo were surprised to see how many children with disabilities were carried on the backs of their parents as a matter of course due to the lack of orthopaedic aids, the exposure that the Games had given was to help promote the country's outlook in future.

> The athletic performance, endurance and standard of these paralysed athletes were also an extraordinary inspiration to the Japanese Government, private organisations and employers to help their paraplegic fellow men in their social and industrial resettlement. Within 6 months after the Games, the first factory, specially built for the paralysed, called Nagano Plant, 70 miles west of Tokyo was opened for 56 paraplegics in an area of many factories producing cameras and communication machinery (Guttmann 1973).

The visionary organisers of the Games had arranged for Japanese people with disabilities to be able to participate in some aspects of the social events with competitors – even if they were not competitors themselves. This shows true foresight for the potential improvement of each individual's self-belief in these circumstances. Public access to competition venues was largely free of charge, and large crowds encouraged competitors to excel. During the Games there was extensive media coverage as well, with much made of interaction between local and international competitors.

When Yoshisuke Kasai and his team of officials returned from that preliminary visit to the 12th International Stoke Mandeville Games in 1962, they had encouraged the setting up of regular regional games for sportsmen and sportswomen with disabilities the next year. But their plans were inclusive of other disability groups rather than only people with paraplegia. As a result, Japanese national games were held following the 13th International Stoke Mandeville Games in Tokyo, accommodating other disability groups. What then transpired was of note for the future of multi-disability sport: competitors from other countries showed interest in travelling and taking part! The organisers agreed to invite participants from Austria, France and West Germany, but in the end only competitors from West Germany could participate.

Technical, titular and regional developments

Reorganisation was needed in the way wheelchair basketball competitions were run at the International Stoke Mandeville Games. Wheelchair basketball had been separated into two 'classes' for some time, one for complete spinal lesions and one for incomplete lesions. The idea was to ensure that no players were greatly disadvantaged at having to play against others possessing significantly more mobility. But by the 1965 International Stoke Mandeville Games, the numbers involved meant that the classes needed to be combined. A points system was recommended, such as the one that had been successfully employed in the United States. At the next Games the points system was lauded as a great improvement, and added to the excitement and enjoyment of the appreciative spectators.

The International Olympic Committee, watching the Paralympic Movement with interest, contacted the International Stoke Mandeville Games Committee to object officially to its use of the word 'Paralympics'. This did not seem to cause too much consternation within the close-knit group of dedicated individuals on the Committee, and even Ludwig Guttmann saw no need for blood to be spilt over this. It was agreed that they would officially avoid calling their quadrennial events 'Paralympic Games', and pay homage to the birthplace of their competition by calling their celebrations in the Olympic Year the International Stoke Mandeville Games. At least this was the official position – it could not affect the athletes' choice of terminology. These same Committee members would take on the struggle for freedom of use of appropriate terminology at a later time.

Another important phase in the growth of the Paralympic Movement was the establishment of various forms of Regional Games. The Pan-American Wheelchair Games organised in Winnipeg, Canada in 1967, was the first of these, opening up new opportunities for many thousands of athletes with a disability. Later the success of regional and world zone games would eventually see the demise of the Commonwealth Paraplegic Games, as the regional arrangement would make for much greater levels of participation because costs of travel were significantly reduced compared with participation in events in the far-flung parts of the Commonwealth. Of course, this also meant that many countries could develop higher levels of athletic competition through regionally organised events. This initiative remained rather disconnected for a while, but it would ensure the growth of access to competitive situations for increasing numbers of athletes with a disability, and it would encourage people to seek integration of events for different disability groups. Commonwealth Paraplegic Games were held in Perth, Australia (1962), Kingston, Jamaica (1966), Edinburgh, Scotland (1970) and Dunedin, New Zealand (1974).

There was a small-scale European Games held at St Etienne in 1966 that sought recognition from the International Sports Organisation for the Disabled – ISOD was not altogether sure that it wanted to give patronage. The Commonwealth Paraplegic Games were very successfully held in Jamaica in 1966. The previous games held in Perth in 1962 had drawn some 100 participants, but the Jamaican Commonwealth Paraplegic Games attracted nearly 200 athletes.

Mexico off, Israel on: 1968

Observers from Mexico attended the Tokyo1964 Paralympic Games to assess the organisation of such an event in their own country four years later. With growing discussion among scientists, the United States offered to send delegates to Mexico City to investigate the possible effects of altitude on sportsmen and sportswomen with spinal injury paralysis. Representatives of the International Stoke Mandeville Games Committee would have planned to travel to Mexico, as a matter of course, to have discussions with the organising committee there for the next Games. But in 1966 the Committee received a letter from Mexico to say that it definitely would not be able to host the Games there. The Mexican Government cited technical difficulties as the reason for not being able to host Paralympic Games in conjunction with the Olympic Games. This was very disappointing, and it broke the youthful 'tradition' of Games held in the Olympic year being located in the same city or country as the Olympic Games. But there were ongoing problems of political stability in Mexico, human rights concerns, and from the competitors' point of view, not was enough known about the effects of altitude on persons with disability.

Arieh Fink, President of the Israeli International Stoke Mandeville Games Committee, and an official of the Israeli government, attended the 1966 Games in Aylesbury to officially extend Israel's invitation to hold the 1968 International Stoke Mandeville Games in Israel. This pleased Guttmann enormously, as the sequence of Games being held outside Stoke Mandeville in the Olympic year could, at least, be maintained – even if the sporting celebration could not take place in the same country as the Olympic Games themselves. He was also quietly pleased to have the opportunity to take the Games to Israel, the home of his religious roots. There had been long-standing associations between Guttmann and Israeli medical specialists working with people who had received spinal injuries, and Israeli teams had travelled to Aylesbury since 1954. Dr Spira, who had spent some time as a Medical Officer at Stoke Mandeville Hospital, brought a team of war veterans to the International Stoke Mandeville Games. Facilities for staging the 1968 Paralympic Games were offered by the Israel Foundation for Handicapped Children (ILAN) in Ramat Gan, a short distance outside Tel Aviv.

As the plans for the Tel Aviv 1968 Paralympic Games began to take shape, it was obvious that this would be a time of great celebration: the 20th anniversary of the founding of the Stoke Mandeville Games was to coincide with the festivities connected to the 20th anniversary of the founding of the State of Israel. At the Opening Ceremony on 4th November, more than 10 000 spectators packed the stadium of the Hebrew University in Jerusalem, and watched the athletes and escorts enter the arena and take their places to form a unified community for the duration of the Games. Yigal Allon, Deputy Prime Minister of Israel, declared the 1968 Paralympic Games open. This third event held in the cycle of quadrennial Games in the Olympic year brought together 750 athletes representing 29 countries.

Athletes, escorts and coaches were accommodated in the Maccabean Village in Tel Aviv, while the members of the International Stoke Mandeville Games Committee stayed in a Tel Aviv hotel. Each day a very well organised system transported the participants by a brief bus ride to the events at Ramat Gan. The Director of the ILAN Sports Centre, Gershon Huberman, directed the sports programme, now expanded further to include lawn bowls, women's wheelchair basketball and 100 m men's wheelchair race for the first time. The events were: archery, athletics, wheelchair basketball, dartchery, fencing, lawn bowls, powerlifting, snooker, swimming and table tennis. Classification systems had been adjusted and were applied in swimming, wheelchair basketball and athletics.

The Australian swimmer Lorraine Dodd made a particularly great impact on the capacity crowds at the pool as she powered her way to three wins. But the newspapers agreed with the spectators and other participants at the Israel Games that the most astonishing accomplishments came from Roberto Marson (Italy), who had previously found success in athletics field events in Tokyo in 1964. In Tel Aviv, Marson scooped up nine gold medals across three different sporting disciplines: three in his home territory of athletics, then also three golds in swimming and three more in fencing. In team events it was the wheelchair basketball that brought the biggest crowds. In particular the news media built up the early successes of the Israeli team, so when they reached the final – to play against the United States – something resembling pandemonium was beheld as several thousand local people struggled to gain entry to the sports centre. It was a rivalry worthy of the attention of so many sports enthusiasts, and the team from the home country eventually pulled away from the United States team to win 47 to 37.

The scientific meetings associated with the International Medical Society of Paraplegia continued with three days of meetings, one day at the Hadassah University Medical Centre in Jerusalem, and the final two days' meetings held in Tel Aviv. Volunteers helping to make the Games a success numbered more than double those of the competitors, coming from schools, colleges and the junior cadet force. There was a large contingent of military personnel helping at all venues.

Was the Stoke Mandeville Influence Waning?

As the Commonwealth Paraplegic Games of 1970 were being prepared for Edinburgh, Scotland, it was hoped that teams travelling from greater distances would take the opportunity of competing in both these and the International Stoke Mandeville Games earlier in July. Many teams did just this, but the organisers in Aylesbury were extremely unhappy that the Australian authorities had decided only to give their attention to the Commonwealth Games. Questions began to be asked at Stoke Mandeville about the possible loss of sway and magnitude of the International Stoke Mandeville Games within the disabled sport movement. They felt strongly enough – and were worried enough – to circulate a request for organisations and nations to steer clear of the timing of the International Stoke Mandeville Games, as they were the event with precedence and should be respected. This was just a touch haughty, and would stir up predictable reactions from people around the world who had begun to feel that they did not need the Stoke Mandeville 'brigade' to lead them by the hand every step of the way. But the Stoke Mandeville Committee did need to reassess its prospects for the future; discussions had to include opening access to other disability groups through ISOD, and the encouragement of regionally coordinated competitions to operate in harmony with the calendar for International Stoke Mandeville Games.

The International Stoke Mandeville Games Committee had consistently come under fire from people involved in various aspects of sport for people with disabilities, including some of those directly involved with the sports movement for individuals with spinal injuries. The lack of democratic structure was one factor that gave cause for concern, as an inflexible structure that showed few signs of changing. But the domineering attitude of Ludwig Guttmann produced the most reaction, although people respected him for all his pioneering work to open up the world of competitive sport. Guttmann never seemed to give up his stance as a medical expert first and foremost – with all athletes treated as patients. Sport was subjugated to being one of a range of rehabilitative processes. Guttmann's strong and belligerent character, so essential in overcoming so many apparently insuperable obstacles in the earliest years, was not able to step back and adopt a calmer, more egalitarian attitude. In the climate of cooperation and growing openness of the late 1960s and into the 1970s, Guttmann's autocratic approach was beginning to affect the progress of the Paralympic Movement.

MAKING PROGRESS: 1972–1980

'1000 Competitors, 1000 Winners': the 4th Paralympic Games, Heidelberg, 1972

The 4th Paralympic Games were held in Heidelberg, Germany. Although Ludwig Guttmann travelled to meet with Willi Daume, the President of the German Olympic Committee, he had been unsuccessful in persuading him to help change the decision so that the Paralympic Games of 1972 could be held in the same city as the Olympic Games. The plan for the City of Munich to convert the Olympic Village into private housing could not be altered or even delayed, and the German Disabled Sports Association (DSV) tried in vain to overcome the logistical nightmare of locating temporary accommodation for the participants. Walther Weiss, a member of the International Stoke Mandeville Games Committee, had proposed Heidelberg when the Munich option was closed to them. So it was that the President of the Federal Republic of Germany, Dr Gustav Heineman, opened the Paralympic Games in Heidelberg, taking the opportunity of presenting Ludwig Guttmann with the Federal Republic of Germany's 'Gold Star of the Great Cross of Merit'. This must have been quite a moving occasion for Guttmann, honoured by the country from which he had sought exile almost thirty years earlier.

In Munich, the sporting phenomenon of the Olympic Games brought wonder and adoration at the marvellous achievements of individuals such as Mark Spitz (USA), Shane Gould (Australia) and Kornelia Ender (East Germany) in the swimming pool, Olga Korbut (USSR) in the gymnastics arena, and the powerful sprinter Valeri Borzov (USSR), all capturing the hearts of sports enthusiasts around the world. But the Olympic Games had also been visited by great tragedy as the Arab terrorists from the Black September Movement took hostage and later killed eleven members of the Israeli Team. The political use of the Olympic Games was more focused than ever before. The Olympic Games would take many years to recover from this outrage, with some scars remaining permanently.

The Institute of Physical Training of the University of Heidelberg was provided as a suitable venue for the sporting events of the Paralympic Games, and expertise was already on hand to support the extremely able band of technical officials brought in by the International Stoke Mandeville Games Committee. Volkmar Paeslack, Director of the Spinal Injuries Centre in the Orthopaedic University Clinic, was the Chairman of the Games Organising Committee.

This was to be an occasion on a monumental scale, with over a thousand competitors from 41 countries – many more than had been represented in Israel. Events were offered for the first time for quadriplegic athletes. The limitations experienced by the organisers prevented the proposed competitions for amputees being staged in Heidelberg. The other significant departure in Heidelberg was that demonstration events were held for blind athletes: goalball and 100 m track event. The positive responses to these demonstrations led to the full inclusion of medal events in the next Paralympics in Toronto, four years later. The sports programme otherwise remained the same as for the previous Paralympic Games. After the exciting men's wheelchair basketball final in Tel Aviv four years earlier, tensions mounted as the same two countries seemed to be lining up to play off again for the top two positions. In the true way of sporting endeavour, the team from the United States nosed past the team from Israel to lift the gold medal with the closest of margins – the scoreline was 59 to 58.

As the Heidelberg 1972 Paralympic Games closed, the meeting of trainers and coaches agreed that more extensive technical input could be offered if each of the sports involved in the International Stoke Mandeville Games formed a sub-committee – effectively a sports technical committee. The first to do this was swimming: the International Swimming Training Association for the Paralysed was founded just before the Heidelberg Games, and other sports sections followed. Although limited by being so strongly attached to the International Stoke Mandeville Games organisation in its terms of reference, these sport-specific bodies would set a precedent for sports technical committees later in the history of the Paralympic Movement.

The 4th Paralympic Games ended with rapturous acclamation for the City of Heidelberg and the Organising Committee. This would be the last time that the Paralympic Games would be held under the banner of the International Stoke Mandeville Games Federation.

Regional and 'World Zone' Games take on Greater Significance

The Commonwealth Paraplegic Games held in Dunedin, New Zealand, in 1974 were an excellent example of the benefits to a country of hosting such an event. With his typical missionary zeal, Ludwig Guttmann toured the country seeking time with as many key people as possible – he would persuade politicians of the dreadful provision their country was making for people with spinal injuries in comparison with a number of other countries. He would tug at the pride of these important people, shaming them into either supporting the smooth running of the forthcoming competition, or into redirecting public or corporate money to longer-term service (or both). The nation of New Zealand embraced the Commonwealth Paraplegic Games willingly, and much positive awareness was created through the more visible presence of people with disabilities. Direct intervention of this sort by Guttmann may have had some influence on the completion of the Spinal Injuries Unit at Burwood Hospital, Christchurch. But the Dunedin Games were to end the sequence of Commonwealth Paraplegic Games. Success was still being found in this formula, but the participating countries had been discussing the very best way that athletes with a disability (in this case those athletes with spinal injuries and polio) could be offered opportunities in sporting competition. The arrangement of the Commonwealth Games caused problems of a greater magnitude for persons with a disability than for other athletes, particularly as the travel was seldom easy or cheap. The Commonwealth Paraplegic Games Committee recommended to the International Stoke Mandeville Games Committee – as the supreme authority in this matter – that 'World Zone Games' should be established. This was a very significant moment in the development of the modern Paralympic Movement; the timing of this proposal was good for it but it did not entirely suit the International Stoke Mandeville Games Committee's plans. This was to be a defining moment in the shift away from prominence of Stoke Mandeville.

People who had been involved in the Paralympic Movement from Singapore, Japan and Australia met in Singapore in April 1974 to consider preparations for regional competitions in South East Asia and the Pacific. Their initiative resulted directly from the wish to build on the successful nature of international competition for people with disabilities, but with an eye on bringing the rivalry closer to home. The Far East and South Pacific (FESPIC) Games for the Handicapped Arrangement Committee was constituted at this April meeting. Appropriately for the time, this organisation would look straight-away at a more extensive range of sporting opportunities, multi-disability regional championships, but under the umbrella of ISMGF and ISOD.

First Winter Paralympic Games: Örnsköldsvik, Sweden 1976

Fourteen countries sent teams to participate in the very first Winter Paralympic Games, hosted by Sweden in Örnsköldsvik. This was a truly adventurous project, although there had long been enthusiasm for the people with disabilities whose main competitive sports were winter sports to have access to opportunities on the same public stage as those catered for by the Summer Paralympic cycle. Those attending the Örnsköldsvik Games fared better than their counterparts at the Innsbrück Winter Olympic Games, where almost a quarter succumbed to influenza-related ailments.

As part of a steady progression, the first Winter Paralympics included events for blind athletes and amputees, as well as a demonstration of the sport of sledge racing. A total of 136 medals were awarded, and the Federal Republic of Germany topped the 'Medal Table', with Switzerland, Finland and Sweden in order behind them. Although the number of participants would not grow inordinately until the Winter Paralympic Games in Lillehammer, Norway, in 1994, the size of the Games in Örnsköldsvik was just right for the ambitions of the organisers. Bengt Hollen acted as Chairman of the Organising Committee, ably supported by an effective team. Classification was the key conundrum that would need much work before the next Paralympic Winter Games in Geilo.

Torontolympiad, Canada, 1976

In 1975, the International Sports Organisation for the Disabled worked together with the International Stoke Mandeville Games Federation to prepare for the Paralympic Games in Toronto, Canada. The effectiveness of their cooperation was secured because of the presence of Ludwig Guttmann as President of both organisations at the same time; this certainly paved the way for effective working practices that would act as an example a few years later, when these two organisations were to be involved in discussions to extend coordination to other international organisations of sport for persons with a disability. Guttmann was keen that the Torontolympiad should be a great success, as he could envisage these Games setting a new pattern for the future: he gauged the inevitability that more disabilities would be added to the Paralympic Games, and to him the only feasible management of such diverse competitions would be via cooperation between ISMGF and ISOD. At this stage Guttmann had not expected that other disability sports federations would need to have a hand in the administration of the Games. In 1980, the same 'double act' would cooperate in the organisation of the Arnhem Paralympic Games.

The Toronto Paralympic Games were also referred to as the Olympic Games for the Disabled, or the Torontolympiad. They saw the introduction of many new events, arising from the inclusion of visually impaired and amputee athletes. Competition rules and classification systems had been agreed within ISOD, and preparatory trials had taken place – Stoke Mandeville had laid on what it called the World Multi-Disability Games in 1974 to test some of the regulations and to familiarise officials who would then be present in Toronto. Dick Loiselle was appointed Executive Director of the Organising Committee and Bob Jackson took the chairmanship. The Montreal Olympic Organising Committee would not permit the use of the Olympic facilities to the Paralympic Movement, just as had been the case in Munich, but remarkable support was pledged from the Toronto and Ontario governments. The Olympium, a new Athletics stadium, was built for the Games, and would be used in conjunction with the stadium at Centennial Park. By the time of the Opening Ceremony, attended by some 25 000 people at the Woodbine Race Track, the uncertainties of whether the Toronto Paralympic Games could actually take place were well behind.

The issue had been apartheid in South Africa, and this was the first real interference of global political matters impinging on the Paralympic Movement. A multi-racial team from the South African Sports Organisation for the Disabled was entered for the Toronto Games. Perhaps the Movement had so far not been 'important' enough to be affected by world politics, and perhaps politics now touched more people in every part of their lives. But just as sport can be an escape from the real world, it also takes place in the context of the real world. The problem stemmed from the logic that admitting a team from South Africa was to give implicit approval for its government's attitude towards segregation and racism. The Olympic Games in Montreal would suffer mercilessly from the boycott of 25 countries – sparked by a New Zealand rugby tour to South Africa. In January 1976, the Canadian Federal Government withdrew its very considerable financial contribution (Canadian $500 000) from the Paralympics on the basis of the acceptance of the South African team's entry, with the start of the Games due in August. Matching amounts of funds were also likely to be pulled out by the metropolitan government if it could not be persuaded otherwise. Guttmann and Bob Jackson worked tirelessly to convince the different levels of government that they should honour their promise and continue the flow of resources to the Organising Committee for the Torontolympiad. They were mostly successful in their endeavours, and any plans to scale down the Paralympics were shelved. Unfortunately, a number of teams withdrew from the Torontolympiad on the same basis that boycotts took place in Montreal. These nations were threatened with exclusion from future events should they fail to comply with the ISMGF Executive Committee's decisions. After the Games, the opinion of the IOC was sought to try to find a joint policy that might prevent this happening again.

Vast numbers of new records were established at the Torontolympiad – many as a result of the additional categories of disability: visually impaired and amputee athletes. New crowd-pleasing events were seen on the track: extending the wheelchair racing to include races for 200 m, 400 m, 800 m and 1500 m. Goalball moved to medal status for the first time, as well as rifle shooting being introduced following very successful trials at Stoke Mandeville. These two sports would thrive in the context of the Paralympic Movement, giving many thousand athletes access to high levels of competition over the years. But the additional numbers of competitors requiring classification nearly overloaded the medical teams at the Games. Accommodating the 1600 athletes was a headache for the Organising Committee. The adjustments that had to be made as a result of the reduction in funding meant that there was no single athletes' village, but participants had to be housed in separate batches. In some unfortunate cases this led to national team members having to be apart. Although the sporting events, and some social opportunities, brought them together, the athletes were largely accommodated by disability – this was expedient use of resources, but it did not integrate the different disabilities as much as was desirable.

Increasingly heard around the competition venues, and in the numerous additional meetings of experts, was the call for a single supreme body to oversee such a complex and expanding phenomenon. The valiant efforts of ISMGF and ISOD were greatly appreciated, and yet this was the beginning of the end for this style of management.

Arnold Bolt, a Canadian teenager, was acclaimed the outstanding athlete of the Toronto Paralympic Games. He won gold medals in both the long jump and the high jump. The most remarkable wheelchair athlete of the Games was the United States' David Kiley, who set world records in sprint and longer distance wheelchair races, taking gold in the 100 m, 800 m and 1500 m events. The multi-talented Kiley was also a member of the winning wheelchair basketball team that again bettered the Israeli basketball team in the 1976 final: 59 to 46. Toronto saw the greatest media coverage of the cycle of Paralympic Games so far, with the daily television and radio coverage serving to attract even more spectators to the sports venues to watch athletes' achievements 'live'.

Apart from minor complications caused by failure of the computer system, the rest of the administration of the Torontolympiad went well. Some readjustments had to be made as a result of the teams that withdrew over the South African team's participation, and the financial uncertainties were well in the past. This was the first Paralympic Games to be marred by political disruption, and it was the first Games of its size and scale – with a welcome to blind and amputee athletes.

Geilo, Norway 1980

The first Paralympic Games to include all locomotor disabilities was the winter competition held in Norway, prior to the summer Paralympics in Arnhem. The small Norwegian resort of Geilo hosted the 2nd Paralympic Winter Games, under the enthusiastic direction of the Norwegian Sports Organisation for the Disabled, and over 350 competitors represented 18 countries. There were some concerns about the extreme cold conditions, and the sports were thought to have some real safety issues to resolve. The top of the Medals Table was occupied by Finland, with Norway coming next, just ahead of Austria. Downhill sledge racing was seen as a demonstration event, and the giant slalom would be introduced in the next Winter Games, in Austria in 1984. While the American speed skater, Eric Heiden, was winning his five gold medals in the Winter Olympic Games at Lake Placid in 1980, Doug Kiel from Alaska was receiving his two gold medals for slalom events in the Geilo 1980 Winter Paralympic Games. Kiel went on to help establish the Challenge Alaska foundation, bringing opportunities to many thousands of people with disabilities.

Waiting Patiently for a Reply from Moscow, and the South African Question

In his usual independent way, immediately after the Torontolympiad, Ludwig Guttmann had tried to make contact with various individuals within the Government of the Soviet Union, to draw them on the issue of holding the next Paralympic Games in conjunction with the Moscow Olympic Games of 1980. Even his usually persuasive techniques had evinced no direct response from them, and Guttmann had to acknowledge defeat. Jean Stone suggests that the official view of the Soviet Union was that there were 'no disabled people in the Soviet Union'. Of course the organisation of the next Paralympic Games had to proceed, and it was with joy that the invitation arrived from the Netherlands Sports Organisation for the Disabled to hold the Paralympics in Arnhem; this was accepted. In addition to the Netherlands, bids had been received from the federations in Denmark and also South Africa. Soon after having its invitation accepted, the Dutch Organising Committee established the Foundation of the Olympic Games for the Disabled. This would eventually have a longer-serving involvement in supporting the sports movement for people with disabilities beyond the Arnhem Paralympic Games.

The racial question was not going to diminish in importance for people involved in international sport. The International Stoke Mandeville Games Federation tried to maintain an ethically supportive position, acknowledging that success was being achieved within the context of sport for people with disabilities in South Africa. In 1977, the Jamaican Paraplegic Association proposed that the International Stoke Mandeville Games Federation should exclude South Africa from future Games. The motion was defeated. Some contact was made with the South African Non-Racial Olympic Committee (SANROC) in 1978, and in March of that year a number of representatives of ISOD and ISMGF travelled to Cape Town to attend the South African Sports Organisation for the Disabled championships. This trip was also an opportunity for the two organisations to investigate the situation in South Africa, and to see for themselves whether the claims of the authorities were accurate: that there was no racism practised within sport in that country. At the ISMGF Council Meeting of 1979, there was extensive discussion on the subject of South Africa in relation to the preparations for the next Paralympic Games in Arnhem. The International Stoke Mandeville Games Federation issued a press release in support of the UN and all those working against racism in sport. In particular, ISMGF made a strong statement commending South Africa for the progress being made. A resolution was unanimously passed:

> The ISMGF Executive Committee, knowing its South African member organisation to have suc-
> ceeded in its struggle against apartheid in sport, being the first organisation in South Africa to send
> multi-racial teams chosen on merit alone to compete in international sports events, unanimously voted
> to support the inclusion of South Africa in the 1980 Olympics for the Disabled in Holland.

As might have been expected, though, this would not be the end of the matter.

The Passing of Ludwig Guttmann

The Arnhem Paralympic Games would mark the turning point for the Paralympic Movement: in order to move positively towards some sort of multi-disability international umbrella organisation, the International Coordinating Committee would be established; there would be four distinct sports federations involved; athletes with cerebral palsy would be involved for the first time. The Stoke Mandeville influence would be reduced conspicuously by the spread of disability groups – each having a discrete constituency to look after. But Joan Scruton has commented that her 'heart was not really in these Olympics'. The major change in mood was to one of sadness at the death of Ludwig Guttmann in 1980. He had suffered a heart attack in October 1979 and died on 18th March. Guttmann had dedicated his life to the medical rehabilitation of spinally injured people and on the way he had given the greatest gift to people with disabilities: hope and an opportunity to believe in self-worth. 'Poppa' Guttmann had been a tough adversary, but in the tradition of many pioneers he had been able to cut through previously impervious barriers to make progress. No one could question the contribution made by Guttmann to the Paralympic Movement, acknowledging that his caustic approach to opposition was part of his constitution. The time was right for the Paralympic Movement to move on to grasp the global view: truly multi-disability Paralympic Games organised by a cooperative group of representatives with expert knowledge of the particular characteristic needs of their own disability groups.

Arnhem Hosts the 1980 Paralympic Games

The South African question almost toppled the Arnhem Paralympics altogether. The International Stoke Mandeville Games Federation's Executive Committee had shown unanimous support at its 1979 Council meeting for the participation of the South African team at the Arnhem Paralympics. But there was pressure from a number of sports organisations in the Netherlands against the Organising Committee, as well as the negative standpoint of the Dutch Parliament. Meetings with the representatives of the South African Non-Racial Olympic Committee produced no solution – public and official opinion was against the inclusion of the South African team. Things accelerated as the time of the Games drew closer. The media feasted on the controversy, interviewing and seeking statements from all quarters. A joint delegation from ISOD and ISMGF met with the Dutch Organising Committee almost without interruption over a period of days. The Dutch Parliament would hold the deciding card: they would vote on whether to permit the Games to be held should the South African Team be admitted. In October the decision went against the South African Team, and they were informed that they would not be allowed to participate. The Paralympic Movement had to accept that it was operating in a real, and political, world.

Papendal National Sports Centre, in Arnhem, was the venue for most of the sports programme of the 1980 Olympics for the Disabled. The De Vallei 50 metre swimming pool at Veenendaal provided the setting for the swimming competition, although there was also a training pool at Papendal. The Arnhem Rijnhal indoor facility hosted the wheelchair basketball and the two volleyball competitions. These were each some distance from the accommodation provided by the army at the Oranje Barracks in Schaarsbergen, but there was no great consternation at having to travel between facilities.

Although much of the publicity relating to the South African participation had been negative, it did succeed in outing the vocabulary of the disabled sports movement into the minds of many people who would not otherwise have considered the subject at all. The Dutch organisers also increased visibility through their fundraising: Telebingo was a very important success, building a fund that would hold a surplus years after the Games. This would naturally find its expression in the International Fund Sport Disabled, supporting the future of the Paralympic Movement in the 1980s.

The Opening Ceremony was held on 12th June, with more than 12 000 participants. Her Royal Highness Princess Margriet of the Netherlands, as Patron of the Games, declared the 1980 'Olympics for the Disabled' open. For the first time, athletes with cerebral palsy would join blind, spinally injured and amputee athletes at the Paralympic Games. Everyone appreciated the wonderful spectacle of so many athletes joined together for the purpose of competing in high-level sport, even if only wheelchair athletes actually participated in the parade of athletes at the Opening Ceremony due to the size of the Papendal setting.

A problem that would remain for a while was the vast number of medals on offer: some 3000 medals were awarded as a result of the entirely separate classifications. It was a puzzle to many members of the public, and the ceremonial proceedings slowed their enjoyment of the event to some extent. The rationalisation of medal numbers would not find a definitive solution for a few years, when classification systems would be altered to integrate athletes. Even in June the weather was very unkind, and rain was prevalent throughout the Paralympic Games in Arnhem.

Sports at the Arnhem Games were archery, athletics, basketball, fencing, goalball, lawn bowls, powerlifting, shooting, swimming, table tennis, volleyball (sitting and standing) and wrestling. Trischa Zorn (USA) came to the medal rostrum to collect a fantastic seven gold medals for her swimming achievements, and Arnold Bolt (Canada) was back again, taking the high jump title and lifting the world record even higher (1.96 m).

Joint Study Group Explores the Way Ahead

There was support for exploration of some sort of coordinating group to represent all international sports organisations in dealings with the International Olympic Committee and the organisation of the four-yearly Games in conjunction with the Olympic Games. Guttmann, as ever, had posed the awkward question of what people wanted the future to be. At the 1977 General Assembly of ISOD he had insisted that members should address this issue.

Joan Scruton, Secretary General of ISOD, wrote a discussion paper for circulation to prompt responses from member organisations. In her 1978 document she wrote:

> There is a real desire and pattern to develop international sports organisations for individual disabilities. I think the time has come for ISOD to recognise this and consider whether it should not assume the role of an overall umbrella organisation, coordinating the work of the individual international organisations. In effect, ISOD would become the coordinating committee of sport for all persons with a disability, like the International Olympic Committee, and in the Olympic years would act as overall organisation for the individual sports organisations. This, I feel, would overcome much of the confusion and conflict which now exist, particularly on a national basis, where often there are several organisations acting independently of each other.

This personally expressed paper held no surprises, but stated some important issues that needed to be addressed before long – chaotic fragmentation would inevitably follow unless there was careful planning.

The next major contribution towards stability came from a joint study conducted by Guillermo Cabezas and Arieh Fink, and submitted to member organisations of ISOD in April 1979. The Executive Committee of ISOD had asked for this study, looking into the present organisation and ways of structuring future operations. It was not difficult for members of ISOD to accept Cabezas' point that there already existed a significant amount of cooperation and directly coordinated activity, and there was even duplication of posts held on different bodies by the same people. But the paper went on to propose a move towards the establishment of a single federation. It was appropriate for ISOD to be the forum for this planning as various branches of the working structure of ISOD were practised in bringing different international organisations together. The Technical Committee and the Medical Committee each had representatives from international organisations who shared specialities relating to their particular membership and needs, but worked together on specific projects. The Executive Committee was a noticeably broader example of representation and cooperation. The Cabezas-Fink paper was essential at the time, considering the increasing number of organisations and the possibility of a more diverse future rather than a unified one – resistance to any change would always be present due to the potential for loss of identity and control. Individuals in any situation like this might feel that they could be ousted from positions they had worked hard to aspire to and achieve. These were not unreasonable concerns, but the main anxiety at this time was that the discernible practical benefits must outweigh the danger of representing their own constituency less well. In this context it was the ISOD itself that stood to lose its identity if further disability-specific international organisations should be established, but it would also suffer if a new umbrella organisation supplanted it in its coordinating role – unless ISOD could become that umbrella organisation.

The Cabezas-Fink paper encouraged the setting up of a Study Group charged with finding a way forward. The Study Group, in action by July 1979, had representation from the International Sports Organisation for the Disabled, the International Stoke Mandeville Games Federation, Cerebral Palsy-International Sports and Recreation Association and the World Council for the Welfare of the Blind. At the first meeting, a resolution was passed that set out their intentions:

> In considering the future role of international sport for disabled athletes, it is proposed that ISOD be established as an umbrella organisation for sport for the disabled, called the *International Sports Federation of the Disabled (ISFD)*. The members of ISFD shall be the existing and potential accredited international sports organisations of individual disabilities (such as the International Stoke Mandeville Games Federation (ISMGF), Cerebral Palsy-International Sports and Recreation Association (CP-ISRA) and international sports organisations for amputees, blind, deaf, and mentally retarded). These international member organisations for individual disabilities shall retain their full autonomy as at present. The international sports organisations shall have as members the accredited national sports organisations for the specific disability in any country who must undertake to obey the rules of their international organisations.

A very lengthy meeting of the Study Group made great headway in June 1980 in Arnhem, during the Paralympic Games. Over three sessions, the representatives tried to work through the intricate problem of how to bring together sport for persons with a disability on an international level in a single unified way: a phenomenon that, on a national level, was represented in two different ways. This puzzle was made more difficult because ISOD had to examine its own future – and it was made up of national representatives and not international disability organisations. With the existence of other international organisations, ISOD had for some time found its main purpose in representing amputees and 'les Autres'. Marcel Avronsart, presiding over the meetings, indicated that in the interval between the second and third sessions there had been informal discussions between some members and a proposal had been formed that might satisfy all those assembled. Bob Jackson outlined the proposal:

> To create a Federation of International Sports for the handicapped as a federation of accepted international sports organisations for individual disabilities with the purpose of bringing unity and mutual cooperation in the field of sport for the disabled and to coordinate international and regional games that involved more than one disability group in agreement and cooperation with the international sports organisations concerned.

A General Assembly would bring representation from disability organisations with the actual eligibility for delegates enabling each country to be represented. After due consideration of this proposal it was resolved that the name of this organisation should be the International Federation of Sports Organisations for the Disabled (IFSOD). With international sports organisations for individuals with spinal cord paralysis (ISMGF) and those with cerebral palsy (CP-ISRA) already in existence, and with blind sport about to be formalised under the International Blind Sport Association (April 1981), IFSOD was to operate on behalf of all other disability groups until a time came when they founded their own international organisations for their disability group. Although the International Federation of Sports Organisations for the Disabled had a relatively short existence, it did give rise to the wider-reaching International Coordinating Committee.

CONCLUSION

Excitement and apprehension would have been in the minds of the officers of the international disability sport federations, as they recognised the inexorable move towards some sort of unified body. These individuals were experts in the needs of their particular membership. In some cases they had been responsible for their largely independent progress over the past twenty years and would not welcome the loss of autonomy, or of the status that came with their position. For others, they were at the helm of a very young federation looking to carry out a newly defined mandate. These factors would lie behind many fiery discussions between them, and it is sometimes surprising that so much was achievable so quickly. The spectacular progress of the infant Paralympic Movement between 1960 and 1979 was one characterised by the 'big events' rather than by the security of the international federations, or their willingness to work together effectively. The last few years had given some limited opportunities to step outside the relatively 'safe' environment of ISMGF running the major quadrennial celebration of disability sport, with others catered for on a less magnificent scale – or so some would perceive it. The period was one of realisation of what the Movement could develop into. Participants realised that the Paralympics, by any name, were here to stay. The Paralympic Movement had to shrug off the symbolic bonds of paternalism and begin to take responsibility for the larger community of athletes with a disability. The Study Group was to lead to the establishment of the International Coordinating Committee that would bring the international federations around a single table to discuss how to manage the Paralympic Movement for the future. It would take a number of years to do this, and it would not carry everyone along with it. But it would open up opportunities to thousands more of the world's athletes, giving hope and meaning to many people who were to benefit from these developments.

CHAPTER 4

Fair, not Equal: 1980 to 1988

OVERVIEW

Before looking at the detailed progress over the next eight years, it is worth providing a brief outline of the major issues that will feature in this chapter. The next step forward in the creation of a true Paralympic Movement was to be along the route of globalisation: acknowledgement that the different international sports organisations for athletes with a disability must effectively draw together to achieve the greatest rewards. The United Nations declaration that the 1980s would be the Decade of the Disabled gave hope to everyone involved. There was the acceptance that some organisations could not survive without the financial and moral support of larger bodies, and the chance of latching on to the United Nations or the International Olympic Committee could mean significant security. But there was also a need for the Paralympic Movement to grasp the sticky problem of heritage: the overwhelming influence of individuals such as Ludwig Guttmann had tended to polarise attitudes among the representatives of the international federations. Decision making was restricted to a few people, and seldom involved the athletes themselves: 'it seems fair to typify the prevailing international-level organisation as being somewhat patriarchal and European dominated' (Miller 1984). An exciting period of forward projection follows, with the International Coordinating Committee being established by the Study Group of the International Sports Organisation for the Disabled (ISOD) and the International Stoke Mandeville Games Federation (ISMGF). The position of the new International Coordinating Committee (ICC) needs to be assessed within a context of increasing calls for a democratic means of organising sport for people with disabilities. This first organisation was considered by some to be the ideal structure for the secure future of the Paralympic Movement. By others it would be seen as a temporary tenancy, and the search for permanence was to begin. The establishment of this organisation was proposed by Jens Bromann at a General Assembly of ISOD and then established by the ISMGF/ISOD Study Group. It was to set off on a worthwhile course, and it would be effective in its duties. But the International Coordinating Committee was to have the tough job of harmonisation across established 'brick walls' of disability groups.

As these years went on the International Coordinating Committee had an increasing influence as truly representing sport for athletes with a disability. But as its influence grew, a number of additional questions manifested themselves. The wish for the ICC to speak with a united voice necessarily meant that it must represent the whole community of organisations. The prize would be recognition and approval from the International Olympic Committee, and also the public association of the Paralympic Movement with the International Coordinating Committee. In order to 'service' a wider membership, the ICC would effectively have to keep a paternal eye on more than just the Paralympic Summer and

Athlete First: A History of the Paralympic Movement   Steve Bailey
© 2008 John Wiley & Sons, Ltd

Winter Games, because the organisations not involved in the founding of ICC were as yet also not involved in the Paralympic Games. The Comité International des Sports des Sourds (CISS), representing sport for deaf athletes, would either retain its existing major events, or at least would not integrate immediately into the Paralympics. Two organisations provided for athletes with intellectual disability: the International Association for Sport for Persons with Mental Handicap (INAS-FMH) and Special Olympics Inc. The latter had been established in 1968 and had already received recognition from the International Olympic Committee. Special Olympics had its own major world championships, and would need good reason to align itself with ICC – but then which of the two organisations for athletes with intellectual disability, INAS-FMH or Special Olympics Inc., should have prominence, as the IOC insisted on only dealing with one organisation representing its constituency?

Financing major events such as the Paralympic Games, as well as the operation of the ICC itself, was aided by the generous help of the International Fund Sport Disabled, which had arisen from the Arnhem Paralympic Games of 1980. But the flow from this source slowed to a trickle and then stopped during this period, waiting to see what would happen to the umbrella organisation of the International Coordinating Committee.

National representation would come on to the agenda in the 1980s, with members of the ICC considering that this would help to strengthen the structure. But the issue of national representation directly on to the International Coordinating Committee was anathema to the separate international sports federations. At the same time, when this debate opened up, it would see the demise of the ICC itself, but in order to give birth to the next generation of organisation – the International Paralympic Committee.

An important seminar in 1985 looked ahead to the future wanted by the member organisations represented on the International Coordinating Committee. The seminar's participants confirmed their wish for a single world organisation to bring them all together; the representatives wanted integration with the sporting programmes of the international sports federations for people without disabilities, so that athletes with a disability could compete in the programmes of each sporting world championship. The delegates at the seminar also recognised that there was a need to combine classifications for locomotor disabilities so as to reduce the number of events, and thereby increase the attraction of the competitions. In 1987 the next ICC Seminar would appoint an Ad Hoc Committee to construct a suitable draft constitution to update the structure of an international coordinating organisation, for ratification in 1989.

As this chapter examines the details of the 1980s, we will see that the decade was a period of seminal change: the dominance of the International Stoke Mandeville Games under Guttmann's direction and control diminished and it shifted to an independent but isolated existence. There was then some haphazard interaction, in preparation for the beginnings of cooperation and coordinated progress. It was time for a disability-focused approach to give way to a sports-focused approach. Tensions underlay every exchange between different international federations, born of the struggle each had had to identify itself in an already unwelcoming environment. They had to be convinced that things would get better before letting go of their hard fought positions.

THE INTERNATIONAL COORDINATING COMMITTEE IS ESTABLISHED

Progress of the ISOD/ISMGF Study Group

Joan Scruton led the third meeting of the Study Group on 6th December 1980, just before the joint meeting of the Executive Committees of ISMGF and ISOD later that day. Representation was always going to be a complex issue and precision was crucial to the feeling that constituents were going to be well served. At this meeting of the Study Group it was agreed that in the proposed confederate body, 'each national group in each country in bona fide association with ISOD, ISMGF, CP-ISRA, and IBSA will have the right to send one voting representative to the General Assembly'. The Executive Committee's constitution also generated lengthy discussion, and with almost full approval the following was agreed: 'The President, Treasurer and Secretary General to be voted for by disability groups to be on the Executive Committee and ex-officio Vice Presidents of IFSOD. Four members to be elected by the General Assembly from three nominations each of the individual disability groups.' This formula would enable each group to have a significant involvement in its own representation. There would be some modification of this structure in practice, leading to representatives appointed by organisations, and effectively those already holding offices, rather than representatives elected for the explicit purpose of working within the umbrella organisation. The perceived lack of democracy was to hamper the standing of the International Coordinating Committee in the minds of the people they were to represent.

When the joint meeting of ISMGF and ISOD took place later in the day, Bob Jackson, President of ISMGF and in the chair for the meeting, urged those in attendance to take a good long look at the draft constitution that would be sent to them subsequently, and 'to see if they could fit into it'. He said that the Study Group had done as it had been asked: 'they had tried to consider the needs of large and small, the developing and the well-developed; they had tried to consider the longstanding disabled sports groups, such as the spinal cord paralysed, and the newly developed blind sports and had tried to put them together in a workable solution'. Jackson circulated a draft soon afterwards, and comments and suggestions from members of the Study Group and from the Executive Committees of organisations led to some revision. A further meeting was needed in order to tidy up the changes and prepare a second draft, so the Study Group met again at Stoke Mandeville in July 1981. Marcel Avronsart took the chair and guided the meeting through the list of suggestions that he and Bengt Nirje had recorded. Great care was taken to cover all points fairly and the group worked towards a paper to be put out for consideration. It was initially suggested that the title of the new body should be the Confederation of International Sports Organisations for the Disabled (CISOD), but it would become known as the International Coordinating Committee. A General Assembly was to be held every four years, with representatives from member countries of each disability group. The Executive was to have half of its members elected by the General Assembly (the President and eight 'members at large'); the four Presidents of the international disability sports federations would be Vice Presidents of CISOD; the Medical and Technical Committees would elect their own Presidents; and the Secretary General and Treasurer would be members of the Executive Committee but without voting rights. Such a structure, had it come into play, would have gone some way to address the complaints about democracy, and the predominance of existing office holders of the international federations.

It was to take longer than people realised to come to a workable structure that could be fundamentally acceptable to every group. There would be some practical delay in formally constituting any new umbrella organisation because each respective federation would have to ratify decisions at its own General Assembly, and these were not phased at conveniently close times. The first of the international organisations to hold its General Assembly was ISOD. It is not altogether surprising that the members at the General Assembly were not in complete agreement that a new umbrella organisation should be created at all, when there had initially been the proposal that ISOD itself might serve in this capacity. But the representatives of ISOD confirmed that there were good grounds for closer, sustained cooperation between individual disability sports groups. The ISOD delegates who assembled in Paris in December 1981 agreed that IBSA, CP-ISRA and ISMGF should be invited together to discuss the creation of 'a Cooperative Committee of the international sports organisations for the disabled'. There was much to gain from working in harmony, and there was obviously significant benefit in having a formal structure for coordination between the different international organisations when planning Paralympic Games, regional and world championships.

The Birth of a New Umbrella Organisation for Disability Sport

In March 1982, the Second World Championships in Winter Sports for the Disabled was held at the beautiful resort of Leysin, Switzerland. Many of the key participants in discussions about the future of the Paralympic Movement were in Switzerland either with national teams, or officiating and representing their federations. This opportunity gave rise to the founding meeting of what was to become the International Coordinating Committee of World Sports Organisations for the Disabled (ICC), on 11th March 1982. This important occasion brought together the following officers of international disability sports organisations:

ISOD: M. Avronsart, H. Lindström and C. Sugny
CP-ISRA: A. Cameron, L. Sorensen and Mrs M. Malstrom
IBSA: H. Pielasch, J. Bromann and J. Molberg
ISMGF: H. Poole, Miss J. Scruton and A. Tricot.

Marcel Avronsart, displaying characteristic modesty, explained that the precedence of the chair only fell to him for this initial meeting because ISOD had extended the invitations. The discussions were lively and extended, but there was complete agreement that 'a cooperative committee' should be formed between ISOD, CP-ISRA, IBSA and ISMGF. The spirit of cooperation was evidenced by the insistence that the chairmanship should rotate among the Presidents of the four organisations. It was at the next meeting that the title was changed to the International Coordinating Committee. This second meeting was held at Stoke Mandeville, with Archie Cameron in the chair, on 28th July 1982. The business of the ICC was sport for people with disabilities, and they got right down to business.

Great interest was shown in the proposal by a number of benevolent people in the Netherlands to establish a fund that could be directed towards the backing of disability sport. When formally constituted in June the next year this was to become known as the International Fund Sport Disabled (IFSD), and it proceeded to serve the needs of many organisations, events and people according to the philanthropic intentions of its benefactors. All members of the ICC joined in their enthusiasm for this much-needed and timely innovation, and member organisations contacted the Executive Committee of IFSD to express encouragement and pledge support – eventually all were to become involved in the detailed functioning of the Fund's activities. In the New Year's meeting of January 1983, each member organisation of the ICC agreed to put together a paper that would try to project the direction that the International Coordinating Committee might take, and how its work might be organised. A 'Declaration of Authority' was settled at this third meeting, formalising the interaction of the representatives.

WORKING TOGETHER TOWARDS INNSBRÜCK

First Dealings with the International Olympic Committee

There was a frank exchange of views on the role and limits of the relationship between ICC and IOC at the meeting between representatives of the International Olympic Committee and the International Coordinating Committee on 15th February 1983. Hans Lindström, Secretary General of ISOD, indicated that the group would 'soon become an international organisation' and identified the four disabled sports organisations represented there as constituting the International Coordinating Committee. At this meeting, attended by Juan Antonio Samaranch, President of the International Olympic Committee and Monique Berlioux, Director of IOC, were officers of the founding organisations:

ISOD: Guillermo Cabezas, President; Hans Lindström, Secretary General, Guy Princivalle, Technical Director

IBSA: Helmut Pielash, President

ISMGF: Joan Scruton, Secretary General

CP-ISRA: Arie Klapwijk, Vice President.

Also in attendance were Mario Pescante of Comitato Olimpico Nazionale Italiano (CONI) and Antonio Vernole, Secretary of the Italian Federation of Sports for the Handicapped.

Samaranch, who often took a forceful lead on such occasions, started the meeting by saying that the IOC proposed to 'lend its aid to the disabled as well as to the non-handicapped'. The IOC President emphasised that it would be easier to work together with IOC if agreement could be established between the four international organisations, and they could be seen to be operating as one. Joan Scruton stressed that at the January meeting of the ICC there had been agreement to work closely in concert. According to Samaranch, the IOC was willing to give its official patronage to a four-yearly sporting event, employing the Olympic rings and seeking financial support from IOC. Effectively, this was an invitation into the Olympic 'family'. The IOC would insist that the term 'Olympic' or 'Olympiad' should not be used in relation to this sporting event. This was entirely consistent with the attitude of the International Olympic Committee in protecting the identification of the symbols of the Olympic Games (Bailey 1996). The response of Pielasch was more barbed – that human rights were the issue; equality of treatment was crucial, otherwise athletes with a disability would be discriminated against. He also considered that the athletes would not understand the restriction on the use of the Olympic symbols and language. Athletes with a disability had been using the term 'Olympics' for a long time, he said, and it was important for them to feel that they were having full recognition alongside other athletes. Hans Lindström emphasised also that the meeting concerned the rights of the persons with a disability. He wanted to clarify that the ICC could not be directly compared to (and therefore treated as) an international sports federation. The Olympic concept had more meaning, therefore, to the constituents, and 'thus the ICC was asking to be integrated into the Olympic family'. Samaranch wanted to remain clear that the Olympic Games were a separate entity: 'a unique event and the IOC was thus duty-bound to protect them'. Joan Scruton brought the meeting back to the important focus on athletes with a disability, for whom 'the matter currently under discussion was their only hope'. She had been wondering why the IOC could not 'go the whole way and agree to the employment of the word "Olympics". The people represented by the four organisations were real Olympic athletes.' Arie Klapwijk questioned whether it could really be thought damaging in any way to use the word 'Olympics' for those with disabilities. He believed 'there was really no confusion if one used the term "Olympic Games for the Disabled"'.

Juan Antonio Samaranch suggested that the International Olympic Committee would offer:

1. Patronage
2. Use of the Olympic rings for the disabled main sport event held every four years
3. Financial aid of approximately US$10 000–20 000.
4. The possibility of organising a demonstration tournament during the 1988 Olympic Games
5. To request the National Olympic Committees of the world to try to form a Federation for the handicapped with the same rights as the other federations.

Samaranch stressed the need to avoid using the term 'Olympic', and said that he would be happy to meet again with two or three representatives of the ICC 'once a consensus had been reached'. The proposal could then be taken to the IOC Executive Committee, but this would need to be in time for the autumn meeting in 1983. The ICC representatives were to meet with the IOC again in September.

An interesting twist demonstrates some of the tensions in the relationship between the fledgling umbrella group and those federations and organising committees with specific tasks. Bertl Neumann, as

Secretary General of the Organising Committee for the 3rd World Winter Games for the Disabled in Innsbrück, had received notification from Juan Antonio Samaranch in November 1982 that the IOC had granted patronage to the Games. This gave permission for the use of the Olympic rings on publicity and other material and for flying the Olympic flag. Neumann had heard from Hans Lindström that ISOD 'was not quite happy about our understanding with the IOC'. Lindström was trying to urge the organisers of the 3rd World Winter Games to re-name the event the '3rd Olympic Winter Games for the Disabled'. Neumann did not wish to accede to this request, and wrote to Samaranch (3rd February 1983) to emphasise that his organising committee was honouring the agreement made regarding the 'protection' of the term 'Olympic'. It is heartening to see that Neumann continued to say that he would be delighted if the IOC, in discussion with ISOD and 'its brother associations' could permit the use of the term for the Games. He expressed his own vision that ultimately they could work towards 'the games for the disabled joined to the games staged for non-handicapped athletes, to form a whole unit – The Olympic Games'. It is patent that Neumann was promoting Innsbrück as the permanent venue for future Winter Games, but he was clear that this blending of the two competitive periods would be in keeping with Pierre de Coubertin's Olympic philosophy of: 'games open to everyone who has qualified for the sports events'. The International Coordinating Committee would have to work hard in the coming years to ensure that their different partners would share their principles. However, these earliest days were days of celebration and hope.

Following the meeting with President Samaranch, a press release was issued (PR/5/83). The intention was simply to state that a meeting had taken place between the IOC President and 'representatives from various sports organisations for the handicapped', and to point out that discussions had centred mainly on: 'the methods which could be implemented to encourage increased participation by the handicapped in the international sports movement'. Samaranch's proposals had amounted to more than this statement. Cautious and true to the content of the meeting, the press release was upbeat, but Samaranch did not want to promise more than he could deliver at this stage.

The Presidents of the four organisations drafted a response to the IOC proposal, dated 25th May 1983. Although this draft did not reach the IOC in its original form, it is significant to understand the intentions of the four Presidents at this time – subsequent events persuaded the ICC representatives that a modified reply was most appropriate by the time September came along. With thanks for the interest and offer of support from the International Olympic Committee, the respondents expressed hope that this was the first step along 'a road to solid cooperation and understanding between IOC and the international disabled sports movement, for the benefit of disabled athletes in the world'. The paper identified the responsibility of the organisations represented by the ICC as providing top-level international competition 'for those human beings in the world who, because of a disability, cannot compete in sports with able bodied on equal terms, and therefore are at present denied the rights enjoyed by their able-bodied counterparts to compete in the Olympic programme of the IOC'. With some pride the authors made clear the accomplishments and the dedication of athletes: 'Quite a few of "our" sports have today developed a high level of competitiveness, quality and standards. They are aesthetically performed and contain action, drama and excitement for the spectator. These sports, at least, are worthy of the highest possible status of amateur sports i.e. to be "Olympic sports".' With this point strongly made, the ICC asked that a sixth clause be appended to the proposal of the IOC President:

> To work out a long term plan together with the ICC, with the aim of including some disabled sports events in the IOC Olympic programmes. Until the first of these events are included in the IOC programme, it is agreed that the ICC be allowed to use the term 'Olympics for the Disabled'.

Finally calling for a further meeting between representatives of ICC and the IOC, the paper was signed by Archie Cameron, President of CP-ISRA, Helmut Pielasch, President of IBSA, Bob Jackson, President of ISMGF and Guillermo Cabezas, President of ISOD.

Some negotiations had been taking place behind the scenes, and progress was being made through incidental personal contact. In the final version of the letter of response to the IOC President's proposal, thanks were expressed for the offer to include a demonstration by disabled skiers at the 1984 Winter Olympic Games, and the possibility of a wheelchair basketball demonstration at the 1984 Summer Games. The ICC nominated three individuals to represent them in meetings with the IOC: Cabezas, Jackson and Lindström. Also added was an assurance that the four international organisations were equal partners, yet they were also autonomous in terms of their own particular groupings of athletes with a disability.

There was a wish not to allow things to stand still with regard to the International Olympic Committee, and a meeting took place between Juan Antonio Samaranch, Bob Jackson and Dale Wiley, Chairman of the Board of Directors of the VIIth World Wheelchair Games, on 27th July 1983. They wanted to explore the usage of the term 'Paralympics', in particular, because they had come up against resistance to the use of this title and their logo from the United States Olympic Committee. It is interesting that Samaranch 'saw no problem' in the use of the term 'Paralympics' to describe the Illinois Games. The Organising Committee had incorporated under the name of the VIIth Paralympic Games, Inc., but the United States Olympic Committee had adamantly forbidden the use of the term. As the meeting broke up there was definitely the feeling among the ICC camp that Samaranch's approach to Don Miller, Executive Director of the United States Olympic Committee, would produce 'a favourable answer', although this confidence would prove to be misplaced.

Canadians Offer a National Perspective

While the international federations maintained a disability-related view, there was a regularly expressed concern for other outlooks: either sport-orientated or centred on nations. In a provocative, but very positive action, Bob Steadward, President of the Canadian Federation of Sport Organisations for the Disabled (CFSOD) and Anne Merklinger, Executive Director of CFSOD, submitted a paper to the International Coordinating Committee on 1st June 1983. As Steadward explained, a number of people involved in the Canadian Federation had been putting ideas together since 1981 (Steadward 2004). They were looking for a way of securing the future of international sport for athletes with disabilities, watching the benign development of a single international body to coordinate the actions of major multi-disability competitions. Steadward and Merklinger put forward extensive analysis of the way forward, and the consequences of inappropriate action (or inaction). CFSOD had already proved itself to be a mature and well-organised national federation – an example for other nations. The *Position Paper on the International Disabled Sport Situation* began by congratulating the ICC for the increased cooperation evident between the international federations represented within the ICC. The Canadian structure was similar in many ways to the structure of the ICC: one umbrella organisation (CFSOD) coordinating cooperation between five individual governing bodies of sport (four organised by disability and one sport-specific organisation). The authors of the paper stress: 'Like many countries, Canada has been and remains very concerned about our need to relate to a cooperative *yet supreme* administrative body at the international level'. There was no doubt from the Canadians' view of things that: 'Sport for the disabled has developed to a level of excellence where the long-term competitive needs of our international athletes are dependent on one voice that can provide a coordinating authority for disabled sport development'. Steadward and Merklinger went on to state several tangible areas of concern. They had seen the circulated papers relating to the constitution of the newly formed International Coordinating Committee, and applauded the wish for ICC to oversee the organisation of 'both the Olympic Games and Multi-Disciplinary World Championships'. In particular the Canadians saw it as important for ICC to have responsibility for: bidding procedures and policies;

forming detailed agreements with organising committees; 'the enforcement of international rules'; and the 'preparation of international event calendars'. In steering the cooperation of a number of international organisations, it was essential that autonomy was respected, and a statement to this effect must be in the constitution. Significantly, and in keeping with the general trend for classification to loom larger and larger, the Canadians were very supportive of the establishment of a Medical Commission of ICC. In the light of the fact that classification had: 'become increasingly more complex over time', CFSOD was moving to establish its own national medical bureau – looking to connect seamlessly with the ICC Commission.

An obvious omission in the make-up of ICC so far was the absence of the federation representing deaf athletes – CISS. Steadward and Merklinger emphasised that all efforts should be made to woo CISS, so that the proposed 'Confederation of International Sport Organisations for the Disabled' could truly represent all sports federations for people with disabilities. Relations with the International Olympic Committee were welcomed by the Canadian writers, especially when the possibility of using the Olympic insignia could be part of any agreement with IOC. The practical benefits from patronage and financial support were acknowledged, but CFSOD wished to encourage the dealings with the International Olympic Committee to be 'the beginnings of a series of ongoing discussions', and therefore the present position must be 'the *first but not final* inroad for the world's disabled athletes' acceptance into the Olympic Movement'.

Getting Down to Business

When the representatives of the International Coordinating Committee met for the fourth time, at Stoke Mandeville on 28th July 1983, each of the four federations had drawn up its ideas on a proposed constitution for the ICC, and Arieh Fink was tasked with the job of working together with the Secretary Generals to construct a synthesis of the submissions. Bob Jackson gave a report of his meeting with Juan Antonio Samaranch the day before, and there seemed to be a very positive sense of progress. The debate about the use of Olympic terminology and symbols within the ICC meeting was always going to be lively and yet sensitive. Reporting on the meeting with Samaranch, Bob Jackson emphasised that Samaranch still appeared to confuse the status of the different groups representing sport for persons with a disability. He 'did not seem to understand the difference between sport for the disabled and Special Olympics for the Mentally Retarded, Blind, and Deaf and so on'. It was the International Coordinating Committee's job to remedy this misunderstanding. But on Olympic terminology there were varying opinions: Jackson urged compliance with the wishes of the IOC, Fink did not want to 'close the door' on particular usage, Scruton emphasised that she did not think they had agreed with Samaranch always to avoid the word 'Olympics' completely – this must be kept open. The most forthright opinion belonged to Hans Lindström, who 'thought confrontation might not be a bad thing as it would get publicity and maybe money for our cause'.

An 'Olympic Manual' was needed as a guide for organising the quadrennial games, and the ICC meeting deliberated about plans for this project to be the focus of a Joint Working Seminar of the ICC early in September 1983 in Hoenderloo, near Arnhem, Netherlands.

Jackson emphasised that they must clarify the purpose and intentions of the International Coordinating Committee 'to avoid the confusion that exists in the eyes of the public, in the Governments of the world and in the International Olympic Committee as to areas of responsibility of sport for the disabled'. Evidence of confusion came even from within the Committee itself when discussion turned to an article that had been published in a Danish magazine, co-authored by Jens Bromann of IBSA. The thrust of the article was in favour of the International Coordinating Committee's work, but the English translation apparently gave rise to some unintentional inaccuracies. This emphasised that the greatest care would be needed to push forward effectively towards their goal.

The organisers of the two venues for the 1984 Games in the United States hosted a reception in the evening of the ICC meeting, and they took the opportunity of presenting information about progress on arrangements in New York and Illinois. While discussing the events and classification of athletes for the 1984 Games, some time was taken to examine the problems faced with regard to basketball for those with disabilities. There was an ongoing dispute in the United States about the inclusion of both wheelchair and standing basketball for the Games. The meeting felt that there should not be this degree of uncertainty so close to the time of the event itself – the formality of the bidding process must be tightened up so that local organisers must, in future, accept conditions laid down by ICC, whether to their liking or not. As there was to be a working seminar in September for the Technical and Medical Sub-Committees, the organisers of Summer and Winter Games should probably be included. Unfortunately, as there was still no signed agreement between the New York venue and ISOD, CP-ISRA or those representing sport for blind athletes, the ICC representatives confirmed that there was still 'no firm line of authority established'. Storm clouds were looming on the horizon for 1984.

The Winter Games preparation looked much more positive, although there was a question mark over the status of the downhill sledge event: this was a financial difficulty and additional funds would be needed if the event were to be included. Joan Scruton commented that the ISMGF representative had informed her that there would definitely be no downhill sledge-racing event. The discussion returned to one of coordination of communication and joint negotiations. Helmut Pielasch expressed what had been an obvious problem from the outset of this umbrella group, that the individual international organisations still bypassed the ICC and dealt with external affairs independently, when they would serve everyone better by working cooperatively. Each disability sports organisation continued to have separate negotiations with the organisers of the Games. It was agreed that the forthcoming seminar should serve to clarify the problems and that participants should endeavour to work together more vigorously in future.

Representatives from Korea and Australia were welcomed to the meeting in Aylesbury Civic Centre, and they indicated that their respective organisations were considering bidding for the 1988 Paralympic Games. It was hoped that firm bids would be prepared by October. The ICC delegates were pleased to note that the two indications of interest were entirely within the newly approved formula of ICC – totally inclusive of all disabilities without separation. Guy Princivalle proposed that circulars should urgently be sent to member nations of the four ICC member organisations calling for bids for the Winter Games of 1988.

Hans Lindström took the opportunity of the July meeting of ICC to present a very significant paper on integrated classification. Introducing the paper, Lindström 'hoped they would find that this integrated classification concept might not be so scary as perhaps many thought before'. Bob Jackson outlined the intention that wheelchair basketball was about to change to functional classification rather than that based on the level of lesion, and that this change looked certain to improve the quality of the sport. Application of classification on integrational principles was to be tried in some sports in New York, and these results would merit examination. The Technical Committee would look in detail at Lindström's paper at the seminar at the end of the summer, but this was an important step that was to have noteworthy impact on the future organisation of sports for athletes with a disability. Functional classification was to be employed in swimming at the World Games in Gothenberg in 1986. Following extensive research, the system was used in the Barcelona 1992 Paralympic Games.

The possibility of gaining affiliation to the United Nations was considered. Arieh Fink thought the most effective and non-bureaucratic way would be for ICC to seek membership of a group already associated with the United Nations, whose purpose was the welfare of people with disabilities. There was some uncertainty as to whether ICC was yet in a clear enough constitutional position to bear scrutiny by the United Nations. Lindström agreed to examine this question. They would eventually wish to seek non-governmental organisation (NGO) status.

A groundswell of interest in the work of the International Coordinating Committee was already being generated widely among sports organisations for people with disabilities in different countries, and ICC was approached by the Swedish Sports Federation for the Handicapped (SHIF) to see whether it would be interested in 'incorporating' the International Foundation of Wheelchair Tennis into the ICC 'movement'. A group called 'Wheelchair Marathon' had made a similar approach; the Chairman stressed the need to 'embrace them and communicate with them', but indicated that it was inappropriate for ICC to be involved with groups that operated independently. This important matter was for the Technical Committee to investigate and consider what sort of relationship would be most appropriate. It points to the representatives of the International Coordinating Committee not having a definitive perception of its present and future character at this stage. Already there was no recognition of the benefit that could accrue from being open to a sport-based viewpoint rather than a disability-only perception.

Friendship, Unity and Sportsmanship

When Bob Jackson wrote to Juan Antonio Samaranch in early August to thank him for meeting with Wiley and himself at short notice, Jackson expressed his gratitude for Samaranch's 'empathy and understanding' when discussing the problems that had arisen in wishing to use the term 'Paralympics' for the Illinois Games. Jackson confirmed on paper what had been emphasised in their discussion: 'in using the term Paralympics to describe the World Games of our Federation every four years and the logo of the three intertwined rings, representing the ISMGF logo standing for Friendship, Unity and Sportsmanship, we are by no means in conflict with or infringing upon the Olympic Games and emblem of the IOC'. Jackson formally asked Samaranch to give approval for the use of the term 'Paralympics' and the emblem for the Games to be held in Illinois in July 1984. Samaranch responded to Jackson's letter in a way that is wholly consistent with similar questions relating to the use of the Olympic symbols by other organisations. He wrote: 'the IOC would see no objection to give (sic) approval to your using the term 'Paralympics' and your emblem representing the three intertwined wheels, however, in order to comply strictly with the principles of the Olympic Charter, you should address your request through the United States Olympic Committee'. The reason for this was that each National Olympic Committee had full responsibility for the use of the Olympic emblem within its own country. In this response, Samaranch was either showing his true sympathies for the potential benefit for the ICC's work on behalf of the Paralympic Movement, or he could have been gaining diplomatic ground by offering something he already knew would be rejected by the USOC, who held the key to the decision.

Jackson and Wiley each approached Don Miller, Executive Director of the United States Olympic Committee (USOC), by letter but the reaction was glacial. To Jackson the USOC Executive Director replied with great respect for the work done for athletes in wheelchairs, but Miller went on: 'yet I cannot disregard the profound implications of further dilution in this country of the Olympic marks, upon which our basis of public and corporate support is derived'. He pointed out that the USOC had pledged $100 000 towards the venues for the 1984 International Games for the Disabled. Miller said that he was 'not prepared to permit employment of either the terminology or the mark', in spite of the IOC President expressing his approval. Of course, Miller repeated Samaranch's spelling out that the control of the Olympic symbols within the USA remained with the United States National Olympic Committee. Interestingly, Miller added that he believed Samaranch was expressing a personal opinion and not that of the IOC Executive Committee in this matter. While closing with this firm position, Miller did say that he would present Jackson's letter to the USOC Committee on Sports for the Disabled at its November meeting. The ability of the National Olympic Committee to 'market' the Olympic Games logo and title, as well as the potential effect on sponsorship of the Olympic Games of permitting wider use of the symbols of Olympism were the governing factors in this strategic blockade. Although the United States Olympic Committee was extending very significant financial support, it was also holding back progress of sport for persons with a disability by exercising a less generous, although technically legitimate control of the Olympic symbols and terminology.

Horace Poole, together with Guillermo Cabezas and Hans Lindström, met Juan Antonio Samaranch on 10th October 1983. His notes make for interesting reading as a commentary on the progress of negotiations with the International Olympic Committee. Poole records that the IOC considered it should start with a few events in the Olympics, as had already been established: 'e.g. IOC has decided to include demonstration of Skiing' and one wheelchair basketball event at Los Angeles. They agreed that they should work together to study how it might be possible to 'include disabled in Olympics (on a selective basis)'. Samaranch indicated that he was willing to accept this sixth clause in the document drawn up from the earlier meeting of 15th February 1983. He was showing great willingness to make himself available – planning to be at Innsbrück for the Winter Games, then to find a suitable time in April or May 1984 for a further meeting. In conclusion to the meeting the IOC President said that it was his intention that the 'disabled Skiing event would be a competition and not merely a demonstration. He would arrange for medals to be presented'. However, he also pointed out that these medals would be different from the medals received by the able-bodied competitors in the Winter Olympic Games.

The International Fund Sport Disabled

The origins of the International Fund Sport Disabled (IFSD) are such as to restore faith in philanthropy. In June 1983 a meeting had taken place between nine altruistic men from the Netherlands. They had their sights set on providing the means of encouraging international participation in sports by people with disabilities. The Arnhem 1980 Paralympic Games had provided a significant surplus through the 'Telebingo' fundraising, and this had formed the basis for the very strong position that the International Fund Sport Disabled was in. It invited a representative from international federations already involved in the field to this meeting: from the International Blind Sports Association, the Cerebral Palsy-International Sports and Recreation Association, the International Sports Organisation for the Disabled, the International Stoke Mandeville Games Federation, Comité International des Sports des Sourds, the International Committee of Silent Chess, the International Association of Sports for the Mentally Handicapped and the International Braille Chess Association. This group became an Advisory Board to the IFSD, with Jens Bromann of IBSA as Chairman. The Advisory Board met twice a year to work through the requests for financial support and to project their recommendations to the Board, which was very receptive to the expertise of the Advisory Board. The stated aims of the International Fund were broad enough to ensure that in addition to the individual donors' national organisations, media and other groups were keen to show their support. There had already been a National Fund Sport Disabled in the Netherlands, and it proffered support together with the various Dutch federations involved with sport for persons with a disability. The founders of the International Fund Sport Disabled promoted its purpose as:

Fundraising for sporting activities for the disabled to finance and to support among others:

1. International championships for the disabled on regional and world level and the organisational assistance thereby,
2. Projects in the field of sport for the disabled in developing countries,
3. The development of sporting materials,

4. A joint bureau to elaborate particulars and information,
5. Training of sports officials,
6. Sport technical and medical research.

The foundation can make money available to bring about a better-integrated cooperation between international sporting organisations for the disabled. The foundation can also give support to individual international sporting organisations for the disabled.

Pieter Van Vollenhoven, husband of Princess Margriet of the Netherlands, was the first President of the International Fund Sport Disabled. In practical terms, countless events have been secured by grants from the IFSD Board, guaranteeing back up and providing the status of recognition. Conferences, seminars and workshops were supported, and publication of materials also financed by IFSD meant that things were achieved that might not have seen realisation otherwise. The reality is that the IFSD was also demanding of the international federations by insisting that they should draw more closely together in their cooperative efforts. The insistence of the Fund on certain conditions being met prior to money being released set on edge some dealings that it had with international federations seeking support for their respective championships, and especially caused tensions between the Fund and the International Coordinating Committee.

ICC MEETS AT THE 3RD WORLD WINTER GAMES FOR THE DISABLED, INNSBRÜCK, 1984

The 3rd World Winter Games for the Disabled in Innsbrück, Austria also provided the location for the fifth meeting of the International Coordinating Committee on 20th and 21st January 1984. The Holiday Inn's scenic and comfortable setting suited the representatives of the world's organisations for sports for people with disabilities. For very practical reasons the agenda was shuffled – Guy Princivalle, as Technical Officer to the Winter Games, had to be free to oversee the downhill competitions, so items relevant to his participation were taken early on. Princivalle reported on the organisation and progress of the 3rd World Winter Games, saying that there had been enormous effort on the part of the organisers, in particular their Herculean effort to ensure that the Nordic skiing events could proceed despite difficult snow conditions. The only way of surmounting the problems had been by military patrols constantly transporting snow day and night! On the more negative side the Games had been affected by the later deletion of certain events, and some significant difficulties in effectively classifying blind competitors. Guy Princivalle also gave the very good news that there had been three unofficial declarations of interest for possible venues for the next World Winter Games: Winter Park, Colorado, USA; Calgary, Canada; and the Federal Republic of Germany – if West Germany was unsuccessful it had indicated that it would bid for the 1990 Winter World Championships.

The maintenance of a joint sports calendar was a good way of demonstrating the cooperative outlook of the member organisations, and it was agreed that ICC should provide this. The calendar would also promote foresight and courtesies with regard to precedence and clashes. A characteristic of each meeting of the ICC was to be the presentation of updates and alterations to the joint calendar.

Marjolijn Hillegers, attending as an observer and Director of the International Fund Sport Disabled, presented the progress report to the ICC on the construction of the Olympic Handbook. The IFSD had made a financial subvention for its completion, and Mrs Hillegers had taken on the role of Coordinator, working together with an Ad Hoc Committee of representatives from the four disability sports organisations to complete the Handbook. The Ad Hoc Committee working on the Handbook was given authority to make further adjustments.

This meeting of the International Coordinating Committee proposed that the International Fund should be asked whether it would establish and finance a Secretariat in the Netherlands. A function of the Secretariat would be to help produce and distribute publicity material, but it would obviously be a great boost to the aims of the ICC to have an office and permanent staff, while also fitting the objectives of the Fund. This administrative support would cement the immediate future of the International Coordinating Committee, as well as providing a direct line between the ICC and the International Fund with regard to fundraising. It was not very much later that an office was furnished in Arnhem. The singularly unusual feature of the IFSD was that all funds had been raised from within the Netherlands itself, and although there were attempts to widen the fundraising base, it remained a Dutch pheno-menon. The unparalleled charitable support from IFSD for the work of the International Coordinating Committee continued well into 1987, when attention naturally turned to the next organisation that was to emerge: the International Paralympic Committee.

Events due to be part of the 1984 Summer Games in Illinois and New York took some attention at the Innsbrück meeting. Some difficulties about the wheelchair marathon needed solutions. The Illinois organisers had wanted a wheelchair marathon using an integrated classification system, as had been discussed at the previous ICC meeting. Joan Scruton informed the Committee that ISMGF had decided to hold a marathon for its classes only in the official programme, and that in addition the local organisers would administer a wheelchair marathon 'open to all locomotor disabilities' as a demonstration event only. This laid the question to rest, except for Harald Natvig's call for the Technical Committee to discuss a wheelchair marathon with sticks – currently used as good training for winter sports. The ISOD Medical Officer wondered whether there could be two classes in the wheelchair marathon, with one to include the use of sticks.

Hans Lindström gave a round-up of progress of arrangements for the 1984 International Games for the Disabled in New York. Something like 48 countries had entered competitors so far, including a good number of countries participating for the first time. Lindström was confident that all those entered could be accommodated within their events. Plans seemed to be going well. Joan Scruton had a report from Champaign, Illinois, where the 1984 World Wheelchair Games (VIIth Paralympics) were due to be held. She said that the facilities were 'absolutely ideal', and that there were some 1600 entries from almost 40 countries. However, in a more downbeat delivery she said 'that there are some financial problems, but hoped that they were going to be solved'. Storm clouds were gathering.

Cooperation with the International Olympic Committee was now a regular topic for each meeting of the International Coordinating Committee, and Guillermo Cabezas gave a summary of recent business. They had confirmed demonstration wheelchair events for the Los Angeles Olympic Games: 800 m for women and 1500 m for men. The demonstration events were to involve the eight fastest competitors regardless of disability, in an integrated event. Apparently the IOC President had been hesitant when asked in February 1983 about the inclusion of athletes with a disability in the Sarajevo and Los Angeles Games, and wanted it put off until the 1988 Olympiad. But he had agreed to accommodate the earlier request. A highly significant statement by Cabezas was that Samaranch 'said that he expects that, in a very short time, the ICC shall be included in the IOC as one more sub-committee'. Predictably, there was a lively reaction to this information from the representatives in Innsbrück.

Unfortunately the updated IOC Directory had omitted CP-ISRA's details, but had included IBSA, ISOD and ISMGF. Cabezas could not explain why there was this omission. The jealous protection of each international federation's identity and status was highlighted in this exchange. Jens Bromann highlighted the lack of truly broad representation in dealings with outside groups: it was ISOD that had been negotiating with the organisers of the 3rd World Winter Games. There were obvious implications for the future cohesion of the ICC in all dealings – in particular, to appear unified and representative of all member organisations, it had to widen the allocation of individuals attending negotiations for major events so that balance was matched by logical representation. It was agreed that each organisation should be able to nominate a representative to participate in any future delegation to meet with the International Olympic Committee. Pielasch lamented the absence of opportunity for blind athletes to participate in the proposed demonstration events in the 1984 Games, but Lindström stressed the fact that the events for Sarajevo had been decided by the IOC together with the International Ski Federation (FIS) and the Sarajevo Organising Committee. Guy Princivalle had promoted the cause of blind athletes at the meeting with Samaranch, but this had not helped. In a very outspoken manner, Guillermo Cabezas later made use of a press conference at the end of the 3rd World Winter Games for the Disabled to express his disappointment at the provision of events for blind athletes, and he stated to the world's press that 'if in 1988 no blind people are permitted to participate, no other will come either'. A worthy pronouncement, but close to over-stepping his bounds as President pro tem of the International Coordinating Committee. Pielasch was full of praise for his fellow ICC members in their show of solidarity on the subject of equal opportunity for blind athletes.

At the Innsbrück meeting, Hans Lindström once again wanted to stress the need to be in control of the situation with regard to the IOC. Lindström cautioned that they must not be 'overwhelmed', and that the representatives must not agree to anything in the next meetings until the IOC 'makes a commitment for future events for disabled within the IOC programme'. Joan Scruton also agreed with Lindström: 'It is important that the athletes agree with what is done'. Anything that is 'given away' must be in agreement with the athletes. Scruton, courteous as ever, thanked Cabezas for all that he had done. Cabezas was entirely of the same mind, observing that the main focus must be the athletes with disability: 'we will disappear, but they will remain'. The athletes themselves would not find automatic participation or entitlement to representation in the administration of these federations for a while longer, but the heart of these principles is evident here.

'The Hoenderloo Seminar was one of the best seminars she had ever attended' – so Joan Scruton declared, seconded by Jens Bromann. All organisations were appreciative of the shared knowledge and spirit of cooperation during the meetings that took place from 1st to 4th September 1984. The consultation was intended to work towards an 'Olympic Manual' for the organisation and administration of Olympic Games for the Disabled. Marjolijn Hillegers found the process very arduous as there were no true guidelines, but the communication between all the various people and committees had proved very fruitful. The document evolving from the seminar had merit, but in the opinion of Jens Bromann 'it was very broad and at present too extensive in relation to what the Olympic Games for the Disabled are in reality'. Others agreed; it was a 'tremendous work' but more exertion would be necessary before it could be sent to all nations and organisations involved in sport for people with disabilities.

Marjolijn Hillegers presented some of the questions that the Hoenderloo Seminar had thrown up, for consideration by the Innsbrück meeting of the ICC. These were absolutely fundamental building blocks for the future definition of the role of the International Coordinating Committee, and the direction that sport for people with disabilities could take. These included subjects such as: classification; the educational role of ICC; the provision of a Secretariat; a consultative body of the ICC to function during the Games; greater collaboration between technical, administrative and medical wings of ICC; what adaptations might be permitted in equipment or 'of the athlete himself'; whether ICC has responsibility towards recreational sport; public relations – all were raised at the Seminar but needed further discussion and some decisions at the ICC meeting. Was the International Coordinating Committee 'in principle following the able-bodied Games' in relation to the bidding process? What were the criteria for decision making should there be several bids? In particular, it was important to know whether the ICC would take the bid from a country that had successfully been awarded the able-bodied Games in preference over other countries that were not hosting the Olympic Games in that year. Emphatically the representatives of the four international organisations agreed that if all bids were of equal preference the ICC would accept the bid from the country 'which is arranging the Olympics for the able-bodied'. There could be no doubting that the true wishes of the senior officers of the international disability organisations shared Ludwig Guttmann's belief in a close association with the Olympiad.

While the meetings were proceeding at the Holiday Inn, two telexes had been received confirming the bid from Korea to host the 1988 Paralympic Summer Games. The ICC delegates agreed to accept this bid in principle and that Hans Lindström, Joan Scruton and Guillermo Cabezas would pursue the details. The Seoul Paralympic Games would be the beginning of what would be considered the 'Modern Era' for the Paralympic Movement.

The Closing Ceremony for the 3rd World Winter Games for the Disabled had an emotional effect on many of those attending; those involved in mapping the future cooperation of sports organisations for people with disabilities wondered what that future would hold as the Olympic flag was lowered. The second day of the ICC meeting started with a positive look to that future. Arieh Fink drew the members' attention to his draft constitution for the ICC – a successful collaborative achievement. The representatives agreed with him that it was more appropriate to designate the final document an Agreement rather than a Constitution, and the meeting confirmed that the most appropriate title for the committee should be the International Coordinating Committee (ICC) of World Sports Organisations for the Disabled. They trudged through the document item by item, and with minor alterations to Fink's version, the Agreement was distributed to member organisations, with a further copy sent to the President of the International Olympic Committee.

Klapwijk referred to a seminar he had attended on recreational and leisure activities for people with disabilities in Japan in April 1984, called RESPO. Klapwijk and Natvig proposed that they should have an ICC mandate to meet with the organisers of Rehabilitation International (RI). The question of whether ICC should be involved in recreational rather than elite sport was unclear still, but the dialogue should continue. Lindström pointed out that another organisation had now been created in opposition to Rehabilitation International, called Disabled People's International (DPI). There had also already been some communication with this group via the ISOD. Lindström was encouraged to keep channels open with DPI while Natvig and Klapwijk forged links with RI.

As the members of the four organisations closed their two-day meeting at Innsbrück they realised how far they had come in such a short time: true cooperation was evident although there were many obstacles still in their path.

GROWTH: PROGRESS AND PROBLEMS

The Collapse of the Illinois Games

The VIIth World Wheelchair Games for spinal impaired athletes had been planned at the University of Illinois at Champaign, Urbana from 19th June to 4th July 1984, under the auspices of the International Stoke Mandeville Games Federation. Other types of disabilities were successfully catered for in multi-disability games in New York. But in the middle of February 1984, the University of Illinois took action after becoming convinced that there was the possibility that the ineffective fundraising would leave the University with a deficit. The University terminated its contract with the Board of Directors of the VIIth World Wheelchair Games. In the end the Wheelchair Games had to be relocated to Stoke Mandeville, without doubt resulting in a setback to the development of the international disability sports movement.

Back in 1980, the United States National Wheelchair Athletic Association (NWAA) had proposed a bid for a competition limited to those athletes who were eligible to compete under the rules of the International Stoke Mandeville Games Federation. The official report into the collapse of the Illinois Games is clear in tracing the enthusiasms and actions of the participants. Ben Lipton, then Chairman of

NWAA, considered that it would be too big a management venture to offer to host a multi-disability event. In addition, the National Wheelchair Athletic Committee (NWAC), which controlled sports other than wheelchair basketball, wheelchair tennis and road racing, agreed that it was not beneficial to be encouraging joint games with other organisations. Five members of the NWAC were nominated to form an Ad Hoc Steering Committee to focus on bringing about the 1984 Paralympic Games. The representatives were Seymour Bloom, Patricia Karman, Stan Labanowich, Robert Szyman and Dale Wiley, who was to act as Chairman. Ben Lipton remained a participant as an *ex-officio* member of the Ad Hoc Steering Committee while he was Chairman of NWAA. They identified a need for answers to three vital questions: site selection, budgeting and fundraising. Firstly, though, they set about working on a 'prospectus' that would form a basic plan for the organisation of the Games regardless of venue. The first meeting, during the Olympiad for the Disabled in Arnhem in July 1980, permitted discussions with the organisers of the Arnhem Games, Colonel Decking and Captain Meyer. They learnt that the opinion of the organisers was that the multi-disciplinary nature of the Arnhem Games had allowed some events not to be 'up to world class standards'. But it was accepted that there were great benefits for participants competing in a multi-disability environment – the opportunity to appreciate other people's disabilities and to share the problems faced. On their return to the United States, the Ad Hoc Steering Committee met again in September and started to discuss fundraising. A complicated period followed, with the enlistment of two professional fundraisers, considerable disagreement, and redrafted and rejected contracts. Personal funding was provided by some of the Committee members in order to make sure that the services of the professionals were retained, but the damage in the Committee had already been done. Labanowich and Wiley were asked to construct articles of incorporation with the advice of an attorney, Thomas Strohm. These articles were accepted in February 1981. When formally incorporated, the organisation was called 'the VIIth Paralympic Games, Incorporated'. It then only remained for the Ad Hoc Steering Committee to set up a Board of Directors and wind up the Committee.

Dale Wiley wrote to William Simon, President of the United States Olympic Committee, to inform him that the VII Paralympic Games Corporation had come into existence, expressing his hope that it could work together with USOC. While the United States Olympic Committee indicated that it would 'continue to follow with interest' the progress of plans for games, it could not possibly pledge support when it had heard from the national organisations for other disability sports organisations (cerebral palsy and blind) that they were also making plans. All three groups were member associations of the USOC, and agreement was needed between them before USOC would assist. Don Miller, Executive Director of USOC, also made the obvious connection between the use of the term 'Paralympics' and fundraising efforts of USOC for the Los Angeles Olympic Games: 'the term would tend to cause confusion with the Olympic Games' (Miller 1981).

The progress towards organising the Games from the technical angle was good: regular meetings of Board members with technical knowledge made this an area of confidence. However, the financial angle was deficient in producing the desired results by 1983. There was a rift blooming between Wiley, as Chairman of the NWAC and Chairman of the Board of Directors of the VIIth Paralympic Games, and Tim Nugent, who was Executive Director of the Games. The differences were serious enough for a Board meeting on 1st September 1983 to insist that a meeting had to be held between Nugent and Wiley in order to clarify their positions and to find a way of working towards the final goal. Another area of growing tension was the conflict between the organisers and the United States Olympic Committee on the use of the term 'Paralympics', and of the employment of the three-wheel symbol. While the communications with USOC continued, other pressure was brought to bear, and Kenneth Clarke, Director of Sports Medicine for the United States Olympic Committee and appointed liaison for USOC to its Handicapped in Sports Committee, attended the Paralympic Games Board meeting of 14th February 1983.

His purpose was quite obviously to persuade the board to change the name of the corporation in order to avert further problems with USOC. The resulting discussion on the issue revealed the fact that the University itself, as represented by the Vice-Chancellor Stan Levy and the Chairman of the Host Committee, Tim Nugent, was eager to do away with the name Paralympics. It was stated by Levy during the meeting that 'if you want to hold the games at the University, you'll have to change the name' (Final Report 1984)

The Board changed the name from the VIIth Paralympic Games, Inc., to the VIIth World Wheelchair Games Inc. This was not the end of the matter, and squabbling over the use of Olympic terminology continued in many arenas. It is very likely that the wrangling had a negative effect on the Board's ability to secure meaningful financial backing, and in the face of a lack of general exposure to an event of this sort in the United States, publicity focused on the negative side of a sensational failure rather than on the much-needed raising of positive awareness for athletes with a disability.

When the University of Illinois concluded that it must protect itself from losses that might be incurred due to the lack of funds or guarantee of funds from the Board of Directors of the Games, it terminated the contract. This happened in February 1984, four months from the opening of the Games. Stan Labanowich met Juan Antonio Samaranch at Beit Halochem in Tel Aviv on the last day of February, and raised the subject of the calamitous situation the World Wheelchair Games found itself in. He subsequently wrote to Samaranch (5th March 1984) to plead for support from the International Olympic Committee in trying to keep these Games on track. Labanowich stated his case strongly and tactfully, suggesting that the athletes had prepared themselves mentally and physically for competing in Illinois: 'To eliminate any possibility of conducting the Games at Illinois and wrench the competitions from the United States will undoubtedly demoralise them and plunge the movement into disarray. I fear that these developments will cause irreparable damage' (Labanowich, correspondence, 1984). His view was that, while Stoke Mandeville could certainly host the events, 'the facilities and arrangements at Stoke Mandeville . . . are inadequate to serve the expectations of the athletes of the member countries in this Olympic year'. Labanowich coolly asked Samaranch to help secure a guarantee of funding from the Los Angeles Olympic Organising Committee to the tune of US$1 million. The answer from Samaranch, in a letter dated 16th March 1984, was regretful of the possible cancellation of the Games, but he was also non-committal about underwriting the Games, and unemotionally said: 'With regard to your query, I shall forward this to the LAOOC for their consideration' (Samaranch, correspondence, 1984).

Notice of the intention of the University of Illinois to cancel its contract to host the Games led John Grant, Vice President of the International Stoke Mandeville Games Federation, to request an urgent meeting with the Chancellor of the University. This took place on 16th March 1983, but the Board of Directors of the VIIth Paralympic Games, Inc. was not informed of the meeting and was not invited to be part of this obvious rescue attempt. This was considered discourteous, and at worst might have been unhelpful. There was no effective way out of the financial difficulties, and the University of Illinois finally issued a 'Breach of Contract and failure to perform' notification for 31st January 1984, and withdrew its facilities from involvement in the Games. The Executive Committee of the International Stoke Mandeville Games Federation produced an appraisal of the reasons for the failure of the Illinois Games. These were summarised by Joan Scruton:

1. Composition of Board, whilst providing prominent technical expertise, failed to have adequate business management and financial expertise
2. Professional fund raisers failed
3. Possible scandal associated with bankruptcy of associated organisation frightened away possible donors
4. Board of Games – for reasons not clear, lacked credibility in the Corporate Boardrooms
5. Internal conflicts developed in the Committee which were harmful
6. Conflict with US Olympic Committee over use of term 'Paralympics' was detrimental to cause

7. University of Illinois had no confidence in ultimate success of on-going fund raising and was afraid of *debt*. Would have been prepared to go ahead with credible Corporate Board
8. Serious fund-raising commenced too late. Little activity in '81 & '82

Note: There is no evidence to suggest any criminal mismanagement of funds.

1984 International Stoke Mandeville Wheelchair Games

The VIIth World Wheelchair Games were to be moved to Stoke Mandeville, UK. The press release was suitably upbeat:

> The traditional Wheelchair games must go on. The Executive Committee of the International Stoke Mandeville Games Federation at their meeting on 4th March 1984 has adopted a resolution pledging firm support for the re-instatement of the VII World Wheelchair Games originally scheduled to take place in June 1984 at the University of Illinois, Champaign, Ill. USA. At the same time provision is being made to relocate the Games if organisational and financial problems in the USA cannot be solved. In that event the VII World Wheelchair Games will be transferred to Stoke Mandeville under the auspices of the British Paraplegic Sports Society.

Seymour Bloom was able to record a very impressive report of the 'Paralympic Games held at Stoke Mandeville': approximately 1100 athletes competed, representing 41 nations. There were initially limits of 900 placed on entries, but in the end these were lifted – a fact that countries appreciated. Venues were more impressive than in the past, using the best amenities available in the vicinity of Aylesbury. Table tennis and weightlifting were held in the town itself, while the swimmers made use of excellent facilities at High Wycombe. Local schools provided good competitive areas for archery and fencing. Bloom predicted that there could be a 50% increase in entries due to the fast development of the Paralympic phenomenon. Labanowich was almost certainly correct in his assessment, however, that the Paralympic athletes now needed Olympic-class facilities rather than high-quality local ones. He was making a crucial point to the President of the International Olympic Committee that the Paralympic Movement had grown up considerably.

Some 400 athletes were examined for classification at the Games, a number not dealt with before at Stoke Mandeville. One problem encountered by the team of doctors on hand was the late arrival of teams. This affected the ability to get through the volume needed. It was certainly frustrating for officials still to be involved with classification examinations after the Opening Ceremony had taken place. But this was to be a feature of the expanding participation levels. The particular circumstances facing the hosts at Stoke Mandeville made this pressure even less desirable. Looking towards the 1988 Paralympic Games in Korea, Cairbre McCann, Chairman of the Medical Committee of the International Stoke Mandeville Games Federation, recommended that at least one Korean doctor should be co-opted to the Medical Committee. Korean doctors should be introduced to the detailed requirements of the classification process as soon as possible. An educational programme should also extend to physiotherapists and medical support staff in good time.

Bob Jackson, by this time retired as President of ISMGF, wrote on 7th September 1984 to express his deep anxiety that he saw the ICC 'in danger of collapsing if recent events are allowed to go unrecognised and unchallenged'. He firstly stressed that his retirement had been planned from 18 months before and was unconnected to any events or persons. Jackson, from his department of orthopaedic surgery at the Toronto Western Hospital, identified several vitally important problems:

- the 'geographic separation of the Games in the USA, and the collapse of the paraplegic games at the University of Illinois';

- 'a fragmented and, at times, aggressive approach to the IOC', which Jackson saw as 'harmful to . . . efforts to integrate sports';
- a lack of 'common sense' in regard to the demonstration of wheelchair racing at the L. A. Olympics.

Jackson asked a pertinent question: is it the Executive of ICC which wants joint games for different disabilities, or do the athletes actually want this as well? He wondered whether the Olympic year was the right time to hold the most significant expression of elite sport for athletes with a disability. Also, Jackson questioned whether it was going to be feasible to serve the ever-expanding numbers of dedicated sportspeople – raising qualifying times and standards 'so that only the truly elite athletes can participate, thus reducing the numbers to workable levels'. These criticisms were not new, but it was significant that a credible former servant of the movement authored them.

The Camaraderie of Teamwork, the Thrill of Competition

The 1984 International Games for the Disabled, Nassau County, New York, were opened by Ronald Reagan, President of the United States, at the new Mitchell Park Athletic Complex on 17th June 1984, almost a month before the Los Angeles Olympic Games were to begin. In his opening speech he told the assembled athletes that: 'By competing in these games, each of you is sending a message of hope throughout the world. You're proving that a disability doesn't have to stand in the way of a full and active life, and you're showing all of us just how far a man or woman can go if only they have the dedication and the will'. Just as important as the communication of motivational messages to others, was the understanding of what it really meant to have strived to achieve the elite levels of the competitors:

> I think I can appreciate . . . what these games must mean to you. There will be the camaraderie of teamwork, the thrill of competition, the sheer joy of meeting other athletes who love the sport as much as you do. Roger Bannister, the first runner in history to break the 4-minute mile, once said, 'Running has given me a glimpse of the greatest freedom that a man can ever know, because it results in the simultaneous liberation of both body and mind.' Exhilaration of mind and body, that's something that all athletes understand. Yet there's something each of you understands that no-one else can ever fully appreciate, something that has to do with courage, with willpower, and with the utter refusal to give up that has enabled you to rise above your disabilities and compete.

Frenetic activity preceded the International Games for the Disabled. There was a very large stock of thousands of volunteers who needed guidance and allocation of duties, and while this was a very labour-intensive job for the experienced technical experts, it also enabled the extensive competitive pro-gramme to have the support it needed. Classification was an inevitably complicated business, and plans to have only a cursory check on those who had recently competed in Denmark were eventually shelved because it was simpler to employ the same routine with everyone. The classification group of 'les Autres' was considered to be very helpful because a number of athletes in the CP-ISRA sports events were considered to be ineligible and were shifted to the 'les Autres' group. In soccer there was a regulation that teams must include at least one player from Class VI, but those teams fielding more than one player from this class were evidently at a disadvantage, and the technical report would call for further regulation to even up the composition of teams in future. An interesting observation was that long jump had been categorised as a field event but the particular circumstances of this athletic event within sports for persons with disabilities suggested that emphasis was more on the run-up – future consideration should be given to thinking of long jump as a track event. Harald Natvig, Medical Officer of ISOD, was sure that the time had come to be establishing procedures for doping testing for the 1988 Games.

The sports programme was extensive. Visually impaired athletes were divided into three classes, and competed in athletics, goalball, swimming and wrestling. Athletes with cerebral palsy, in eight classes, competed in archery, athletics, boccia, cycling, dressage, football, powerlifting, shooting, swimming and table tennis. 'Les Autres' athletes were placed in six classes, and competed in archery, athletics, basketball, powerlifting, shooting, swimming, table tennis and volleyball. Amputees were divided into nine classes, and competed in athletics, lawn bowls, powerlifting, shooting, swimming, table tennis and volleyball. Exceptional athletes at this high-level competition included Charles Reid, an American powerlifter with cerebral palsy. Mustapha Badid (France) won the 200 m wheelchair race, and Jim Martinson (USA) established a new world record in the 100 m wheelchair race. The athletes came from 45 countries, bringing their enthusiasm and camaraderie together in a fiercely competitive atmosphere. As Michael Mushett, Games Director, noted, the athletes were not very interested in the theorising about the psychosocial benefits derived from their involvement in this world-class athletic event; they had the same determination and vigour as any elite athlete competing at Olympic level in their sport (Mushett 1984). Mushett quoted Janet Rowley, a blind American athlete competing in the athletics field events: 'I hate to see newspaper headlines that read: "Rowley Overcomes Blindness." We disabled athletes go in for Athletics for exactly the same reason as nondisabled people. We have fun in athletic competition and we need an outlet for our competitive instincts.'

Venues were all superbly close to the hub of the Mitchell Park Stadium, with the exception of the equestrian events, having to be located further out. The trials for the demonstration events to take place at the Los Angeles Olympic Games were held on 29th June, when eight competitors and two reserves were selected for the men's 1500 m and the women's 800 m wheelchair races.

The practical administrative aspects of the Games were slow to get into gear, but seemed to work up to a functioning operation. Accommodation was considered to have been of a very high quality, in a tented 'city' named 'Olympic Plaza'. Entertainment followed the established tradition of the 'beer tent', this time nicknamed 'Cabaret International'. Food was plentiful and the quality was high: described by Kristian Jensen of the Dansk Handicap Idraets-Forbund as 'tasty, nutritious and abundant' – but with no provision for kosher food. Marjolijn Hillegers was appreciative of the efforts made by the organisers, but she found that many people considered the Opening and Closing Ceremonies to be too long and unstructured. Speeches seemed to go on and on, and content might have been too specifically targeted at a limited audience 'in the know'. Transport was adequate, but there was a shortfall in information about bus times and in availability of transport for athletes attending receptions outside the Olympic Plaza itself. As can be expected, a great deal of further thought would be required before being able to claim to provide the perfect system for the particular needs of the athletes and officials. Golf carts were available for movement around the Olympic Plaza, but these were soon used less by competitors and officials – they did provide some fun for the policemen and volunteers. The Executive Director of ICC found it difficult to be very positive in her report. She said: 'it is inevitable that for me the organisation of these Games was very disappointing'. The future would have to include a determined effort to scrutinise all the observations and recommendations from various quarters, and to strive to improve for the next Olympic year.

Hans Lindström was constructively critical in his report of the 1984 Games in New York. He felt that the Organising Committee was under strength: 'there were too few responsible for too much'. A criticism of the organisation of the Games was that the volunteers seemed to be involved only for relatively few hours each – not enough to ensure consistency of support. In hindsight the official verdict was that there were far too few people involved who had experience in either high-level sports officiating or in sport for persons with a disability, or both. Officiating came in for particular attention from Lindström. He commended his own sport of swimming for having highly capable officials, although he didn't agree with the tendency to ignore such transgressions as unconcealed coaching from the poolside during races by over-enthusiastic coaches. Lindström did not think it right for medal ceremonies to proceed while a protest was under consideration, or for awarding additional medals when medals had been awarded to competitors who were later the subject of an upheld protest – instead of withdrawing the originals. Reportedly it was not possible to ratify certain world records in athletics due to questions about the level of qualification of the officials. Overall Lindström decried the perceptible attitude towards the athletes of: 'don't disqualify, after all they are disabled'. Scathing as some of his criticisms were, Lindström was as consistent as ever in putting them in a context of 'how to do it right next time'. He provided extremely clear action points for future organisers.

The women's goalball was scheduled for a hall that was unsuited for its purpose, with floor tiles instead of a wooden floor playing surface. As the problem was identified, the competition had to be relocated to share the men's facility. This led to an inevitable rescheduling of both programmes. Table tennis competitors were certainly not appreciative of the well-worn equipment provided for competition. The tables appeared to be damaged and of questionable quality, and the playing arena suffered from overheating and significant draughts. The competition was fierce all the same, and athletes thrilled at the opportunity of pitting their skills against each other. There was a rather rigid and unimaginative arrangement for the different disability groups to compete in swimming and athletics on different days – wholly devaluing the integrative potential of holding multi-disability games. The athletes with Cerebral Palsy competed on one day, the blind athletes on the next day, the amputees on the third day, and all others on the fourth day. Media attention outstripped both Arnhem and Toronto with a New York public relations company, Carl Byoir & Associates, managing the distribution.

The International Coordinating Committee Meets at the International Games for the Disabled in New York, June 1984

This sixth meeting of the ICC was held at Hampstead, New York on the occasion of the International Games for the Disabled. This had been a difficult period for the International Coordinating Committee, with the split venues for the quadrennial Games, but in particular with the emergency relocation of the Games to Stoke Mandeville after the disastrous collapse of the financial base for the Illinois Games. Archie Cameron chaired the meetings, and took the assembled representatives through the terms of reference for the Bureau being set up in Arnhem for the International Coordinating Committee, with Marjolijn Hillegers agreeing to take on the administrative role there. The programme for the 1988 Games in Seoul formed a major portion of the meeting's agenda. The next ICC seminar, planned for January at the Papendal Sports Centre in the Netherlands the following year, was also outlined. This second seminar would continue to work on sharing technical and medical expertise while working towards unified principles that were acceptable to each of the four member organisations. The seminar should also try to formulate a 'philosophy' of sports for persons with a disability as well as setting out what representatives believed relationships should be with able-bodied sports organisations. The latter was pertinent because of the announcement that FIBA, the international governing body of basketball, was to set up a committee for basketball for persons with a disability. Administrative and operational questions needed to be tackled at the seminar, as well as discussing ways of working together with 'able-bodied sports organisations'.

The International Coordinating Committee needed to agree a format to proffer when faced with other sports organisations seeking membership. It was decided that the organisation should be asked its reasons for wanting membership of ICC; and the conditions for membership were agreed to be:

1. Organisations must be involved with sports for the disabled
2. They must demonstrate a democratic structure
3. There should be a minimum number of member countries (as decided by ICC).

A delegation from Korea attended the ICC meeting and a provisional contract was signed for the 1988 Paralympic Games. The proposed starting date for the Paralympics was 10th October 1988 but the use of the facilities for the Olympic Games prior to the Paralympics gave strong confidence to the ICC members. All were agreed that the ICC must be fundamentally involved at every stage with the successful planning and execution of the Games in the light of the disappointment over the 1984 Illinois Games. This was a proving ground for the International Coordinating Committee, still heading towards maturity. There had been an Ad Hoc Committee for matters pertaining to organisation of the Games, and this was given a formal footing as the Olympic Committee of ICC.

The Agreement pieced together by Arieh Fink for the constitution of ICC was put before the Presidents and signed by Cameron (CP-ISRA), Pielasch (IBSA), Poole (ISMGF) and Cabezas (ISOD). This finally settled the prescribed interaction between the four member organisations for cooperation – now a formality because their relations had been highly successful already. The formal arrangements helped reassure their respective members of retained autonomy as well as making dealings more straightforward with other bodies such as the International Olympic Committee.

Scrutiny of some details of the Agreement help to clarify the intentions of the delegates from the four international disability sports organisations. Under the subheading of 'the Role of the Committee' the preservation of individual identities shows through clearly: 'To be responsible for coordinating the joint activities of the various subscribers to the agreement, always paying full regard to the autonomy and the constitution of the individual organisations in membership'. Prominent in the Agreement is the agreed role of ICC acting as 'the joint authority to control the organisation and programme of Olympic Games, joint World Championships and cross-organisational major events involving more than two member organisations', and 'To be the representative organisation of sport for the disabled to negotiate with such bodies as the International Olympic Committee and United Nations'.

Broad and explicit aims hold no surprises: 'To endeavour at all times to further the development of sports for the disabled in all parts of the world', 'To promote friendship and unity amongst disabled athletes and cooperation amongst international organisations (sports disabled)'. Also evident are the expected statements insisting on encouraging widest practice of sports among athletes with a disability and unbiased inclusion without discrimination.

The structure of the Committee was logically related to its evolution: three delegates appointed by each of the member organisations (CP-ISRA, ISOD, ISMGF and IBSA as 'founder members'), with the chairmanship of the Committee rotating between the Presidents so that their period of office lasted from the close of one meeting to the close of the following. In this way the burden of implementation of action points from the meetings did not fall on any one President or the Secretariat of any one organisation. But the lack of elected representation, along with the impossibility of any national or regional representation, were to be weaknesses in the International Coordinating Committee as it moved beyond its honeymoon days. The method of voting within the ICC was by majority, with each member organisation having a single vote to cast. To avoid unnecessary delay in decision making there was a policy of having papers prepared and circulated in time for each member organisation to be able to discuss the implications for its members; papers were to be posted by registered mail at least 35 days in advance of each meeting. Providing this timeframe was employed there should be some confidence that delegates had the mandate of their organisation.

Problems were going to continue with recognition of national disability sports organisations because they were not directly catered for by ICC's structure – and they could remain under-represented if they had no other recourse. One such example is that of the Austrian Federation of Sports for Disabled Persons, which had been refused admission to the Austrian National Olympic Committee in 1984.

Olympic Scientific Congress, Eugene, Oregon, July 1984

Eight days in July saw more than 2000 people, from some 100 countries, meeting for the Olympic Scientific Congress. The College of Human Development and Performance of the University of Oregon hosted the conference, with help from volunteers drawn from the cities of Eugene and Springfield. As a theme 'Sport, Health, and Well-Being' was adopted, and national and international organisations sponsored the programmes of the disciplines and sub-disciplines at a congress like this for the first time. The structure of the eight day period was also groundbreaking: mornings were for sub-disciplinary presentations and afternoons were directed towards cross-disciplinary and interdisciplinary exchanges. Evening keynote lectures rounded off the official programme. Many international organisations held their business meetings during this important congress. Stan Labanowich coordinated and chaired the part of the congress devoted to 'Sport and Disabled Athletes', while Claudine Sherrill edited the Proceedings as one part of a nine-volume set. Among the papers presented in this division at the Eugene Congress were thought-provoking presentations of original research in many areas of biomechanics and exercise physiology; extensive treatment of history, philosophy, sociology and psychology; and a separate section on the ever-present classification debate. The Olympic Scientific Congress was important not only for its vigorous exchange of ideas and information, but also because it was to see the beginnings of prominence of the International Council of Sport Science and Physical Education in the organisation of pre-olympic scientific congresses in future. It was to struggle regularly with the International Olympic Committee over the use of the word 'Olympic', just as the Paralympic Movement was to expend so much time on this same issue.

At the Olympic Scientific Congress held in Eugene, in July 1984, the International Association for the Research of Sport and Exercise for the Disabled (IARSED) was founded. Its aims were: 'to facilitate research, education and communication amongst individuals who are involved in the sport and exercise sciences with physically disabled populations'. It was intended that the organisation would promote the first World Congress on 'Sport, Research and Exercise for the Physically Disabled' in April 1986 in Banff, Alberta, Canada. As a result of this planning, the Congress Coordinator, Leanne Squair, wrote to ICC asking for patronage and any financial assistance that might be forthcoming. A prime mover in the new organisation, and in the preparations for the Congress, was to be Bob Steadward. Here was a clear move away from the medical model of disability: the learned gathering of professionals to focus on sport first rather than disability first, as in the International Medical Society of Paraplegia. In reply to the request for patronage, Marjolijn Hillegers sought further details for the ICC members to look at about the Congress, while pointing out that the International Coordinating Committee also had a Research Sub-Committee. It was of importance for the ICC to remain fully informed about the newly established international organisation. As she put it, ICC was 'very curious and indeed eager to have more information'. An umbrella organisation needed to ensure that it could retain its coordinating role with specialised bodies as they sprang up – in this case with potentially damaging effects for ICC unless the other organisation could be persuaded to work in conjunction with ICC.

Demonstration Events at the Los Angeles Olympic Games

More than 90 000 spectators filled the Olympic Stadium in Los Angeles to enjoy the spectacle of the demonstration wheelchair events at the Olympic Games on 11th August. There had been worrying difficulties for the administration of the ICC, with a complete lack of communication from the Los Angeles Organising Committee: there was no information about accreditation, accommodation or identity cards. Eventually the decision was taken to fly Marjolijn Hillegers to Los Angeles three days ahead of the main group in order to resolve the difficulties. With the help of Walther Tröger, Sports Director of IOC, most problems were ironed out, but with the drastic step of replacing the appointed coordinator. The other main criticism made by Jens Bromann and Marjolijn Hillegers was that almost all publicity before and during the Games centred on the athletes with disabilities from the USA only, rather than on the work of ICC and sport for athletes with disabilities more broadly.

The demonstration events were met with enthusiastic support from all dignitaries who attended: the King and Queen of Sweden, Juan Antonio Samaranch, President of IOC, and Primo Nebiolo, President of the International Amateur Athletics Federation (IAAF). Queen Silvia of Sweden presented medals to the first three competitors in each event (Women's 800 m: Sharon Hedrick, USA, Monica Säker, Sweden and Candace Cable, USA; Men's 1500 m: Pol Van Winkel, Belgium, Randy Snow, USA and André Viger, Canada). After the presentation of medals, Samaranch indicated to the ICC delegates that he would welcome future demonstration events. There was a flurry of activity to arrange for the athletes to have the opportunity of participating in the Closing Ceremony, but many had already departed on the Sunday afternoon. It was reported that a number of Australian and Danish athletes with a disability joined their counterparts in the Closing Ceremony, but unofficially. The wheelchair demonstration events had generated 'a wave of goodwill', but the ICC representatives were bitter that the local organisers appeared not to be able to set aside their partisan interests to promote the cause of sport for people with disabilities more globally.

The 1984 Los Angeles Olympic Games were to be the most profitable Olympic Games ever. The city of Los Angeles had established a contract with the International Olympic Committee that permitted significant marketing opportunities. This would attract a high level of corporate interest, and leave a massive multi-million dollar surplus for the organising committee after the Olympic Games were over. Peter Uberroth headed up the Los Angeles Olympic Organising Committee (LAOOC) as a major business concern. Most outstanding performances at the Olympic Games were seen from Carl Lewis, the American sprinter and jumper; Michael Jordan took the US Basketball team to gold. But in spite of the Soviet boycott reducing the competitive range, in retaliation for the US boycott in Moscow in 1980, the phenomenon of the Olympic Games was a great success.

Slow Progress at Lausanne, but Some Signs of Promise

Representatives of the International Coordinating Committee met for an hour and three-quarters with Juan Antonio Samaranch at the Chateau Vidy, IOC Headquarters, Lausanne on 10th January 1985. Samaranch was pleased with the progress made over the past 12 months and wanted to review the past year as well as to plan for the next stages. He delegated responsibility to the Sports Director, Walther Tröger, for the ICC's contact with the International Olympic Committee. This indicated the IOC President's serious recognition of the ICC's significance. Tröger had great influence and practical abilities to make things happen directly. The subject of patronage was addressed in the meeting, Tröger requesting that a single centrally agreed list of events should be presented to the IOC for patronage, preferably a plan for the next four years. Jens Bromann formally notified the IOC officers that there was now an official single body to provide this centrality entitled the International Coordinating Committee of World Sports Organisations for the Disabled, with its headquarters in the Netherlands. He informed Samaranch and Tröger that four international organisations had formed the Committee: ISMGF, ISOD, CP-ISRA and IBSA. Samaranch asked about the status and involvement of other disability groups and Bromann replied that 'the International Committee of Sports for the Deaf (CISS), under the Presidency of Mr Jerald Jordan from the USA, and the mentally retarded, which are not grouped into an international organisation, were not part of ICC'. At this the IOC President said that he was to have the opportunity of trying 'to convince Mr Jordan and his organisation to join ICC'. A meeting was already planned between them for 3rd March in New York. Samaranch asked that a copy of ICC Regulations should be supplied to him so that he could prepare for this meeting with the CISS president. There was some discussion about funding both by the International Fund and by the IOC, and Samaranch indicated that he could make a sum of US$200 000 available for the period 1985–88 for patronised events.

Once again the sticking point returned to the use of terminology and symbols: Samaranch reminding the meeting of the IOC responsibilities to protect the identity and symbols of the unique phenomenon of the Olympic Games as identified in the Olympic Charter. He restated that ICC was expected to refrain from using the word 'Olympic'. While agreeing to this restriction both Jens Bromann and Joan Scruton stressed the ICC's 'desire to be treated on an equal footing as the non-handicapped. It is felt that the disabled athletes would not easily understand this restrictive use of the word "Olympic".' The debate went further into the philosophy of the Olympic Movement and its ideals, with Samaranch making it clear that he considered the ICC to be a member of the Olympic family – demonstrated by the IOC's willingness to lend its patronage and offer financial aid: 'The use of the Olympic flag and rings would prove to the world that ICC is part of the Olympic Movement'. Samaranch also wanted to point out his wish for caution that the integration of the ICC into the Olympic Movement should 'proceed gradually and should be in compliance with the Olympic Charter'. His concern was that there might be a negative reaction from the Olympic Movement if any integrative moves were too sudden. There should be time for 'the world of able bodied sports . . . to accept and adopt (sic) to such integration'. Very specifically he insisted that the words 'Olympic Games' should not be used for the events taking place in Seoul in 1988. Samaranch put it plainly that ICC was free to use the term 'Olympic', but in that case, would have to 'go their own way without IOC in future'.

The meeting went on to cover the proposals for demonstration events at Calgary and Seoul, with a need to expand the programme for women and blind athletes. Samaranch wanted to ensure that ICC could 'come up with a program of very spectacular events' for Seoul in particular. The International Olympic Committee would undertake to cover the costs of athletes and officials in Calgary and Seoul, as well as supporting the ICC delegation to visit Calgary two years before the Games. Finally, Samaranch suggested that the ICC should identify some important championships at which demonstration events by athletes with a disability could be encouraged – offering to personally 'intervene with the Organising committees' where necessary. Another helpful move was for Samaranch to agree to send a letter to international federations and National Olympic Committees to help affiliation of the International Coordinating Committee. Cabezas asked Samaranch also to use his influence to help make architectural adaptations for sport for persons with a disability. In these matters Samaranch actioned contact almost immediately with certain groups, asking that they consider ways of furthering the cause of sports for persons with a disability within their own particular movements. He wrote to leaders of international sports organisations in archery, athletics, basketball, skiing, swimming and volleyball, as well as the international federation of sports equipment manufacturers and sports facilities.

Marjolijn Hillegers drafted a series of recommendations by Jens Bromann, Joan Scruton and Guillermo Cabezas following the IOC meeting. This reflects the logical conclusion that support from the International Olympic Committee was worthwhile, and that sacrifices would have to be made in order to be accepted: 'it would not be wise to decline this cooperation and go our own way for many reasons . . . This cooperation could greatly serve the cause of sports for the disabled.' It was also very important to seek a suitable alternative title for 'the event "Olympics for the Disabled" which will express this unique happening once every four years and underline the "Olympic Status" of the event'. The President of the International Olympic Committee was working hard to ensure that the future of the Paralympic Movement was promising. He had the diplomatic skill to proffer very positive ways forward, even when having to say 'no' to some other requests. Samaranch was consistent in his personal enthusiasm for the promotion of sport for people with a disability. It was far more difficult for him to persuade all factions of the Olympic family to share his viewpoint.

Arnhem Hosts ICC Again

The second ICC seminar ran at Papendal from 31st January to 3rd February 1985, at the Papendal National Sports Centre in Arnhem. Delegates arriving at Schiphol Airport travelled by bus to Utrecht and then took the train to Arnhem. Archie Cameron guided discussions fruitfully, and a valuable and constructive debate helped plan for the future role and structure of ICC. He acknowledged that his recent retirement from the Presidency of CP-ISRA rendered him an appropriately unbiased chairman for the discussions in Papendal. Interested in the future of sport for athletes with a disability, some delegates had travelled from as far as Australia and Korea to attend the ICC seminar. Originally the delegates were to be separated into workshops, returning to deliver a summary of their findings later. But almost as one body they insisted on remaining together in seminar form: everyone would hear the opinions of everyone else, and while this was more unwieldy, a more open debate could be promoted. Jens Bromann led off with his view of integration in sport so that athletes with a disability competed alongside other athletes as far as possible. Contributions from the floor delved into the numerous aspects of integration that would need careful consideration: the sturdiness of the existing international federations themselves, before looking more widely at linking up with federations for other athletic populations; whether integration should apply to recreational sport as well as elite; qualification standards for elite events; the meaning of the term 'elite'; and athletes' views. The ICC was asked to remain attentive towards recreational sport for participants with disabilities.

Classification was agreed to be the cornerstone of standards and qualification – but there was a reminder that the movement had swung away from rehabilitation, and was now firmly a 'sports movement'. With this being the case the division between competitive and recreational sport was marked, although athletes were likely to transfer from one system to another. The technical side of classification was described as being 'too haphazard', and needed steady research to find a system that would be most workable while also being appropriate to the aims of competitive sport. It was agreed that: 'The primary requirement for classification is to have athletes competing with a meaningful purpose'; the delegates acknowledged that they must 'never manipulate for administrative purposes unless the situation is such that there is no option due to an inability to accommodate the numbers involved at one venue'. A sensitive discussion took place on the rights of the more severely disabled to participate in 'Olympic level' competitions. Some concerns were voiced about the possibility of ridicule of participants due to their appearance, and it was not fully agreed that a 'right' to participate at this most elite level should exist. While no conclusions could be reached, the relatively young organisation for athletes with cerebral palsy would need to show ways of regulating and monitoring entry standards so as to distinguish sufficiently the very highest standards for competition.

The participants in Papendal agreed that the International Coordinating Committee had a responsibility in the area of promoting workshops in developing countries. Relations with the International Olympic Committee were discussed as well, mainly in the form of an update of information for delegates on the current position ICC held with IOC. Much work was done on the Olympic Manual, and there was a postponement of the deadline so as to finalise procedures for doping control and protests. At this point there were no procedures in place for spot checks out of competition.

Strategic proposals were made for the creation of medical and technical sub-committees, and the ICC at the meetings immediately following the seminar soon enacted these. While it was recognised that the ICC was an umbrella group, the assembled delegates felt that there should be a single international body, acting with sub-groups for each category of disability. At the time there was the expectation that the newly formed organisation for people with intellectual disabilities (INAS-FMH) would seek membership of ICC, and that the sports organisation for deaf people (CISS) would come to work cooperatively as well. This would provide a very strong platform for future strength. The seminar's participants declared: 'Ultimately a federation is a possibility, probably to be formed by the next generation'! It was proposed that a world congress to work on the major restructuring of ICC should be held in good time prior to the 1988 Games. The International Coordinating Committee was not judged by the people at the seminar to be the organisation that would ultimately take the Paralympic Movement into the next century. The ICC would always be seen as an interim measure, except by a small number of individuals who wished to turn it into the single international body representative of all disability sports organisations.

Helmut Pielasch was very ill at the time of the February 1985 meeting, so Jens Bromann, also of IBSA, took the chairmanship when the ICC met during the seminar. Another absence from among the regular participants in the Committee was Archie Cameron, who had retired from his presidency of CP-ISRA by this time. This brought Arie Klapwijk to the position of President of CP-ISRA, and also saw Elizabeth Dendy attending her first meeting of the International Coordinating Committee, representing CP-ISRA. Hers was to be a lengthy association and she would eventually preside over the final meeting of the ICC in Larnaca, Cyprus, in March 1993.

The reports were delivered of the New York Games and the Stoke Mandeville Wheelchair Games that had replaced the Illinois Games. These had significant implications for future events on the world stage – a crucial time either to draw together more firmly or to accept a need for a coordinated but separate series of events. As John Grant urged the Committee members: the 1984 Games were now 'history' and real attention must turn to supporting the success of the 1988 celebration in Seoul, Korea.

This was thought to be the right time to approach the International Olympic Committee to request formal recognition 'as a member of the Olympic family'. The minutes of the seventh ICC meeting, held on 3rd February 1985, declared that the delegates considered that good progress had been made with IOC towards 'full integration'. This does not seem to have been the agreed goal of all in attendance, but there is no dissent recorded. The members also proposed that in future the Games held in the same years as the Olympiad should be known as Paralympic Games. On this point there was complete agreement from the assembled members of the International Coordinating Committee. With regard to the 1988 Olympic Winter Paralympics, Jens Bromann suggested that the Administrative Sub-Committee should consider approaching the International Olympic Committee about a co-operative effort, as the ICC had not as yet received a bid for these Games.

Also in keeping with the growing responsibility of the ICC as an umbrella organisation, there was a request from Mr Choudhuri, of the Sports Organisation for Disabled in Bangladesh, for support for a project to advance sport for persons with a disability in developing countries. Members undertook to gather proposals for support and suggestions for projects, sending them in to the ICC Bureau in the Netherlands – John Grant, for example, would gather information from his contacts in Kenya. The work of the International Coordinating Committee in the field of developing countries was to be known as Project 001. The ICC managed to support a workshop in Algeria between 19th and 30th April 1985, but then turned attention to Mr Choudhuri's proposal of holding a workshop in Bangladesh in 1986. Unfortunately the plans, although well advanced, had to be set aside because of a change in governmental situation with corresponding withdrawal of available funding. The working group moved its resources to Malaysia and held the next workshop between 13th April and 24th April 1987.

Through particular communication channels in the International Fund Sport Disabled, the interest of agencies of the United Nations was aroused. The United Nations had expressed interest in the idea of a 'chain of workshops' in developing countries, dovetailing well with the Decade of Disabled Persons. It was hoped that IFSD would be able to apply to the trust fund of the United Nations – AGFUND – once the proposals had been formalised. From the United Nations Decade of Disabled Persons (1983–1992) had come the encouragement to promote the spread of specialised knowledge and skills that would help developing countries. The United Nations General Assembly in 1982 had passed resolution 137:

> The importance of sports for disabled persons is becoming increasingly recognised. Member States should therefore encourage all forms of sports activities of disabled persons, inter alia, through the provision of adequate facilities and the proper organisation of these activities.

Adjustments were essential to the structure of the ICC so that it could extend its efficient functioning: Administrative, Technical, Medical and Youth Committees were established. Each member organisation could decide whether to appoint one or two delegates to the Technical and Medical Committees but only one vote would be extended to each organisation. A Research and Classification Sub-committee was later set up, with a questionnaire about participation as the first project. These committees would need structural revision, but they would help take the burden of more specialised groundwork away from what would become an Executive Committee – allowing policy decisions to be taken more effectively.

A newsletter was being constructed for ICC members, giving information on events and progress in negotiations. With support, the newsletter would become an important public face of the work of the International Coordinating Committee.

Grant Explores the Olympic Family

John Grant attended the International Olympic Committee's gathering for the Federation of International Sports Organisations for summer events on 29th May 1985. This was a very illuminating opportunity for Grant to see how members of the Olympic family operated with specific reference to the regulations governing their relationship with the International Olympic Committee. He explained that the International Coordinating Committee had first been accepted with observer status, alongside the international federations for baseball, orienteering, ten-pin bowling and water-skiing. Grant had only praise for the obvious energy and commitment of Juan Antonio Samaranch: 'a man clearly set apart to lead such an organisation as the International Olympic Committee. He is a person with a very obvious concern and interest in the disabled sporting movement and wishes to see the disabled sporting movement advance.' Grant urged that ICC should immediately familiarise itself with the intimate workings of the Olympic movement – the Olympic Charter and the organisational structure – and establish regular contact with key people, in particular Walther Tröger.

The Olympic Solidarity movement was given emphasis in John Grant's report. He could see a significant benefit accruing to ICC's aims from involvement in Olympic Solidarity's activities. Grant reported that the Olympic movement had difficulties with the excessive size of its events; urgency would be essential in moving towards decisions on disability demonstration events for Olympic Games. Samaranch had asked the international sports federations to look into the possibilities and respond by including their ideas in the submission of their programme requests for the Olympic Games. Another important emphasis was on time: the summer Games federations were being asked to look six years in advance for their planning, so ICC would immediately be under pressure. It would soon become essential for the International Coordinating Committee to be seen to work in synchronisation with the planning orbit of the International Olympic Committee. Other useful contacts were made during this journey for John Grant. He discussed membership of the General Association of International Sports Federations (GAISF) with Luc Niggli, the GAISF representative, as well as discussing sport for persons with a disability with the leaders of the international federations for orienteering and volleyball (both attending as observers), and for archery, badminton, equestrian events, wrestling and yachting. As an aside, and perhaps as an amusing illustration of the International Olympic Committee's impressive attraction, Grant described a moment taken at the meeting for the IOC to be presented with 'over three hundred televisions and video recorders' for their member federations. Grant speculated whether one of these machines might be forthcoming to ICC!

Comité International des Sports des Sourds Starts to Climb Aboard, August 1985

Another retirement from a leading role within one of the member organisations was that of Bob Jackson, who yielded his position as President of the International Stoke Mandeville Games Federation to John Grant. Grant therefore took the Chair at the eighth ICC meeting, held at the Civic Centre in Aylesbury, UK, on 4th and 5th August 1985, when Jerald Jordan, President of the Comité International des Sports des Sourds (CISS), observed proceedings. Jordan, whose organisation was the oldest of all international disability sports organisations, stated that his group intended to apply formally for membership – an important further development in the profile of the International Coordinating Committee.

There is no doubt that Jerald Jordan's meeting in March with the President of the International Olympic Committee will have helped nudge the CISS towards participation in a collective representation of disability sports groups at the international level, but with some anxiety over what might be lost of its long-established identity and expectations. John Grant also pointed out to the other ICC members that welcoming CISS as members would in turn please the International Olympic Committee's President, and would probably help 'give an impetus to our move towards full membership of the IOC'.

Jordan wrote to Samaranch soon after returning to Washington DC, where he was based at Gallaudet College. He described the discussion at the CISS Congress relating to joining ICC: reportedly 'in the end the members voted to give it a try'. This was not a wholehearted endorsement of an exciting new venture for the CISS! In his letter to Samaranch, Jordan also commented that he had sensed a very cool reception from the representatives of the international sports organisations at the International Coordinating Committee: 'I must admit that the announcement was greeted with less than wild enthusiasm'. Jordan emphasised that the acceptance of CISS into the International Coordinating Committee was largely due to the efforts of Arie Klapwijk. The umbrella group had rejected the request for sign language interpreters and escorts to be funded by ICC for its meetings, and Jerald Jordan feared that this might cause a lower level of attendance. However, Jordan pledged that CISS would enter into its side of the relationship with full commitment. Samaranch responded to Jordan's letter encouraging perseverance and stressing that there would be no change to CISS's receipt of IOC recognition for events; just that it would 'be much better for all handicapped organisations to work together as far as the Olympic Movement is concerned'.

Although the CISS had applied for membership of ICC, the Aylesbury meeting did not formally consider its application because one major sticking point remained – the organisation for sport for the deaf wanted to retain its own dealings with the International Olympic Committee. There was no surprise in this outlook: the CISS was the most senior disability sport organisation, and had received recognition from IOC long before most other organisations had been in existence. The lengthy and regular communication between Robey Burns and Avery Brundage in earlier years gave authority to the precedence of CISS's standing with IOC – now reasonably to be defended as a measure of its status, identity and independence. But at this crucial time, the International Coordinating Committee had to try to work towards its aim of providing one voice for communication with the International Olympic Committee, and so ICC kept CISS at arm's length until it became prudent to be more inclusive. Of course, it was also essential for international organisations to be treated with due respect and to acknowledge the great service that had been done to their particular population. It is certainly possible that some reluctance on the part of ICC to include CISS was also seen as insulting to this latter organisation in the paucity of regard given. Travel costs to meetings of ICC (and costs of sign language interpreters if not otherwise funded) would have to be wholly justifiable to the Executive Committee of an international organisation, and this would depend on an assessment of whether CISS was going to get 'value for money' from the actual ICC meetings themselves. Some doubts that this would be the case had been expressed in CISS Executive Committee meetings. The Committee was unlikely to favour directing resources to a venture that might reduce its own influence on the world 'stage', and damage the effectiveness of the CISS as an organisation working for its membership. Jerald Jordan was unhappy that his organisation was being made to feel like 'second class' citizens because of the identification within ICC of 'founder members' – obviously excluding CISS and INAS-FMH, which had not been involved in the initial setting up of the International Coordinating Committee.

A logo for the ICC could not be agreed at the August meeting of ICC, but it was thought that members might wait until after the Seoul Paralympics 'with a view to asking permission to use their logo'. Another seminar was proposed for 1987, with a theme of either the future of ICC or the future of sport for persons with a disability – each an ambitious undertaking. There had still not been any formal bids for the 1992 Paralympic Winter Games, although France, the Netherlands (Amsterdam) and Spain (Barcelona) had tendered bids for the Paralympic Summer Games.

Carl Wang, Vice President of ISOD, put a discussion document before the meeting suggesting that ICC should move towards regional or continental committees. Wang's input was to have a fundamental effect on the rational restructuring of the International Coordinating Committee, and later he would help draw out the new principles of the International Paralympic Committee. The success of ICC's efforts so far had been acclaimed at both the ISOD seminar in Poland in April 1985, and by the General Assembly held in Norway in May. Wang commended the 'fusion' of medical representatives from the four member organisations into one ICC Medical Committee as the sort of positive progress that should be encouraged further. But he also pointed to the tendency for all international organisations to encourage the clustering of national bodies into continental groups. His own organisation had recently agreed to head this way, as had IBSA. Importantly, Wang put forward the idea that the International Coordinating Committee should seek the same reorganisation in order to form continental committees, thereby 'slowly taking the place of the ECISOD and FESPIC, and possibly other continental/regional commit-tees'. Carl Wang's proposal was that the establishment of continental or regional committees should preclude each of the four disability sports organisations from needing to establish their own. Efficiency of operation and communication would be significantly greater from a central hub, and cost should also be reduced.

The Administrative Sub-Committee met in Copenhagen, Denmark, in October 1985 and straight-away acted on the lack of bids for hosting the 1988 Winter Paralympics by writing to those member organisations with which they had already had some contact. So as to avoid a repeat of the earlier tension, the Sub-Committee agreed that it would be a good thing to write to selected countries inviting bids for the 1992 Paralympic Winter Games. At the same time it was confirmed that the Seoul Paralympic Committee had approved the use of its emblem as the ICC logo; Marjolijn Hillegers and Joan Scruton were asked to find out on their visit to Korea whether the Seoul organisers had a 'Paralympic hymn'. Even in the Tokyo 1964 Paralympic Games there had been songs composed specifically to honour the Games, and the mirroring of the Olympic Games is quite clear.

Requests for recognition of sporting events by the International Coordinating Committee was an important aspect of the umbrella group's rising profile as a worldwide influence, so some sort of judicious structure for providing recognition was established. Organisers of major competitions might be better able to secure local corporate financial support with ICC recognition, and the ICC would climb the ladder of recognition as an organisation of substance with each request. The format suggested was for 'patronage' to be the highest level of official acknowledgment the ICC should offer, with the Paralympic Games fitting this category. The ICC would offer to 'sanction' an event of the next level down – national or regional competition, giving support and technical expertise where needed. A third category – 'approval' – would offer legitimacy to smaller events operating within the regulations of the ICC member organisations, such as invitational competitions. Support might be given along varying lines: administrative, technical, medical and even financial. Approaches to potential sponsors and other supporters were more likely to meet with success if the contest organisers could produce these kinds of acknowledgement from an international organisation such as ICC. The Administrative Sub-Committee decided that the starting point of requests for recognition must be for the relevant international federation to give its approval to the event, and the national organisation must oversee the conduct of the competition. The ICC would then consider the level of recognition it would offer.

The Winter Games Rule Book was ready for the printers in October 1985 but there was concern that ISOD had indicated it would not accept it, and IBSA had also raised some questions. It appeared that it might not be the right time for formal production of this publication, so the Administrative Sub-Committee agreed to shelve the idea of going to print, in favour of working to the rules of the appropriate member organisations. It might have been too much at this moment to force the issue of moving to a centralised document governing all member organisations. The International Coordinating Committee had confidence in the document but had no need to invite confrontation and division.

The International Fund Sport Disabled considered expanding its activities to establish parallel funds in other countries – the benefits to those countries were obvious, but the IFSD could also broaden the fundraising base and therefore generate larger sums for distribution. In late November at its regular meeting, the IFSD Board was advised by the ICC members of the Advisory Board to be careful not to 'try to export the Dutch system' to other countries, but to closely examine each country and assess the most suitable structure that might be encouraged. The wishes of the national organisations, as well as of their needs, would have to be considered when leading a drive of this sort. There was some conflict brewing between ICC and the International Fund Sport Disabled: one group saw its role as an independent philanthropic organisation that could make things happen, while the other saw itself as the coordinator of sport for people with a disability and therefore the seat of decision making about what events should be supported. For the International Fund to start up 'branches' in other countries could be confusing for the national organisations, and could reduce the developing influence of the International Coordinating Committee.

Sport for Athletes with Intellectual Disabilities, February 1986

Sport for athletes with intellectual disabilities had remained outside the influence of the International Coordinating Committee, and the youthful International Association of Sports for Persons with Mental Handicap (INAS-FMH) was discussed when the ICC gathered for the ninth time, in Barcelona on 14th February 1986. Guillermo Cabezas chaired meetings that explored the broadening of membership to enable the ICC's aims. There had been several difficulties in bringing about unity of representation for several reasons, but one problem for ICC was that only one organisation should represent persons with intellectual disabilities, as both INAS-FMH and Special Olympics Inc. operated in this area. Robert M. Montague Jr, Executive Director of Special Olympics Inc., had written on 5th August 1985 to ask ICC to consider an application for membership. It had just celebrated the European Summer Special Olympic Games in Dublin in July, with over 2200 athletes. INAS-FMH was a newly formed body, and did not have an established background yet, and ICC members were unsure about the wisdom of including it in their organisation. The constitutions of both INAS-FMH and Special Olympics Inc. were to be scrutinised by ICC members before further progress could be sought. This would continue to be a difficult area for any umbrella organisation in times to come, and perhaps one of the thorniest aspects of collaboration for different disability sports organisations to balance adequately. But there appeared, on the surface, to be agreement that the way forward was to work towards welcoming both INAS-FMH and CISS into membership of ICC. Special Olympics was already strongly established and well-funded. It was also very North American in its focus of administration, in contrast to most other sports organisations for individuals with disabilities – it did not seek a role in the Paralympic Games. Perhaps the younger organisation would be more malleable, and would serve the aims of the ICC better in the future.

It was not long before Jerald Jordan (CISS) expressed dissatisfaction with ICC's commitment to its new member organisations. Arie Klapwijk had sent some papers to Jordan in April 1986 and Jordan wrote on 28th April to acknowledge receipt and to pass on some of his observations, prior to a CISS Executive Committee meeting to be held in May. Klapwijk had seen that Jordan would be disappointed with the way their membership had been 'handled' – Jordan had not been made to feel that CISS was at all welcome in ICC, and he was critical of the attention paid to him in Aylesbury. Only one issue seemed to dominate at this meeting: why CISS could not adapt the long-established CISS Games to fall in the Olympic year and fall into line with the Paralympic Games, and why, 'if we are so able-bodied, we do not compete in the Olympics and disband our Games'. Jordan felt that the invitation to attend the Barcelona meeting had arrived so late as to appear as 'an afterthought'. He could not possibly make himself available with such short notice. The papers that Klapwijk had sent to Jordan served to clarify the wish of ICC to welcome CISS into the fold, but they also seemed to cement in Jordan's mind that ICC was: 'actually an organisation for the locomotively disabled. Other groups do not fit in and the ICC is not certain how to include them.' He was perceptive in commenting that ICC might not be moved to give serious consideration to the inclusion of persons with other types of disabilities 'were it not for the fact that IOC requires it'. Jordan could understand the position, and he also admitted to his members the value of truly valid membership of ICC in its umbrella function. He would not endorse the idea of CISS being admitted to ICC as an associate member rather than a full member, and called on the ICC to acknowledge the need to be more fully embracing of its purported identity as an umbrella organisation – broadening its horizons in order to achieve its stated aims.

Planning for Seoul

When the delegates of the International Coordinating Committee eventually did meet with the Secretary General and representatives of the Seoul Paralympic Organising Committee (SPOC), on 14th May 1986, there was a need to delicately rebuild bridges in their relationship. ICC had been worried about the lack of response from SPOC over time, and had started to consider that alternative arrangements could be needed once again in order to ensure that a celebration of the quadrennial games went ahead. Il Mook Cho, Secretary General of SPOC, explained that following its own National Games in October 1985 it had consulted participants and organisers about the timing of the event. The view was that October was a challenging time in Seoul due to the climate. Unfortunately July and August were the hot and rainy months, and the Organising Committee of the Seoul Olympiad itself and the Ministry of Sport dismissed May because facilities and even some venues might not have been completed. The Seoul Paralympic Organising Committee then spent time exploring the possibility of using alternative facilities and accommodation nearby, but this proved unworkable. It had returned to October 1988 as the time for the Paralympic Games to take place – with the advantage of being able to make use of existing facilities from the Olympic Games that would have just finished. Dates were agreed between SPOC and representatives of the ICC, and at this stage it was intended that accommodation would be within the Olympic Village, as the contract had insisted. In the end it was necessary for the organising committee to arrange for the construction of a Paralympic Village, including 14-storey apartment blocks capable of external wheelchair ramps in case of emergency. The Seoul City Government was responsible for this, and its representatives later visited Stoke Mandeville and West Germany to study appropriate accommodation.

Terminology

Identity and terminology continued to be of great importance to the members of the ICC. At its Executive Committee meeting in September 1985, the ISOD had voted to recommend that another name should be found for the Paralympics, establishing an unquestionable and unwavering identity for the major summer and winter events in the calendar. The ISOD Executive considered that the Seoul Games had acquired clear association with the title 'Paralympic', and felt that a new name was needed. Hans Lindström wrote to ICC members in December 1985 to ask a small group of people to investigate a suitable alternative name. The Barcelona meeting of the International Coordinating Committee threw around some ideas: Handyilympic, ICClympic, and a return to Winter/Summer Olympic Games for the Disabled. But there was a strong attachment to the name Paralympic Games.

'Every Handicap is Ours'

The founding meeting of the International Association of Sports for Persons with Mental Handicap had only taken place at the end of January 1985. But its membership was fast expanding with vigorous leadership. At the tenth meeting of the International Coordinating Committee in Gothenburg, which began on 6th August 1986, INAS-FMH had been asked whether it could meet the criteria for membership as amended, and Joseph Paul Kieboom replied that, although a young organisation, he considered that it did fulfil the requirements: it did have an international programme that had 'a competitive character', and its rule books were still in development. The members of ICC debated the nature of INAS-FMH competitions and worked through some doubts about their exact parallel to the programmes of other existing organisations, but they eventually agreed unanimously that INAS-FMH should be accepted into membership of ICC.

At the same time it was agreed that CISS had now overcome its reluctance to acknowledge the International Coordinating Committee's representative authority. Jerald Jordan accepted that CISS could recognise ICC as 'a body for mutual interest and joint authority, but that the sports programme of CISS would of course differ from that of CP-ISRA, IBSA, ISMGF and ISOD'. CISS would not seek to be involved in Paralympic competition as it had its own very successful Silent Games. Towards the end of this discussion there were several calls for clarification of the voting rights for the two new member organisation; existing members wanted to ensure that CISS and INAS-FMH would not be able to vote on matters relating to Paralympic Games. The vote to accept the two organisations into membership of ICC was precipitated by a knock at the door to say the champagne ordered to celebrate the momentous induction was ready! Arie Klapwijk was heard to exclaim that ICC could finally realise the assertion made in its objectives: 'that every handicap is ours!'

Jens Bromann wrote proudly to Samaranch to inform him that both CISS and INAS-FMH had been inducted as members of ICC, at the same time writing to the United Nations and the European Economic Community to complete the picture. Of course, the membership of the International Coordinating Committee was going to be marked by disruption, but for now the full spectrum of disabilities was represented. When the Administrative Sub-Committee proposed amendments to the criteria for membership in the Agreement maintained by all member organisations, while CISS and INAS-FMH were added to the list of organisations in membership, the control of the Sports Programme remained within the domain of the other four 'founding members'.

There was some confusion later relating to the transcripts of the discussion in Gothenberg, with disagreement of exactly what had been agreed about voting rights for the two new member organisations of ICC. Hans Lindström wrote to all ICC members to clarify the fact that membership had been agreed with the condition that INAS-FMH and CISS did not have voting rights in matters relating to the Paralympic Games. Joan Scruton had proposed a 'good old English compromise' in Copenhagen in January 1987 by qualifying the voting rights to be inoperative until after the 1988 Games. But the deep-rooted concerns remained that these new members had substructures that did not fit neatly into the original principles for international competitive sport for athletes with a disability drawn up by ICC. CISS expressly wished to remain separate from Paralympic competition, and to retain its much older Silent Games, but the corresponding lack of involvement of CISS in any discussions relating to the Paralympics necessarily held it at arm's length from the other federations.

With regard to the status of ICC with the International Olympic Committee, Hans Lindström was concerned about the time lag in having sporting events accepted into the Olympic Programme. He urged the ICC members to act now so as to be in a good position for 1992. The timing was crucial because the International Olympic Committee would announce the country to host the 1992 Olympic Games on the 17th October 1987, and ICC was considering approaching the organising committee concerned as soon as possible after the announcement, to discuss both demonstration events and full medal events. The International Olympic Committee had urged ICC to only operate through the IOC, but this could slow progress. There were two directions identified as possible ways forward for ICC to have full events included in the Olympic Games. One was to work with the international sports federations to have particular events proposed by them for inclusion as part of their Olympic Programme. This process had a lead-in time of four years. The other tack was to get the IOC to accept that the International Coordinating Committee was actually an international federation itself, and as such was entitled to propose a programme for inclusion in the Olympic Games. Lindström knew that the IOC President thought that the international sports federations were not 'ready yet' for this input.

Now that ICC represented six disability sports organisations it was with greater confidence that Hans Lindström proposed the second route to the ICC representatives in Gothenburg. He made it clear that he felt it was most important to seek full medal status events, what he called 'real events for disabled sports', rather than just demonstration events. Lindström felt that for this it was worth sacrificing the use of the term 'Olympic' in the quadrennial games for athletes with a disability. There was not full agreement; John Grant felt unable to go along wholeheartedly without being able to consult his International Stoke Mandeville Games Federation members, even if his personal opinion was aligned with Lindström's proposal. Guillermo Cabezas felt that without the support of the international federations, the sports events for people with disabilities would not be accepted within the Olympic Programme, so they must be contacted first. The debate went forward to agreement that Hans Lindström would prepare a letter for Samaranch, to announce that the International Coordinating Committee wished to be considered an international sports federation. In effect this was a reaffirmation of the purpose of ICC, although tactically it was thought to be the most effective way of moving towards the inclusion in the Olympic Programme of events for athletes with a disability. Lindström described his sense that Samaranch, for no clear reason, seemed to be a strong supporter of the sports movement for persons with a disability. There was the prospect of innovation that by the end of his presidency Samaranch might wish to be seen as the one who had opened up the world of sports to individuals with disabilities. In Lindström's opinion this inclination might give their interest group an advantage over 'others knocking on the door'. For now, the ICC need not declare more than its claim to identity as an international sports federation.

The International Coordinating Committee had to face requests for help from all quarters. Nadas Pal, President of the Sports Committee of the Association of the Hungarian Disabled wrote to Marjolijn Hillegers to describe the problems his association was having because the Ministry could pay only for membership of one international organisation – at present it was ISOD. As a result the Hungarian athletes with a disability were not given access to competitions under the auspices of CP-ISRA and ISMGF. The sensible plea was aimed at the International Coordinating Committee unifying its member organisations to ease the financial burden on national associations suffering real financial difficulties. This had certainly been done with regard to membership fees of umbrella organisations such as the International Council of Sport Science and Physical Education, with temporarily reduced membership fees for developing countries and others with overt problems with resources.

The First World Games for Disabled Youth had taken place in Nottingham, UK, in September 1986, the beginning of a great festive celebration of sporting promise and high-level competition. The timing of this event had been moved to allow for the emergency relocation of the Illinois Games to Stoke Mandeville. There had been generous sponsorship from the National Westminster Bank, and the British Sports Association for the Disabled directed the event. Arrangements for competitors and officials were thoroughly planned, and 'it was stated more than once that the provision at the Polytechnic was equivalent to the best that had been provided for International and World competition'. The World Games was established around the idea of providing high level concentrated coaching for young sportspersons with disabilities, preceding the competition, which then ran for the last few days. The future of the Youth Games needed to be secured. To this end the Technical Committee of ICC recommended that the Youth Committee set up to help with these Games should be disbanded and that a sub-group of the Technical Committee should be established to formalise the place of the World Youth Games in the umbrella of ICC. The 2nd Youth Games were to take place in Miami, USA in 1989, and the next in St Etienne, France in 1990.

The Sixth Clause

As had been agreed at an earlier ICC meeting, Hans Lindström wrote to President Samaranch in September 1986, signifying that the International Coordinating Committee had fully digested the Olympic Charter. Indicating that the letter was also being circulated to all international sports federations, Lindström had constructed an argument aimed at ICC applying for recognition as an international sports federation in its own right. Doing so, Lindström cited Rule 43 and Rule 44 of the Olympic Charter. The argument was that ICC, as an international federation, could be considered to be representing sport for persons with a disability as a whole. This was supported by the fact that some disciplines within ICC's competitions had no international federation of their own – goalball was given as an example. 'Further, it cannot within a reasonably near future be expected that other international federations (IFs) than ICC will be able to handle the more specific requirements for sports for people with disabilities, like the definitions of minimum handicaps and other medical and functional classification matters.' Other specific requirements for facilities and sports equipment could not be expected of international federations; close cooperation would be needed, but 'ICC's role as an IF for sports disabled is obvious'.

Lindström pushed further the importance of including events for people with disabilities in this same letter to Samaranch, quoting the United Nations Declaration on the Rights of Disabled Persons (no. 3447, December 1975). He stressed that the title 'Olympics for the Disabled' had been used for the quadrennial Games although the word 'Olympics' had become a concept in its own right, 'although solely connected to the IOC and its policy'. Lindström argued that the United Nations declaration states: 'Disabled persons, whatever their origin, nature and seriousness of their handicaps and disabilities, have the same fundamental rights as their fellow citizens of the same age, which implies first and foremost to enjoy a decent life, as normal and full as possible'. The line of argument Lindström employed was one of equality of access:

The 'fellow citizens' of the same age who have no functional limitations because of disability enjoy the right to become elite athletes within the conception 'Olympic Athletes', and this right should consequently also belong to disabled athletes. Just as the physical quality of muscle mass on the form of bodyweight is the basis for admitting Olympic events in power sports, so can the physical quality of functional events for disabled.

Expressing the opinion of numerous participants and organisers in disability sports, as well as representatives of international organisations within ICC, Lindström articulated the point that many 'value the word "Olympic" even higher than support from and affiliation to the IOC'. For this reason in particular it is essential that participants and organisers can see 'that disabled athletes are given space in the official Olympic Programme in a few events'. This highly compelling analysis was followed by a straightforward application for recognition of ICC as the international federation for sports for persons with a disability, but also applications for specific sporting events to be included in the XVI Olympic Winter Games in 1992 and the Games of the XXV Olympiad in the summer of 1992. Lindström was moving towards full medal status events rather than demonstration events for athletes with disability.

Administrative Overload, 1986

Arie Klapwijk and Joan Scruton met representatives from Rehabilitation International (RI) in Papendal on 13th September 1986 to discuss future areas of cooperation between RI and the International Coordinating Committee. Originally, Respo '86 was to have been organised by Rehabilitation International in the Spring of 1986, but financial limitations meant that it asked ICC to take it over, and the Bureau picked up the traces. Arie Klapwijk was determined to focus on three themes: recreational sports; the severely disabled; and developing countries. The vehicles for involvement were through medical symposia, sports technical workshops and presentations on organisational structures. In each category there were distinctions between contributions from developed and developing countries, giving the particular slant that affected the lives of those individuals living and working in very different environments. Some 212 participants attended, representing 43 countries (over 35% from developing countries). Financial support was found for some participants to attend who could not otherwise have afforded the travel costs. Publicity was strong and public awareness was heightened by the media coverage. A direct impact on funding that arose from the seminar was the interest of the European Economic Community (EEC), whose representative helped secure EEC financial participation in the International Fund Sport Disabled. The recommendations of the organising committee following the conclusion of Respo '86 were far-reaching. It called for: the International Coordinating Committee to take responsibility for organising Respo as a week long conference every four years (between the Olympic years); encouragement of the training of teachers in physical education to have expertise in provision for pupils with functional limitation; encouragement of the ICC to be involved in the development of new sports and games for those with disabilities, with ICC as a coordinator of initiatives; and support for production of wheelchairs and other accessories in developing countries as well as establishing an International Wheelchair Exchange Fund. Finally, the committee recommended pooling of research information so that 'cross-cultural' research could be set up and that work should be towards 'the creation of an Interdisciplinary Science of Sport for the Disabled'.

Administration of the International Coordinating Committee was becoming more taxing, and the Bureau came under fire as the volume of regular duties began to prevent effective operation of the office. Joan Scruton explained to the Administrative Sub-Committee at the end of November 1986 that she was worried about the coordination of preparatory work for the 1988 Paralympics; she proposed that a special sub-committee was essential to be able to keep everything flowing well. Sensitivities had been raised because Hans Lindström had implied criticism of the Bureau's efficiency in a letter. He was adamant that the criticism had not been directed towards the abilities of the Bureau staff but towards the systems of operation within the whole organisation, and also the shared duties that they had: towards ICC and IFSD (Lindström 1986). Marjolijn Hillegers, understandably protective, expressed her frustration that Board Members might feel 'matters are beyond their control' not because of the Administration, but 'because of the political situation, in which few decisions are taken'. But Jens Bromann expressed his concern more strongly: that 'in the name of democracy ICC paralyses itself'. In his assessment, there was a preoccupation with excessive consultation: 'everybody wants to be an expert on all levels, which is of course not possible'. It was time to assess the working structure of ICC, but for now the immediacy of providing support for the Paralympic Games organisation must take precedence.

. . . And Then There Were Six, January 1987

When Jens Bromann welcomed the delegates of the International Coordinating Committee to his hometown of Copenhagen, it was to an evening meeting on 30th January 1987, marking the eleventh time the Committee had gathered. This meeting saw the largest assembly of its kind, representing six international organisations for athletes with a disability: IBSA, CISS, CP-ISRA, INAS-FMH, ISMGF and ISOD. After a lengthy slog tidying the minutes of the Gothenberg meeting, the delegates set up their work for the following day and adjourned at 10.00 pm. The following morning Korea was a focal point. There was justifiable concern that effective systems must be in place for scrutinising the progress of arrangements for the 1988 Paralympics, and there was agreement that a committee should be made up of four members of the Technical Sub-Committee, two members of the Administrative Sub-Committee and one member of the Medical Sub-Committee – this group was to be called the Paralympic Sub-Committee. This smaller, discreet band would have the flexibility to travel to Korea, communicate efficiently, and keep up a steady overview of the approaching Games.

The working group that had been preparing the second workshop for developing countries reported on the arrangements for its event in Malaysia. Project 001, as it was labelled, had already proved to be one of the most worthy initiatives of the International Coordinating Committee. The first workshop, in Algeria, had taken place between 19th and 30th April 1986. The fundamental coordination was between ICC and the Algerian Federation of Sport for the Disabled (Fédération Algérienne des Sports pour Handicapés et Inadaptés). The Algerian Ministry of Youth and Sport was helpful, and vital financial support came from the United Nations Centre for Social Development and Humanitarian Affairs in Vienna. Participants from 14 countries in the region attended the first workshop, with observers from another four. A training manual was produced following the workshop, translated into five languages. This was to prove an asset to participants and trainers returning to their home countries. Media attention was significant, and awareness of the sports movement for athletes with a disability was heightened measurably. A by-product of the Algerian workshop was a momentum to form a provisional coordinating committee for sports activities for persons with a disability in the African region.

As had been the situation in Algeria, the Malaysian Government had agreed to finance the board and lodging of participants in the second workshop. The principal contact in Malaysia was Daoud Amin, the IBSA Member. John Grant asked what had happened to the idea he had put forward of holding a workshop in Kenya. He explained that he had taken trouble to visit Kenya and make good contact with people and organisations who indicated that they were willing to support such a venture. He had even met with the President of Kenya, who was receptive and who indicated that there was a possibility of financial support. The group tasked to work on Project 001 explained that it had seemed appropriate when concluding the Algerian workshop for the Asian region to be the locus for the next event, rather than holding another workshop relatively close to the first one. John Grant was reassured that his extensive effort would be acted upon. With further discussion of the Malaysian workshop, representatives of INAS-FMH requested involvement for their members in the programme of events. Marjolijn Hillegers explained that the timescale for the project was well advanced and that the sports programme had been fixed already, and that financial and logistical arrangements would rule out modifications at this point. Although it was regrettable that INAS-FMH could not be accommodated within the programme this time, the principle was accepted that future workshops would have to take into account that there were six international organisations represented within the International Coordinating Committee.

With a generous, but rushed lunch the meeting reformed to welcome four delegates from Korea. Koh Kwi Nam, President of the Seoul Paralympic Organising Committee, described his pleasure at the receipt of preliminary entry forms from 49 countries. He also explained that the Korean Government had asked the number of participants to be reduced from 4000 to 3000 due to problems in finding suitable lodgings. When pressed further he was asked to honour the signed agreement that Seoul would accept 3000 competitors and 1000 escorts. Koh asked for the understanding of the assembled representatives for the problems being faced in Korea: pressure had been brought to bear on the Paralympic Organising Committee from the Government – caused both by financial and facility limitations. The ICC members expressed their considerable disquiet at this unexpected turn. John Grant proposed that the representatives of the Seoul Paralympic Organising Committee should discuss the matter with the Government on their return to Korea, asking them again to respect their signed agreement with the International Coordinating Committee.

With the ICC representation now extended to six organisations, it is interesting to observe the response to the application for membership by Special Olympics Inc. It had asked to be allowed to attend the meeting in Copenhagen, and was seeking full membership of ICC. Owing to the existing admission to membership of INAS-FMH, it was considered appropriate that Special Olympics should be refused membership in its own right, and that it should be pointed towards an arrangement for INAS-FMH to represent it. Although there was logic in this decision, it was also not difficult to understand that Special Olympics might see this as a significant insult to its much more mature and securely established organisation. Robert Montague wrote to Marjolijn Hillegers on 21st November 1986 to complain that ICC had accepted INAS-FMH 'while apparently not acting on the application for membership by Special Olympics'. Special Olympics considered that its application, acknowledged by Arie Klapwijk on 26th February 1986, was still pending when the ICC accepted INAS-FMH. Therefore the acceptance of INAS-FMH was offensive to Special Olympics. As Montague put it: 'Special Olympics International is the world's largest program of sports training and athletic competition for individuals with disabilities. We are larger, better and more financially secure than any of the sports for the disabled organisations that are ICC members'. Montague was Chairman of the United States Olympic Committee section on Sports for the Disabled, and had only learnt of the acceptance of INAS-FMH into ICC from another of the representatives at one of the USOC meetings in the United States. Again the International Coordinating Committee had proceeded with less tact than should have been employed. The bumpy ride was set to continue.

Rift Develops with the International Fund

A fairly prickly problem for the January 1987 meeting in Copenhagen was the request for observer status from the International Fund Sport Disabled. This was not really welcomed by the delegates, but a pragmatic approach was essential. The Chairman of the International Fund Sport Disabled had warned that the Board might 'have to reconsider future financial assistance'. The Fund provided the lifeblood for ICC and any damage to relations would endanger the future of ICC's functioning – the Bureau was completely financed by IFSD, which also provided significant financial support for many ICC sanctioned events and initiatives. There had been unfortunate accusations about the wielding of power through the International Fund. John Grant expressed his horror on behalf of ISMGF at the idea of such accusations, but André van Emden had stuck by his allegation: he claimed that the IFSD had been referred to as the 'Dutch Mafia' by some people present at ICC meetings. Hans Lindström was careful to point out that his own comments had been misconstrued – he had said 'the money had power, not the Board members; and that power was the basis for the political background of the work for the disabled'.

The Chairman of the International Fund had proposed that he should himself become one of the Vice Presidents of ICC, and that the President pro tem of ICC should be acting Vice Chairman of IFSD. He had arrived at this proposal after first considering that there should be an exchange of observers. It was certainly time for the IFSD to formalise its relationship and its status with ICC. Jens Bromann suggested that the ICC try to find an indirect way of responding to the question, rather than just refusing. Guillermo Cabezas put forward the idea that the President pro tem may invite an observer from IFSD when discussing matters of finance pertinent to IFSD. He also suggested that a positive move would be to encourage the ratified minutes of ICC meetings to be sent to IFSD. This compromise was accepted, although without full approval from INAS-FMH and CP-ISRA. The issue was not to be brought to a head, as there was already considerable groundswell for major changes within ICC that would lead to the eventual emergence of the International Paralympic Committee. The next ICC Seminar effectively set this in train. These proposals were bound not to match the ambitions of IFSD, and understandably so.

Bids from Barcelona and Albertville

Demonstration events for the Calgary Winter Olympics in 1988 were accepted, along with agreement over arrangements for ICC sanction of the World Games in Assen in 1990 – Hans Lindström described this bid as 'rather fantastic'. Of great significance was the acceptance of the official bid from Barcelona for the Paralympic Summer Games in 1992, and the notice that an official bid had also been received from Albertville, France, for the Paralympic Winter Games. This was most important because it represented the first time that the Winter Paralympics would take place in the same venue as the Winter Olympic Games. The French authorities had indicated that they would offer free accommodation for the athletes, and that no entry fees would be raised. Barcelona had indicated that its bid was dependent upon its success in gaining the acceptance of the IOC for its bid for the Summer Olympic Games. All the countries bidding for the Olympic Games also provided bids for the Paralympic Games this time.

The Technical Sub-Committee presented a four-year schedule of international events that would form a regular cycle of sport for athletes with a disability:

Year 1:   International and Invitational Games
Year 2:   Winter Paralympics
          Regional Championships, for example, FESPIC
          Pan American, African, European
Year 3:   World Championships
          International and Invitational Winter Games
Year 4:   Paralympic Summer Games
          Winter Regional Championships

Doping control at international events required immediate attention; the officials at the ICC-sanctioned World Games in Gothenberg had dealt with athletes failing tests. Sixty-five athletes had been tested, with three positive tests made; two under the auspices of ISOD and one under ISMGF. The substances found in the tests were varied (amphetamine, phenylpropanolamine and dextropropoxyphene), as were the countries (Israel, Canada and the Federal Republic of Germany). The medals were to be withdrawn from those athletes, while the Medical Sub-Committee was tasked with the establishment of an official ICC anti-doping policy for sanctioned events. However, protests were later upheld on procedural grounds and sanctions had to be withdrawn. There was urgency for secure doping procedures that could be replicated with the utmost integrity in any environment, just as had been established for sport for those without disabilities. In fact Harald Natvig had received a communication from Prince Alexandre de Mérode, Chairman of the IOC Medical Commission on 28th April 1987 proposing that there should be a universal approach to doping control throughout the sporting world – a much more straightforward approach for everyone, but not easy to achieve.

An Illusion of Unity

The imminent shift of presidency of ICC was discussed. As the coming year was the Paralympic year, it was proposed that the cycle should be interrupted to ensure that the President and Vice President were representatives of international organisations that were participating in the Paralympic Games. This was an important consideration due to the visibility offered to ICC on these occasions. John Grant was duly acknowledged as President pro tem, but Guillermo Cabezas was to take the position of Vice President instead of Jerald Jordan of CISS. As Jordan was not present in Copenhagen, Jens Bromann was to write to him to explain this decision. Under the delicate circumstances of relations with CISS, this was always going to be a difficult moment. The depth of disquiet that was simmering was quite clear in the reply Jerald Jordan sent to Jens Bromann in February 1987. In it Jordan conceded the reasoning behind the decision about the rotation of the Presidency of ICC. He had no intention of accepting the position in any case 'while the present issues remain unresolved'. There was no indication to Jordan among the preliminary documents circulated for the March Seminar of ICC that the 'issues' were to be tackled, so he stated that he believed that CISS might never take the chair of ICC while there was no change to this 'parochial aspect of ICC'. Jordan, in his usual clear and unreserved manner, expressed his sadness that CISS could be thought of as a threat to the success of ICC. The four founding member organisations had their common interests served, but Jordan could not 'understand resistance to change now that change has been thrust upon us'. Magnanimously, the President of CISS assured Bromann that he would keep working towards a satisfactory change in ICC, but he was losing hope.

CISS was watching closely to see in which direction ICC would move, whether to continue in its present representation or to turn towards national representation. The coming ICC Seminar was to shift the direction altogether. When Jerald Jordan wrote to John Grant on 21st April, it was to indicate that he felt CISS should withdraw from membership of ICC. Jordan had looked over the report of the seminar, but could see no future in the relationship between CISS and ICC. In fact the seminar emphasised in Jordan's mind that 'there is no place in the ICC for non-Paralympics participants'. His letter, copied to Lindström, Lovett and Sondergaard, delineated the problems encountered by individual members of CISS who had been forced into undermined positions with loss of financial support for events and weakened autonomy, reportedly due to CISS's membership of ICC. Jordan identified a two-tiered ICC membership: those 'in' and those 'out'. CISS, by virtue of being one of the two 'out' member organisations, had spent thousands of dollars on travel and interpreters for very little tangible benefit. IOC funding to ICC could only be expended on Paralympics – in which CISS did not participate. As Jordan plainly put it: 'Consequently, what can we contribute to ICC other than our name and an illusion of unity? What benefits do we incur from such a use of our name? On the other hand it appears to be causing problems that affect our members in various countries.' It was not possible for CISS to see past the Paralympics issue when it had no intention of giving up its own antecedent Games: 'the mouths kept saying "ICC" and the words kept meaning "Paralympics"'. As the Seminar was steering ICC towards one 'supreme body composed of national members, possibly organised along sports lines', Jordan considered that it would mark the 'end of autonomy' – he was emphatic that CISS would not accept that the new body could possibly offer enough to make it worth giving up its autonomy. In conclusion he felt it was best that they should go their separate ways, 'respecting each other's different needs'.

ARNHEM SEMINAR SHAPES THE FUTURE, MARCH 1987

Although the position of CISS was crystallised by what passed at the ICC Seminar, the meetings were also crucial to the future direction of the International Coordinating Committee, and ultimately to the International Paralympic Committee. The meetings between 12th and 15th March 1987 awakened a renewed vigour in the delegates working towards an effective unity for sports for persons with a disability. The gathering was entitled 'International Seminar on the Structure and Future of Sports for the Disabled'. Bids had been received from Australia and Canada, but it was considered prudent to make use of the administrative convenience of the ICC Bureau by accepting the bid to hold the Seminar at Arnhem. The topics identified for discussion at the Barcelona meeting of ICC a year earlier were: sports programmes for the future; combined classification; relations to 'sports able' bodies; and the structure of the ICC. When the papers were circulated on Christmas Eve 1986, the aim of the Seminar was described as: 'to discuss the future of the Paralympics'. By the time the Seminar took place the emphasis had shifted to place greater importance on the reorganisation of the structure of a world body. Many groups and organisations were represented; 210 people from 52 countries were in attendance. John Grant opened the meetings at the Hotel Haarhuis with the suggestion that an Ad Hoc Committee should be formed to take forward the recommendations of the Seminar. As the meetings got underway the enthusiasm and vitality of the gathered delegates made it clear that there would be no holding back of views – keeping discussion focused and to time was to prove difficult for those tasked with coordinating the events. There were brief position statements that provided plenty of thought-provoking perspectives on the past, present and future. Key discussion papers proposing specific solutions were presented by national bodies: the Swedish Sports Organisation for the Disabled (SHIF), the Spanish Federation of Sport for the Disabled, the Canadian Federation of Sport Organisations for the Disabled (CFSOD), the Australian Confederation of Sports for the Disabled, the Dutch Sports Association for the Disabled (Netherlandse Invaliden Sportbond), the French Federation of Disabled Sport (Federation Française Handisport), the Austrian Federation of Disabled Sport, the Norwegian Stoke Mandeville Games Committee, the Danish Sports Organisation for the Disabled (Dansk Handicap Idraets-Forbund), and the Norwegian Sports Organisation for the Disabled (Norges Handicapidrettsforbund).

Some delegates expected an emphatic support for a world organisation that would serve elite competitive sport, but the seminar voted 25 for and 81 against a motion that the future structure should only deal with Paralympics and elite sport. The assembly categorically wished to promote the establishment of a unified single body to lead sport for persons with a disability. Another strongly felt view was in favour of a formally regularised programme of events in a cyclical calendar as was being developed through ICC. Although not universally endorsed, they wished to explore the subject of integrated sport for athletes with a disability to compete alongside athletes without disability.

The ICC Seminar voted unanimously for an Ad Hoc Working Group to be established. Their agreed mandate (accepted 99 votes to 1) was 'to formulate a constitution of the new organisation that will replace ICC'. Once the process of investigation and consultation had taken place, a 'Constitutional Assembly' would be called to ratify the new Constitution. There was widespread support for proposals to reduce the number of classes in competitions; international organisations were asked to investigate their own pertinent contributions to this development. Integrated classifications were only to be acceptable after rigorous research and communication. The ICC was given the authorisation to continue under its present mandate until the new organisation had been formed. Representatives on the Ad Hoc Working Group came under three categories: continental representatives athletes' representatives, and representatives appointed by the international federations. At Arnhem the following individuals were put in office:

Regional representatives:
Africa: N. Salem (Egypt)
Asia: Y. Chow (Hong Kong)
Europe: C. Wang (Norway)
Middle East: A. Masarweh (Jordan)
North and South America: H. Glynn (Canada)
Oceania: K. Cosgrove (Australia)

Athletes' representatives:
A. Trotman (UK)
D. Bryant (USA)
M. De Meyer (Belgium)

Representatives of international federations:
CP-ISRA: J. Weinstein
ISOD: G. Cabezas
INAS-FMH: J Kieboom
IBSA: J. Bromann

CISS and ISMGF did not identify their representatives immediately. The athletes' representatives were nominated from among those athletes in attendance at the Seminar.

Developing Countries

As new initiatives matured into established 'trademark' projects for ICC, there was still a need to retain a critical analysis of effectiveness in order to remain sharp and worthy of the high regard that was accorded them. As the Working Group for Developing Countries was discussing the results from the highly successful workshop in Malaysia, there were strong words of criticism and advice for the future from Marjolijn Hillegers. Acknowledging the successes and the clear benefits to the participants of these workshops, there had obviously been some difficulties in the outlook of the instructors. Hillegers advised the Working Group to look more closely for particular characteristics when recommending suitable instructors for future workshops – not just technical ability in a particular sporting area. There was an obvious need for an understanding that they were preparing to offer their skills within a developing country – by definition there would be discomforts, and expectations had to be adjusted. It was essential that appropriate attention be paid to local customs and sensitivities. Her list of required personal attributes for the instructors might, however, test candidates for sainthood: 'It needs talent of improvising, mental and physical strength, denial of individualism, and acceptance that the input of every member is different but nevertheless valuable in its own right. Further, it needs sensibility, a sense of humour, flexibility, confidence in [one's] own capacities, and a sense of responsibility for the total happening.'

The Revolution Has Come at Last

Carl Wang, Chairman of the Ad Hoc Committee, reported to the ICC meeting in Aylesbury on 2nd and 3rd August 1987 that two rather poorly attended meetings of his group had taken place. They had an immediate objective of preparing a constitution for 1989, based on a draft that was to be produced for discussion in Seoul during the 1988 Paralympic Games.

Marjolijn Hillegers reported that she disagreed with those who declared that 'the revolution has come at last'. She was also disappointed with the late withdrawals from the Seminar, costing the organisers dearly. Hillegers praised the organisers of the Malaysian workshop for developing countries – Project 001 – which had 90 participants from 18 countries. Unfortunately, despite John Grant's enormous efforts, it looked as though plans for a workshop in Kenya were unlikely to be feasible due to a lack of official recognition from the Government.

In her position as Executive Director of the ICC Bureau, Marjolijn Hillegers was very aware of the delicate balance of ICC with the International Fund Sport Disabled – her own office was fully provided at the pleasure of the Fund. She reported in July 1987 that the Fund 'does not wish to dominate the ICC, nor does it wish to take the role of a Mafia Godfather'. There had been an appraisal of the current state of sport for the disabled and the Fund had concluded that this was a pause for thought. It would harbour its resources, and 'until the world movement has decided on which way to go, it will concentrate on fundraising'. The International Fund Sport Disabled decided that it would take a specific position: to give financial and administrative support to the Ad Hoc Committee but not to fund ICC meetings; and to allow the Bureau to continue to act as a coordinating centre for dissemination of information. In practice this secured the funding of the developing countries workshops, the research project earmarked for Seoul, the preparatory work for the Innsbrück and Seoul Paralympics of 1988, and some finance for demonstration events at the World Athletics Championships in Rome in September 1987. The IFSD agreed that the ICC newsletter should continue to receive its support. Other specific requests for support to IFSD would be considered on the same basis as for other organisations. It was clear that the International Fund was now detached from ICC – no more financial cover of travel and subsistence for ICC delegates to meetings, and no further secretarial provision at meetings. Marjolijn Hillegers concluded her report by suggesting that change did not equal revolution, and that sport for people with disabilities was still in its youth: 'Maturity is the ability to see and understand the other point of view, the ability to accept change, and the ability to realise that one's own view, no matter how important one thinks it is, is not necessarily the only view on any subject'.

The position taken by IFSD was certainly a blow to the International Coordinating Committee, but it was also likely to have been a considered reaction to the proposals made at the ICC Seminar, in which real action was going to be taken to establish a single world body that would eventually become the International Paralympic Committee. Jens Bromann and Björn Eklund of IBSA wrote to Joan Scruton following the ICC meeting to stress that the International Fund Sport Disabled had no right to go on with fundraising in the name (and using the actual names) of the international organisations of sports for athletes with a disability, without the organisations having a direct involvement in the allocation of those funds. They suggested that any new world body should have its own fundraising wing built into its structure. For the time being IFSD should cease its activities until a constitution had been agreed for the new organisation.

In view of the instability of the relationship between the International Coordinating Committee and the International Fund Sport Disabled, it was proposed that the Bureau of ICC should be moved immediately to Aylesbury. As also appeared quite natural, Joan Scruton was proposed as Secretary General. Marjolijn Hillegers was to be asked to resign as Executive Director following the meeting. John Grant, as President pro tem of ICC, wrote to van Emden, Chairman of IFSD, to explain the move of the Secretariat, and to ask for a meeting at his earliest convenience.

The place of demonstration events had vexed people for some time. There was a school of thought in favour of the prominent display of elite sport for athletes with disability in an arena shared with other world-class sportspersons, but there was also a view that demonstration events were demeaning and provided a curiosity value rather than empowering those people with disabilities striving for excellence in sport. At the Aylesbury meeting, explanation was needed of the process by which the events in Rome came to be reduced. Jens Bromann expressed the anger felt by members of IBSA because the 400 m track race for blind athletes had been scratched. Colin Rains described the sequence of events: the International Amateur Athletics Federation informed him on 10th June that the 1500 m wheelchair race for men, 800 m wheelchair race for women and 400 m race for blind runners had been accepted. However, a telex arrived on 6th July to say that only the two wheelchair events had been accepted. The disappointment of IBSA representatives was clear from the motion proposed that ICC would withdraw all demonstration events from the 4th World Athletics Championships. No one seconded the motion and it failed to proceed. There would be demonstrations of two wheelchair events.

John Grant took the gathered delegates through the meeting that he, Guillermo Cabezas and Hans Lindström had attended with Juan Antonio Samaranch and Walther Tröger on 2nd June 1987. The ICC was due to have been represented by Jerald Jordan, but he could not attend due to illness and so Grant had invited Guillermo Cabezas to step in instead. In view of the communication between Jordan and Grant in April it seems strange that Jordan had been expecting to join ICC representatives at all in this visit. The IOC President wanted clarification of the current status of ICC, and was given assurances that the existing structure would obtain throughout any transitionary phase, and until a constitution had been formalised by those developing a single body to represent international sport for athletes with a disability. There was discussion about the challenges ahead, particularly with regard to financial pressures during the next stage of development. With the absence of Jerald Jordan, John Grant felt obliged to express some of the concerns held by the CISS and its members. It is not clear whether Grant told Samaranch about the proposed withdrawal of CISS from ICC, or whether Jordan had already communicated this to Samaranch himself. Overall progress in the meeting was very positive, and with the help of Walther Tröger, there were agreements on demonstration events for Seoul and Calgary, as well as discussion of participation in the opening and closing ceremonies. Samaranch expressed his hope that IOC would be able to assist in the funding of athletes and escorts for demonstration events. The Paralympic Games were discussed in detail and, although Samaranch appeared anxious about the numbers of participants and the financial burdens, he was very positive about the progress the IOC and the ICC had made together.

Calgary is Off, Innsbrück Hosts the 4th World Winter Games for the Disabled

Calgary, successful in its bid to host the Winter Olympic Games of 1988 and the 4th World Winter Games for the Disabled, had 'unexpectedly cancelled' its hospitality to the disabled sports fraternity, citing a lack of officials as the reason. Following complex and extended discussions, the organisers of the 1984 World Winter Games for the Disabled in Innsbrück persuaded the Austrian authorities to host the Games for a second time. Austrian state institutions subsidised the budget to the tune of 15 million Austrian Schillings, added to generous sponsorship from within the country as well. Once this had been settled, the International Coordinating Committee requested that the 4th World Winter Games

Organising Committee alter the name of the event to the 'Winter Paralympics 1988'. This was not a popular move, as the Austrian organisers felt they should be able to retain symmetry with their previous success in 1984. Bertl Neumann wrote to the ICC to say that they wished to keep the emblem, the title and the people involved in running the event exactly the same as for the 3rd World Winter Games for the Disabled. Reflecting on the way that these Games had proceeded, André Raes considered that the organisers of the Innsbrück Games did not pay him and Horst Kosel, as nominated Technical Delegates of ICC, due respect. They were not invited to the Opening or Closing Ceremonies, nor were they able to become involved with the actual operation of the Games as jury members without resorting to their own energies. Owing to bad weather and poor snow conditions, the Nordic events had to be relocated to Seefeld from Natters, meaning that they were held some 32 kilometres from Innsbrück. Alpine events were held in Mutters, but had to be taken above the 1500 metre level in order to find better conditions.

Harald Natvig, as the Chairman of the ICC Medical Sub-Committee, wrote to Bertl Neumann to express his concern at the news of the organisers' reluctance to have 'foreign doctors' involved with classification at the Paralympic Winter Games. He pointed out the clear instruction in the ICC Handbook that medical support and the Organising Committee should provide suitable facilities for physiotherapy, but that classification would be under the auspices of the Medical Committees of the international organisations themselves. Natvig went on to identify himself as the appointed ISOD/ICC doctor in charge of classification at Innsbrück, together with Dr Jonas from the Organising Committee. Dr Duane Messner (USA) was to be responsible for classification of athletes with locomotor disabilities competing in Alpine skiing, while Dr Bjørn Hedman (Sweden) would look after classification in Nordic skiing. Natvig and Cairbre McCann (USA) were to have responsibility for sledge sports, with Dr Luigi di Salva and/or Dr Asbjørn Tønjum classifying athletes with visual impairment.

The blind skater Åke Pettersson had composed a fanfare and offered it for use by ICC. The members were very pleased with the music but felt that it might be necessary for it to be rather longer in order to suit their purposes. Pettersson would be asked to see if he could lengthen his fanfare.

The newest members of ICC, CISS and INAS-FMH, were again to be dealt an unwelcome affront at the Innsbrück meeting. When discussing the representation of ISOD at the Seoul Paralympics, a proposal was made to reduce the places available for official representatives from INAS-FMH and CISS to one each, while the other four organisations were to retain two places each, with one place left to the discretion of the ICC for allocation. Of course, in the ballot for this matter the two affected groups were the only ones to vote against. Less contentious was the decision that ICC should be represented at the Olympic Games by those organisations whose athletes were involved in the demonstration events. However, when planning for the next meeting with representatives of the International Olympic Committee, the delegates agreed that they should seek invitations from the IOC for all six presidents of the member organisations of ICC to attend the Olympic Games, and World Championships. This would remove the problem of ICC prioritising funding, as the IOC should pay the expenses of those they would invite.

Colin Rains, on behalf of the Technical Committee, in the presence of the Seoul Paralympic Organising Committee representatives, reported on the preparations for the Seoul Paralympic Games to the ICC. Entry forms had been received from 53 countries, although there was a complication, with nine countries still having indicated their intention to compete but not yet having submitted entries. As this was the first opportunity for athletes with intellectual disabilities to be involved in the Paralympics, it was decided that the wheelchair demonstration event proposed should have another event added to it. In comparison to the complicated and detailed debate within the International Olympic Committee about protocol and flag ceremonies, the International Coordinating Committee acknowledged that it had been given permission to use the Olympic flag and hymn. SPOC thought that the Olympic flag should be used but with the Paralympic anthem. Other possibilities were that the Seoul fanfare should accompany the approach of athletes to the presentation of medals, and the national anthem of the winning country would be played at the raising of the national flags. Discussion at the meeting of the

ICC Technical Committee, on Monday 20th June 1988, expressed concern for the number of 'victory ceremonies' involved in swimming and athletics, where there might be as many as 40 each day. This was going to hold up proceedings considerably. Some modifications would be necessary to the fanfare and time taken in procedures in order to help expedite matters effectively for both competitors and spectators. The Closing Ceremony should see the raising of the national flag of the country next to host the Games – in this case Spain, with Barcelona due to host the 1992 Paralympic Games.

Looking to the next Paralympic Winter Games, in 1992 in Albertville, the ICC meeting was able to welcome representatives of the Fédération Française Handisport: André Auberger, Claude Sugny and François Terranova. They thanked ICC for the confidence shown in the French organisation by awarding the Games to them. Auberger stressed the importance of this event as the first time that the Winter Paralympics would take place in the same location as the Winter Olympics. Further presentations would be made at future meetings.

Carl Wang gave an update on the work done in the Ad Hoc Committee so far. He conveyed the worry that people seemed to be showing very little determination to pursue the mandate given in Arnhem, and Wang asked the international organisations involved with ICC to be vigorous in their energies. John Grant suggested that a possible reason for this cooling of enthusiasm was that the Seminar had effectively been the point of revolution; they had agreed that change would come, and the urgency was not there any longer. Grant later asked for these comments to be deleted from the record, and replaced with a statement indicating that he considered that ICC was functioning admirably and that they should submit a proposed constitution of their own in Seoul. He was also careful to emphasise that he didn't feel bitter about the revolutionary nature of the Arnhem proposals in any way. There was further discussion about the continued functioning of ICC, and encouragement for broad discussion in Seoul. The members who would not be represented in Seoul, CISS and INAS-FMH, asked that their views be taken into consideration at another time. One feature of the new organisation was likely to be representation on a national basis, and there was certain anxiety expressed at the ICC meeting that some members of the Ad Hoc Committee seemed to be in favour of the disappearance of the international federations presently constituting the International Coordinating Committee. One member recorded his views that the ICC was on shaky terrain: 'I cannot help but feel that there is little common ground amongst the committee at this time'.

The International Coordinating Committee had continued to make great progress through its workshops in developing countries. The Working Group 001 heard a summary of the successful Zimbabwe workshops when it met on 21st April 1988 in Abcoude, the Netherlands. The actual instruction and participation had gone very well, but the project suffered serious hindrance because the local administration was ineffectual. No national organisation had met its agreed financial commitment, and the Zimbabwean Government had not fulfilled its obligations either, so fundraising had to be carried out on the spot. In all 122 individuals participated in the workshops, representing 14 African countries. The next project was to carry out the planned workshops in Colombia in 1989.

Combined Bids for Olympic and Paralympic Games in Future, June 1988

The IOC President had met with delegates from the International Coordinating Committee on 14th June. Walther Tröger led the delegates through a wide-ranging agenda. The discussions were very positive and included the status of Special Olympics Inc. and the demonstration events at Calgary, along with those planned for Seoul. The International Olympic Committee had made an agreement with Special Olympics Inc., and ICC saw this as problematic because INAS-FMH was the international organisation with delegated responsibility within ICC for athletes with intellectual disability. As a result, this conflicted with the insistence that the IOC had repeated often to ICC: that disability sports organisations should speak with one voice, that of the International Coordinating Committee. Walther Tröger agreed to try to persuade Special Olympics Inc. to work in harmony with INAS-FMH, while asserting that ICC did not need recognition of the sort accorded to Special Olympics Inc., as 'the IOC regarded them as their sole counterpart'. As necessity was to demand, the lure of further financial support from IOC for the work of the ICC was to help keep the relationships between these groups as calm as possible. Samaranch had indicated that he would be reviewing the levels of fiscal support for ICC after the Seoul Games had finished.

Tröger expressed disappointment at the spectator numbers for the demonstration events in Calgary, with major attendance only at the giant slalom. The general view was that the Alpine events were not challenging enough to really show the capabilities of athletes with a disability. They were also held at a different venue from the able-bodied Alpine events. Jerry Johnstone was congratulated on his excellent preparation and attention to detail in organising the demonstration events in Calgary. In fact the delegates involved with the organisation of the events for athletes with a disability chose not to ask for a change of venue because they had watched the regular disruption at the Nakiska venue (some 80 km outside Calgary) due to strong winds. The giant slalom was won by Alexandre Spitz of the Federal Republic of Germany, with Greg Manino (USA) and Fritz Berger (Switzerland) taking silver and bronze respectively. Queen Silvia of Sweden presented these medals, with Juan Antonio Samaranch presenting the medals for the women's event. Athletes were well looked-after, housed together with all other athletes at the Southern Alberta Institute for Technology (SAIT).

The bidding process was reviewed in the light of the unwillingness of the Calgary Organising Committee to host the Paralympic Games – and Innsbrück having stepped into the breach. It was mooted that future bids should be inclusive of intention to host both Olympic Games and Paralympic Games, or that the two competitions should intentionally divorce from one another to aid clarity. When discussion moved on to the inclusion of athletes with disabilities in the Olympic Games, Tröger stated that the IOC was keen for demonstration events to continue as they stressed the inclusion of athletes with a disability as part of the Olympic family.

Relations with the International Fund Sport Disabled had remained in suspended animation; no response had been received from André van Emden to the letter from ICC of 14th May. However, a telex from van Emden was received during the ICC meeting, offering a meeting on 22nd July. This was immediately agreed to, and the delegates were to wait patiently for news of the growing distance between ICC and IFSD. With the severely limited resources now available to ICC, Juan Antonio Samaranch suggested that the International Coordinating Committee might benefit from a meeting with Birgitte Smith of the marketing company ISL. When this happened, the company was not hopeful of making progress in time for the Seoul Paralympics, but with more information about the ICC, the marketing company would work on a scheme and outline the possibilities at a future meeting.

When the Executive Committee of ICC met on 19th and 20th June 1988, once again in Aylesbury, Carl Wang told the gathered members that the draft constitution of the Ad Hoc Committee investigating a new world body had been sent out by the end of May to all the national organisations. The 'hearing' was to take place in Seoul on 23rd October. The paper had not been sent to the international federations, as it was believed that the members of the Ad Hoc Committee would make it available to their own federations, with it being in their interests to discuss it together. The plan was for an amended version of the constitution to be circulated early in 1989 for debate within the general assemblies of the various international federations. Bids would be invited for a country to host the first general assembly of the new organisation. The ICC delegates were planning to hold additional meetings during their stay in Seoul, to facilitate as many opportunities as possible for consideration of the future structure, and to consider the future of the International Coordinating Committee itself.

Zoubir Ketfi, an expert in international law recommended by the International Olympic Committee, joined the July 1987 Ad Hoc Committee meeting, so as to guide it towards an appropriate structure for the new organisation. His excellent presentation opened the eyes of those attending towards the juridical status of international organisations, emphasising that the choice of country in which the headquarters was located was a decisive factor. An 'Agreement of Headquarters' signed with the country would give the organisation the legal status of that country. If the choice of country was matched to the aims of the organisation, the climate could be very favourable for both autonomous operation and legal protection. Interestingly, Ketfi stressed that the International Olympic Committee was not a democratic organisation, but had a structure for absolute power: 'having no representation from the base, and therefore it would not be a good model for the new organisation'. He recommended that each country should create one national federation (Paralympic Committee) to have representation at a General Assembly (thus providing representation at the base level). International federations representing disability sports groups could have representation on the General Assembly as well. The General Assembly would elect an Executive Committee to have absolute authority to carry out its mandate. Affiliation and payment of fees would also be delicately organised: instead of each country paying fees to a number of international federations plus the new organisation, the fees could be paid by the national Paralympic Committee directly to the new body – to then be distributed to the international federations.

CONCLUSION

Just over ten years had passed with the International Coordinating Committee in the driving seat. Not everything had gone smoothly, and not all international federations were working together, but the urgent work of the early 1980s had been tackled bravely and firmly by the ICC – to a great extent it was successful in its role as an umbrella organisation. The meetings that were to take place in Düsseldorf in 1989 and beyond would see the creation of the International Paralympic Committee: the spirit of the future. The 'interim government' of the ICC was appropriate for its time and context. When the ICC began its work it was a time to move to a more global outlook, and for the organisations of sport for people with disabilities to really try to speak with one voice, even if the sounds were still discordant occasionally.

During this period, relations with the International Olympic Committee had improved, while there was concern not to surrender too many of the principles of the Paralympic Movement in an attempt to retain recognition by the IOC. Finances were tight: the International Fund Sport Disabled was holding on to see what would transpire in Düsseldorf, and the International Coordinating Committee had to rely on the International Olympic Committee.

By the end of the 1970s the call of the plentiful participants in the Paralympic Movement was for national participation in the government of their Movement, and for the sports themselves to have a clear representation in any international umbrella organisation. Although this would have been too radical for the late 1970s, it was fundamental to the continued progress of the Paralympic Movement by the beginning of the 1980s.

The Seoul Paralympics of 1988 would take the Paralympic Movement to new heights. As First President of the International Paralympic Committee, Bob Steadward, would comment:

> the 1988 Seoul Paralympics dramatically demonstrated the effects of proper organisation, and the shift from sport as rehabilitation, to sport as recreation, to elite sport . . . The winning athlete was the elite athlete, one at the peak of training and conditioning. Thus these Games are considered the first games of the modern Paralympic era.

CHAPTER 5

Building Bridges not Walls: 1988 to 1992

A hero is no braver than an ordinary man, but he is braver five minutes longer (Ralph Waldo Emerson, 1803–1882)

OVERVIEW

The Paralympic Games held in Seoul, South Korea, in 1988 were to be the turning point for the Paralympic Movement. As the first Games of the 'Modern Era' the Seoul Games took sport for people with disabilities into another dimension.

The work of the Ad Hoc Committee, appointed at the Arnhem Seminar of 14th March 1987, was coming to a close. The two years of extensive communication between national representatives, sport federations for athletes with a disability, athletes themselves, and the International Fund Sport Disabled, had brought everyone to a new departure: to establish a new world organisation. In coming to decisions about the structure proposed for the body it had been necessary for everyone to embrace compromise and to develop tolerance. The key difference in the proposed structure was the centrality of the nations rather than the pre-eminence of the international federations. Although the International Paralympic Committee must wait until after the Barcelona Paralympics before receiving the mantle from the International Coordinating Committee, there was much to do to get ready.

The next phase of growth for the Paralympic Movement would establish a clear parallel between the International Olympic Committee's work and that of the International Paralympic Committee in the bidding for and organisation of the Games. Joint administration by an organising committee that took on the management of both Olympic Games and Paralympic Games might lead to a seamless progression. As Juan Antonio Samaranch would later comment: 'I believe that the Paralympics should be almost like a continuation of the Olympic Games . . . this great celebration the Games represent is a joint celebration' (Samaranch 1994).

SEOUL 1988: THE FIRST PARALYMPIC GAMES OF THE MODERN ERA

The Seoul 1988 Paralympic Games saw a turning point in the meteoric development of elite sports for athletes with a disability. The number of participants included 3053 athletes from 61 countries, and 962 escorts. The Seoul 1988 Paralympic Organising Committee (SPOC) should take credit for helping the Paralympic Movement to advance so decisively in the course of this one event. The Paralympics were to be held in the same city where the Olympic Games had just been celebrated. This had been the stated aim of the stakeholders in the Paralympic Movement, but they had not been able to achieve this goal since Tokyo in 1964. A Paralympic Village had been constructed in Seoul, comprising ten apartment blocks with excellent access for people with disabilities.

Support for the 20 athletes and four technical delegates involved in the demonstration events at the Seoul Olympic Games came in the form of US$72 000 towards travel from the IOC, with the Seoul Olympic Organising Committee paying for board and lodging. But ICC tried to persuade the Organising Committee to extend its provision to help the four coaches as well. The Organising Committee agreed to find two twin rooms, but the costs would be borne by the international federations.

The Olympic Games of 1988 were to be tarnished by the disqualification of Ben Johnson for drug abuse, and doping would largely replace political rivalry to become the bugbear of the Olympic Games. The Seoul Games could have been massively affected by ideological conflict, but this did not materialise: protests were confined to the peculiar image of a South Korean boxer staging a lonely protest against defeat, remaining in the ring for over an hour. But nothing could lessen the impact of the spectacular achievements of athletes Carl Lewis (USA) and 'Flo-Jo' Florence Griffith Joyner (USA), and swimmer Kristin Otto (East Germany).

The participants in the demonstration events at the Olympic Games were to be hosted by the Olympic Organising Committee rather than the Paralympic Organising Committee. But the arrangements did not go smoothly: the athletes and officials had not been met at the airport and were uncertain about their accommodation and payment of subsistence. When Joan Scruton and Jens Bromann arrived in Seoul on 28th September, as part of the 'advance party' for the Paralympic Games, they received a cordial welcome from the Seoul Paralympic Organising Committee. They held a brief press conference and proceeded to the Hotel Intercontinental. But on arrival Joan Scruton was faced with sorting out the problems of the athletes and escorts from the demonstration events. Some had made their own way to the Hotel Intercontinental, but they were booked into the Hotel Lotte. Scruton arranged for the athletes and escorts to be transferred there, after persuading the Hotel Intercontinental that the athletes had mistakenly taken occupancy of rooms there. The officials had been booked in to the Tower Hotel. That evening the Paralympic Organising Committee hosted a marvellous dinner for the participants in the exhibition events in their hotel, the Hotel Lotte. Over dinner Joan Scruton had another complication to sort out: the participants in the demonstration events were due to be accommodated in the Youth Camp for the bridging period between the end of the Olympic Games and the start of the Paralympic Games. But the Youth Camp was now not going to be available, and the costs of ordinary hotel accommodation were well beyond the means of the athletes. The Seoul Olympic Organising Committee were to assume responsibility for them as soon as the Paralympic Village opened. Mr Byun, coordinator of the exhibition events for the Olympic Organising Committee, provided the solution: he suggested that the athletes and their escorts be accommodated within the Olympic Family House where the costs were very reasonable. With the exception of the American representatives, who were looked after by the US Army, all Youth Camp participants moved into the Olympic Family House the next day.

As the Opening Ceremony of the Seoul 1988 Paralympic Games burst into a vibrant musical extravaganza on 15th October 1988, some 75 000 people packed into the Olympic Stadium. The President of South Korea, Roh Tae-Woo, presented the new Paralympic flag to Jens Bromann, President pro tem of the International Coordinating Committee. Athletes with visual impairment joined their counterparts with spinal injury, amputees, athletes with cerebral palsy and 'les Autres'. After much debate and discussion at many meetings, Seoul Paralympic Organising Committee eventually agreed to the inclusion of wheelchair tennis as a demonstration event. Great interest was shown in this spectacle, proving the struggle for its inclusion worthwhile. The sports programme included archery, athletics, wheelchair basketball, boccia, cycling, fencing, football, goalball, judo, lawn bowls, powerlifting, shooting, snooker, swimming, table tennis and volleyball. The participation levels were staggering, as were the sheer numbers of volunteers and staff on hand. The highlights included Trischa Zorn achieving a sweep of ten gold medals in the swimming pool, establishing nine world record times along the way. John Morgan, also from the USA, took eight gold medals and two silver medals in the pool. Connie Hansen was a favourite with the crowds in the stadium, claiming victory five times in wheelchair racing events. In the wheelchair basketball competition the United States took gold in both men's and women's events. The wheelchair basketball had come to represent the biggest rallying point for the national teams, and the spectators and all those living in the Village followed the last few rounds avidly.

The accommodation and provisioning of athletes and escorts were magnificent during the Paralympic Games. It was frequently heard that this whole process should be the model for future events. However, one aspect of the model they would not wish to have replicated was the seemingly endless queues for food within the Paralympic Village. The administrative hub of the Paralympic Games was the Hotel Intercontinental, providing the location for both the ICC Secretariat and the Seoul Paralympic Organising Committee. The apparent calm and outward tranquillity of the foyer, where the trio of house musicians played their cares away was, according to Joan Scruton, deceptive in masking the 'intrigues, assignations, and machinations going on around them'. She thought the environment would suit a playwright researching 'a drama or a farce!'

Joan Scruton described her dismay at the obvious lack of coordinated coverage from the world's press. She heard from a leading journalist that they were all on their way home after the Olympic Games. Had the Olympic Games and the Paralympic Games been closer together in time the whole troupe of journalists would have been inclined to stay for the Paralympic Games as well.

Competitors and coaches were enthusiastic about the organisation of the Games, and they would carry their experiences for the rest of their lives. There was frustration, however, at the frequency with which events were cancelled once the Games had begun – mainly because not enough competitors were entered, or because a classification issue led to withdrawal. Although it was legitimate to scratch events under certain conditions, the decision to cancel sometimes came so late as to prevent the disappointed athletes from switching to other events – their Paralympic preparation was ruined. The International Coordinating Committee issued a statement supporting the athletes, assuring them that everything would be done to minimise the cancellation of events. During the Paralympics, some lines of communication were less clear than they should have been, so that it was sometimes ambiguous who should be contacted to solve a problem or meet an enquiry.

A political demonstration disrupted proceedings at the Seoul Paralympic Games. On 18th October the Iranian goalball team chanted an aggressive 'war cry' aimed at the Israeli team, refusing to play against them, before exiting the competition hall. As a result of the gross misuse of the sporting platform for political aims, the Iranian goalball team were disqualified, and immediately arrangements were made to send them back home. The Iranian team manager, Asghar Dadkhan, made a formal statement of apology the following day, pledging that all other athletes from his country would compete with full regard to the regulations, and would compete against Israeli and any other nation. This was not the first time that an Iranian team had been expelled from international competition of this sort; they had been sent home early from the International Stoke Mandeville Games in 1982 for distributing political propaganda.

A Libyan team arrived at the Seoul Paralympic Games without having gone through the normal entry procedures. The Seoul Paralympic Organising Committee urged the ICC to accept them, and a compromise was reached. The Libyans were permitted to participate as observers, could compete in the marathon event without having any medal entitlement, and would not be accorded official recognition at the Closing Ceremony.

As the Seoul Paralympics drew to a close there was a sense that those individuals who had been involved in officiating in both Olympic Games and Paralympic Games were tired. There had not been enough time between these major events. As a result of the difficulties of attracting the Korean organisers to gain experience at other world-class events prior to the Seoul Games, more technical delegates were required from outside Korea – creating additional costs and administrative arrangements for accommodation, accreditation and logistics. Hasty arrangements had been made to ship Korean officials to events just before the Games, but this could have been avoided.

The foresight of the International Coordinating Committee to establish a Paralympic Committee in the preceding years to manage the preparation of the Seoul Games was certainly rewarded. This group comprised four members of the Technical Sub-Committee, two members of the Administrative Sub-Committee, working together with the Chairman of the Medical Sub-Committee. Many points of detail had been anticipated, and regular communication was maintained with the main members of the Seoul Paralympic Organising Committee. The ICC Paralympic Committee functioned up until the start of the Games, but remained available to reassemble if required. The report of the ICC Technical Sub-Committee agreed that there was no turning back from the high standards of Seoul: 'This pattern of events should be the hallmark for future Paralympics. The principle of hosting the Paralympics programme in the same venue as the Olympic programme should never be violated.'

The Korean Government announced that the heightened awareness of the plight of people with disabilities would lead it to establish a register of persons with a disability following the Paralympic Games. Services mirroring those in other countries could then be set up with the aim of improving the lives of those so far not recognised or helped by the state.

It had been intended that progress would allow for the Ad Hoc Committee to draw all its deliberations together for ratification of a constitution for a new world organisation during the Seoul Paralympic Games. But the impediments were just too much at this time, and no compromise could be found that would permit the separate international federations to release enough of their grip to establish a new body. While many contentious issues were discussed furiously, the real decisions would have to wait a while longer – for Düsseldorf in September 1989.

PREPARATIONS FOR BARCELONA

'Keep the Mentally Handicapped Out of Our Arena' – Copenhagen, January 1989

The sixteenth meeting of the International Coordinating Committee took place in Jens Bromann's hometown of Helsingor, Copenhagen. The delegates gathered on Friday 27th January 1989 at the Marienlyst Hotel to begin their discussions, facilitated by the Danish Sports Organisation for the Disabled. From the hotel the delegates were able to look out over the Sound to the 16th century Kronborg Castle.

Financial constraints had prevented the ICC from being represented at the meeting of the General Association of International Sports Federations (GAISF) in Lausanne in November 1988, a disappointing absence in the light of the need for the ICC to be seen in this sort of forum. Members of the International Coordinating Committee had taken the opportunities provided by the Seoul Olympic Games and Paralympic Games to have several discussions with Juan Antonio Samaranch. He had explained that the number of sports in the Olympic Games would probably be reduced for Barcelona, compared with Seoul, and that this should not affect the demonstration events at all. In fact Samaranch was of the opinion that there should be greater exposure of demonstration events in the Olympics.

Jerald Jordan was praised for the high quality of the 16th World Games for the Deaf in New Zealand, when 1000 athletes participated, and where the Olympic flag flew over the stadium for the first time during games for the athletes with a disability in New Zealand. The organisers had suffered financial difficulties, but the lasting benefits to the deaf population were going to be enormous, as government funding had been intimated for the future. Jordan was critical of the International Coordinating Committee for not ensuring a better spread of financial support for all member organisations, rather than just for those participating in Paralympic Games. He called for greater equity in the dispersal of budgeted funds within ICC. The standing of the World Games for the Deaf was also an issue for Jordan. He suggested that he would seek his own contact with the International Olympic Committee to establish a better status. In order to dissuade the CISS from pursuing its own direction, the ICC members passed a motion to: 'respect the World Games for the Deaf as having the same sports level as the Paralympics'. This was acceptable to Jerald Jordan on behalf of the CISS. But this did not address the financial inequality.

The other aspect of ICC's finances, relating to the International Fund Sport Disabled, came up next in the Copenhagen meeting. A letter had been received from the Chairman of the International Fund dated 6th January 1989, which called for a meeting later in January; should agreement not be brought out of that meeting the ICC agreed that it would officially distance itself from the IFSD. While contact had been made with the IOC's fundraising company, there was no prospect of its help to ICC in the immediate future. Was the reluctance to proceed on behalf of ICC related to the undecided future of a world organisation for sport for persons with a disability, just as with the IFSD?

The Technical Committee had reported that any decision about whether INAS-FMH athletes should be allowed to participate at the Assen Games in 1990 and the Paralympic Games in Barcelona in 1992 should be deferred due to the discomfort expressed by other international federations. Martin Vicente wanted the delegates to reject this proposal, saying that the INAS-FMH athletes were eager to compete in any competition under the ICC banner. Stan Labanowich conveyed the views of the ISMGF sports sections that 'admission of mentally retarded persons to a Paralympic competition would be detrimental to the sports movement of the disabled'. Vicente expressed utter amazement at hearing this. Bengt Nirje was also shocked at this opinion. Labanowich went on to say that 'there was concern from physically disabled athletes that being cast into the same arena as the mentally handicapped affected their participation'. Bromann reminded the meeting that decisions had already been made that demonstration events in swimming and athletics would take place for INAS-FMH athletes in Assen. Representatives of ISMGF proposed that the ICC delegates should return to their membership and discuss the inclusion of INAS-FMH events in Barcelona. But Vicente insisted that a decision should be made immediately, at that meeting. Even with the urging of others that opinions of their members should be sought, the INAS-FMH delegates pushed for a decision, seconded by CISS. Although a vote was taken, with ISOD, CISS, INAS-FMH and CP-ISRA being in favour of athletes with intellectual disability participating in Barcelona, the matter was deferred to the next meeting. The realistic worries of the participants were reflected in this ironic exchange: a wish to safeguard the gains made already in the Paralympic Movement at the risk of discriminating against a distinct group of people with a disability. The fear was that the support of the public – growing enormously with each Paralympic Games – could be affected by the inclusion of athletes whose performance might not appear to represent elite sport in terms understood by them.

Carl Wang gave another update on the workings of the Ad Hoc Committee. As was known by many of those present in Copenhagen, all nations and international federations had been invited at the Seoul meeting to submit comments and amendments to the draft constitution by 21st December. Wang reaffirmed that a final draft would be sent out after their next Ad Hoc Committee meeting in March. An inaugural General Assembly was to be convened in September 1989 at the Congress Centre in Düsseldorf.

Fin Biering Sorensen, replacing Harald Natvig as Chairman of the ICC Medical Committee, told the ICC meeting that there was a need to establish a universal doping committee, and that common protest procedures for classification issues should be adopted for clarity at ICC-sanctioned events. The work already done to develop medical identity cards was now thought to be unnecessary because there was a general acceptance of progress towards 'sports-specific classifications'. An important new avenue for the International Coordinating Committee was the proposal from the Medical Committee for a multi-disciplinary sports science committee. The Chairman of the Medical Committee stressed that this would be a valuable pooling of resources because all energies: 'can be used in one committee instead of committees in each separate federation'.

The newly inaugurated Medals of Honour were bestowed on members of the Seoul Paralympic Organising Committee at the end of the meetings in Copenhagen in recognition of the enormous effort in preparation for the Seoul Paralympic Games. Jens Bromann, President pro tem of ICC, presented the ICC Gold Medal of Honour to SPOC President Koh Kwi Nam; the Silver Medal was presented to SPOC Secretary General Cho Il Mook; while the Bronze Medal of Honour went to Chung Ho-Yong.

As the future of the International Coordinating Committee was still to be decided, there was concern shown within some parts of the organisation that any imminent events could suffer if the ICC was dismantled. The Technical Sub-Committee made plans for continuity of event management to be maintained should the ICC be broken up. When the Committee met in March 1989 there was agreement that the international federations should nominate two representatives each to make up an Advisory Board specifically for the Assen Games in 1990. With the continuing financial difficulties, it was agreed also that the Assen organisers would host the meetings, and the federations would be asked to meet travel costs. This was a sensible arrangement that would ensure that the very best conditions were guaranteed. When the Technical Sub-Committee met again in July 1989, all federations had agreed to these arrangements except ISMGF, which wanted to consult further within ICC. The Sub-Committee spent some worthwhile time discussing the future, in the light of the forthcoming General Assembly in Düsseldorf. Certainly the members were anxious that the operation of two distinct bodies, claiming to be umbrella groups, could 'put sport for the disabled back to where it was 20 years ago'. Fundamentally they asked whether they should plan future meetings at all, and indeed, whether they had any future at all! The positions of the separate federations were outlined: ISOD had recently considered whether it should disband if a new world body was founded, as should ICC; IBSA's General Assembly was reported not to have discussed the implications of a new organisation in great detail – was this out of a wish to remain aloof or had they alternative plans? There was some debate as to whether ISMGF would 'go it alone'. Altogether the different organisations were steeling themselves for forthcoming change.

Classification for fairness

The preparation of facilities for the Barcelona 1992 Paralympic Games were judged to be excellent by John Grant, on his inspection visit. Grant reported in his capacity as President pro tem of the International Coordinating Committee when the ICC met for its seventeenth meeting on 30th and 31st July 1989, in Aylesbury, UK.

The Paralympic 'division' was part of the Barcelona Olympic Organising Committee, COOB'92. The Director of Sport for the Paralympic Division, Alberto Joffre, attended the Aylesbury meeting and delivered a sharp warning to all the delegates: 'The Games in Barcelona must be serious Games; there must be only elite sports and elite athletes . . . ICC must stop arguing among them and work together. In order to have sports for the disabled equal to those of able-bodied the ICC must act as the IOC. The ICC must be a very strong body'. It was agreed that the majority of athletes should be classified before their arrival in Barcelona – leaving no more than 12% requiring classification at the Games. Joffre stressed that functional classification should be introduced in as many sports as possible before Barcelona 'in order to reduce the classes, and to produce spectacular and excellent Paralympics'. Some will have bridled at these words, but the tough talk was invigorating and motivational. In response, members of ICC wanted to reassure the COOB'92 representative that their often frank and lively discussions should not be misunderstood to be internal squabbling. On the subject of classification, it was explained to Joffre that the additional workload was caused by the loss of computer data at a crucial stage in the proceedings, and as computer staff were changing over. Although there was ongoing debate over functional classification as the way forward, it was most likely that there would not be functional classification for track and field athletics by the Barcelona Paralympics. Joffre was obviously affronted by the tone of the ICC responses, and explained that he was a medal-winning Paralympic athlete himself, and understood the problems of such events from personal experience. He shot back with the comment that a gold medal had reduced value when it was won in a competition fought between only three or four people. The insistence that functional classification was used for Barcelona had been discussed at the ICC Medical Committee meeting. The members of the Medical Committee wrote: 'The body conformation of able-bodied people dictates their choice of sport so a classification system cannot be used to make all athletes with a disability into elite athletes in every event. The Medical Committee supports the concept of elite sport for the disabled. Classification is to make the sport fair *not* equal.' With these reservations, it was still agreed that as many sports as possible would work according to functional classification by the time of Barcelona.

After Joffre had left the meeting, discussion took place about the nature and content of the minutes. Unfortunately for those wishing later to follow the discussions more completely, it was decided that only subjects and decisions would be recorded in minutes from this point onwards – perhaps sanitizing the debate for posterity and avoiding similar criticisms about disunity to those of Alberto Joffre. But the very next item on the agenda proved that Joffre had probably been correct in his criticism of ICC. Martin Vicente wished to propose that INAS-FMH should be permitted to participate in the Barcelona 1992 Paralympic Games. However, the ICC meeting was told that the ISOD General Assembly had passed a motion opposing this. The fact that INAS-FMH did not represent all athletes with intellectual disability was important to ISOD, with Special Olympics Inc. still not openly cooperating with it. Likewise, the International Stoke Mandeville Games Federation's Council of Nations agreed that they 'did not wish to participate with INAS-FMH in the Barcelona Games'. But ISMGF wanted to add that its expression of opinion should not be considered to constitute discrimination. CISS, not involved with the Paralympics, abstained from the discussion. However, when the minutes were circulated, Jerald Jordan asked that there be an addition from him: 'CISS felt strongly that INAS-FMH had a right to participate. ICC had had four years to resolve this problem and had chosen to ignore it. If ICC did not think the mentally retarded were fit to take part they should not have admitted them to ICC'. This was a fundamental matter of principle. The IBSA General Assembly did not want to make a full programme available to INAS-FMH competitors in Barcelona, but indicated that it would accept demonstration events from athletes with intellectual disability. The delegates of ICC voted on Vicente's motion for INAS-FMH to be involved, and the motion was defeated. Vicente then asked for a vote on demonstration events only – this was lost as well.

When the ICC delegates discussed their relations with the International Olympic Committee, the mood was very positive. At the most recent meeting, on 8th June 1989, President Samaranch had congratulated the International Coordinating Committee on the success of the Seoul Paralympic Games, and offered his continued help to ensure that Barcelona would be as successful. Samaranch had reservations about the number of events and the consequent 'devaluation of medals'. The IOC President raised the question of the relationship of IOC with the proposed new organisation. John Grant explained how the present situation had arisen: starting out as a coordinating body of sports bodies for athletes with a disability gathering to organise the Paralympic Games, the International Coordinating Committee had become something much more. Grant then described to Samaranch that ICC had mandated an investigation into the introduction of national representation. The Seminar in Arnhem in

1987 had been called to discuss this, and to explore a new constitution. Grant here presented Samaranch with the impression that all actions were being directed towards resolution of problems by modification of ICC – rather than by the creation of a completely new body. Grant had not mentioned the Ad Hoc Committee, effectively helping reinforce the notion of ICC's overall centrality. It is doubtful that either Samaranch or Walther Tröger was uninformed about the true situation, especially as Tröger told the ICC representatives that he was to have a meeting with the organiser of the congress at which the future structure was to be discussed, in Düsseldorf, the following week.

Reassuring to the ICC members was Samaranch's expressed opinion that change needed to come from within ICC itself, thereby retaining the autonomy of the international federations. The way forward was to continue with demonstration events at international competitions and Olympic Games. Samaranch offered to smooth the way with any international sports federation that put obstacles in the way of demonstration events happening. The meeting between the IOC and the ICC representatives also confirmed that, in future, the title of the winter games would be the Winter Paralympics, officially approved by the International Olympic Committee. This was a highly significant recognition for the International Coordinating Committee, as use of the terminology had proved to be such a contentious issue in earlier events.

The Ad Hoc Committee, calling for nominations by 15th May 1989, had established a Nomination Committee. This was criticised by members of the ICC because the 'Ad Hoc Committee had over-stepped their mandate'. A range of opinions were expressed at the meeting, largely wanting to use the circulated draft constitution as a basis for agreement, but including some contrary views. In principle IBSA believed that the proposed structure for the new international body was workable, with some alterations. Discussions within ISMGF were along the lines that ICC should consider modifications to its constitution so as to provide for national representation, thereby being more in compliance with what was wanted as a new organisation. At this point, representatives of IBSA affirmed that they thought it most important that ICC did not appear to 'have a common stand' but should represent its own international federations. CISS could not see any merit in the new structure for its members, stating that it would withdraw from involvement in any new organisation that came into existence with the proposed format. It was sure that ICC could be more effectively, and more easily, reorganised to suit everyone's purposes.

The brittle relationship of the ICC with the International Fund Sport Disabled was reviewed. The Fund had responded to communication from the ICC, and this was discussed together with a letter that had been received from the EEC. Several members felt strongly about the continued fundraising of IFSD 'in the name of sport for the disabled from which the International Federations were not benefiting'. While the federations were struggling to carry out their normal activities, the delegates thought it immoral that 'IFSD was pumping money into the Ad Hoc Committee'. A letter was to be sent to the EEC, to member nations, to the Dutch Government and the United Nations clarifying the 'views of the ICC towards the Fund'. When the European Economic Community replied to the ICC's castigation for its having handed over money to IFSD, the clear response was not what the ICC members wanted: that the EEC had been giving financial support to IFSD since 1986 and no changes were planned.

In the report of the Medical Committee, Michael Riding informed the ICC delegates that there was definitely momentum to gradually develop a 'full sport science coordinating group'. Kathy Curtis, of the National Wheelchair Athletic Association, USA, had agreed to seek the approval of her national association to help 'act as the hub of the co-ordination process'. Behind this positive report was the discontent within the Medical Committee that ISMGF had separately embarked on its own Sports Science Committee. In the face of this, the ICC Medical Committee sought to make use of networking among scientists working in the area of sports for athletes with a disability, using newsletters, a database and symposia at international events. Contact would also be through the International Federation of

Adapted Physical Activity (IFAPA) and national organisations for disability sport. Riding was determined on the subject of doping control. The IOC list of banned substances and procedures must be employed, and any athlete currently taking banned drugs would have to transfer to medication that was not on the IOC list of prohibited drugs – 'a letter from a physician was not an excuse for taking banned drugs at the elite level'. Some modification of IOC procedures would be needed for athletes with a visual impairment and athletes with a physical disability.

At the Executive Board meetings of the International Olympic Committee at the end of August 1989, a letter from UK Minister of Sport, Colin Moynihan, was discussed. The Parliamentary Secretary of State, also a former international oarsman, had written to the IOC to ask that it consider including a clause in the Olympic Charter that would see the co-hosting of the Paralympic Games in the same venue as the Olympic Games. He cited the success of the 1988 Seoul Games, and the discussions following his presentation of a paper on the subject of sport for people with a disability at the 6th Conference of European Ministers in Reykjavik in June 1989. The discussion in the IOC Executive Board was very opinionated: Samaranch was very strongly in favour of supporting the Paralympic Movement in a measured way. Other IOC Members were largely opposed, not always sympathetically. Vitaly Smirnov considered that it would be risky to travel down this road, that the 'Games for the disabled should not obligatorily be a part of the Olympic Games'. He believed that this would open the IOC up to other such claims. He also stated that 'athletes with a disability were not interested in top level competitions, but wanted instead to prove that they could compete'. Dick Pound felt that such a move would impose undesirable organisational restrictions on organising committees. Zhenliang He offered his view that: 'the aim of the disabled was more one of rehabilitation than of seeking top performances'. Juan Antonio Samaranch was in favour of a cautious approach, acknowledging the concerns of others. He pointed out that the IOC already had a relationship with the International Coordinating Committee, but he was anxious that 'the disabled wanted to be part of the Olympic Games at all costs, which was not in the IOC's line of action'.

MOVES TOWARDS AN INTERNATIONAL PARALYMPIC COMMITTEE

Turbulent Times in Düsseldorf, September 1989

Wulf Preising, from the West German Olympic Committee, acted as convenor of the meeting at Düsseldorf to discuss the establishment of a new world organisation for sports for athletes with a disability, held on 21st and 22nd September 1989. The Messe Congress Centre was the venue for meetings, and the 203 participants from 42 countries stayed in four nearby hotels. The hosts were the Deutscher Behinderten Sportverband and the International Fund Sport Disabled, with the Chancellor of West Germany, Helmut Kohl, as Patron. With so much invested and so much at stake, all existing international sports federations were represented, together with a number of additional interested parties. In addition to English, simultaneous translation was provided into German, French, Spanish, Arabic and Sign Language for the Deaf. The Ad Hoc Committee, under the direction of Carl Wang, had circulated draft constitutions in the lead up to this gathering, and comments had been received from a good number of national representatives. There was an understandable tension in the meeting, and some less orderly interruptions soon emphasised the need for restraint and clarity. Some federations that had been very dominant in the administration of sport for athletes with a disability stood to lose their prominence should a new organisation be structured along different lines. The original intention had been for only national organisations to have a voice in agreeing the proposed constitution, but when challenged from the floor, this policy was extended to permit the international federations also to have speaking and voting rights. The procedural details, sometimes left dangerously unclear, had to be firmly established at the very start: each of the international organisations would have six votes. To have excluded the direct involvement of the international federations would have been insulting and disrespectful to those who had been responsible for the current health of the Paralympic Movement.

Joan Scruton described the gathering as 'hours of debate, argument and disharmony', with some worries that there would never be any positive outcome. Emotions were running high and interfering with progress. 'Things were going nowhere and I suggested voting on the main principle and tying up the details after that,' said Bob Steadward. Jens Bromann, President of IBSA, saw a way of pushing past the clutter that had led to the stalemate, and turned this around so as to assist the development process. In order to manage the volume of decisions that had to be made at this crucial but short meeting, a vote was taken on the formal proposal of Jens Bromann, York Chow and André Raes to launch the new world organisation: 'We propose that: ... The founding congress accepts in principle the rest of the articles drafted by the Ad Hoc Committee and go to the item point: "The official founding of ICSOD (International Confederation of Sports Organisations for the Disabled)"'. Once the details of other Articles had been untangled, the organisation was declared to have officially come into being later that afternoon. With the agreement of the majority in each vote, the tasks were to elect an Executive Committee and to agree on the constitution. The original proposals for the constitution were supplanted by several sensible alterations, so that the intentions agreed to at the 1987 ICC Arnhem Seminar could be realised. The name of the new world body was not to be International Confederation of Sports Organisations for the Disabled, but the International Paralympic Committee (IPC). The IPC was to be: 'the only World Multi-Disability Organisation with the right to organise Paralympic and Multi-Disability World Games, as well as World Championships'. Other fundamental identifying principles were that CISS, CP-ISRA, IBSA, INAS-FMH, ISMGF and ISOD were celebrated as 'Founding Members' of the IPC.

The structure was also important because it provided for the desired national representation not provided for before, as well as encouraging greater self-determination from among the athletes:

> A national organisation of sports for disabled representing more than one disability group shall have a number of votes related to the number of disability groups, but no more than six votes. A national organisation of sports for disabled representing one disability group shall have one vote. Each international organisation of sports for disabled (CISS, CP-ISRA, IBSA, INAS-FMH, ISMGF, ISOD) shall have six votes. Every encouragement is to be given to having persons with a disability in the delegations.

Officers of the Executive Committee would have a breadth that was to be welcome: a President, two Vice Presidents, a Treasurer, Secretary General, three Members at Large, a Technical Officer, a Medical Officer – all elected by the General Assembly; plus six representatives of the regions elected by the regions, one representative of the athletes elected by the athletes, and six representatives appointed by the six international organisations of sports for athletes with a disability. Crucial to the evenness of the balance of the International Paralympic Committee was the insistence in the constitution that 'Officers elected to the Executive Committee cannot hold a position in any other Board of the international organisations of sport for disabled'. There was an exception made to this principle later, with Michael Riding being permitted to remain as Chairman of the ISMGF Medical Committee and to lead the IPC Medical Committee. The elected members of the Executive could serve for a period of four years, and could be re-elected for two non-consecutive periods. The Executive Committee is described early on as 'the collegiate body of government, administration and representation ... with executive, jurisdictional and disciplinary power, as well as that of interpreting the Statutes, Regulations and agreements of the Assembly'. This was a highly appropriate declaration for the central participants in the new organisation.

The role of the Executive Committee was specified in the proposed constitution. It was encouraged to: 'initiate studies, and to make decisions on the policy as dictated by the General Assembly'. The organisation was intended to be in the hands of the wider membership, and to respond swiftly to the needs and preferences of the community for which it had been created. More fundamental activities of the Executive Committee were: to set out the rules for 'sanctioning international multi-disability events'; to maintain a calendar of all international multi-disability events, and to 'see that they comply with the established rules'. The Executive Committee should also have a monitoring role – ensuring that events were carried out within the framework of rules laid out by IPC in order to warrant their sanctioning. Administration was to be carried out by a Secretariat, responsible for communication with all members and other organisations. An innovation that was clearly part of the impetus from the Arnhem Seminar was the principle that the full national members of the International Paralympic Committee were to have the right to: 'participate in all international competitions, in all sports'. In the draft proposal this had been phrased slightly differently; that the full national members 'shall have the right . . . to enter their athletes in all competitions run by the IPC'. The difference in wording allows for greater right of entry, while still encouraging freedom of access that would come from combined classification. It was not quite endorsing a blurring of disability groups. The separate international federations retained their rights to organise their Games where these were separate from Paralympic Games and joint championships. That earlier paranoia of loss of identity seemed to play a lesser role, although it was still in evidence.

The new International Paralympic Committee would need its sub-groups, functioning with special-ised tasks, just as the International Coordinating Committee had been operating so far. The draft constitution proposed several committees (including Technical, Medical, Athletes', Membership, Nominating), and the structure was refined to suit the immediate needs of the IPC. There would also be scope to appoint Ad Hoc committees to complete short-term assignments.

Into the newly shaped positions on this Executive Committee came individuals with a wide range of previous experience. Some had already been leaders in the international organisations; others had shown their mettle in planning and carrying out complex arrangements for major international events. But they came together in the rejuvenated spirit of hope that was provided by the Düsseldorf meetings:

President:	Robert Steadward
First Vice President:	Reimer Krippner
Second Vice President:	Zauba Al-Rawi
Treasurer:	André Auberger
Secretary General:	André Raes
Members at Large:	Il-Mook Cho
	Valentin Dikul
	Elisabeth Dendy
Technical Officer:	Hans Lindström
Medical Officer:	Michael Riding

With the euphoria surrounding the initial meetings still evident, the Executive Committee met on 23rd September in Duisberg, not far from Düsseldorf. When they first met, those above were joined by:

IBSA Representative:	Jens Bromann
CP-ISRA Representative:	Jack Weinstein
ISMGF Representative:	John Grant
ISOD Representative:	Guillermo Cabezas
Oceania Representative:	Barbara Worley

West Asia Representative: Akram Massarweh
East Asia Representative: York Chow
Africa Representative: Nabil Salem
America Representative: Jim Leask

No regional representative was elected for Europe; this was a more complicated issue that would need the involvement of the European Committees of both ISOD and IBSA. Also delicate was the position of the Far East and South Pacific Games Federation (FESPIC), whose President, Harry Fang, wrote a statement of complaint. The message was that the timing of the meetings for the inauguration of the new organisation clashed with the FESPIC Games in Kobe, Japan. This meant that some participants had to miss the Closing Ceremony in Kobe in order to present themselves in West Germany. Fang's strongly worded statement decried the 'dictatorial attitude' of those behind the decision to hold the inaugural General Assembly at this time. He also suggested that the FESPIC Games Federation should be the sole representative of its region, as should any other existing regional organisation.

The remainder of the constitution needed to be developed into a fully comprehensive document, and the proposals made in advance by various countries helped form a serviceable instrument of government. The first Executive Committee meeting did not finalise the constitution, but the discussion document displays a mixture of clear thinking and pipe dreams. An important practical objective of the International Paralympic Committee was the immediate claim that IPC would become the sole 'representative liaison body' with the International Olympic Committee and other such groups. It was assumed that the IPC would take over management and control of the Paralympic Summer and Winter Games from the International Coordinating Committee. Also foremost was the stated aim of seeking 'integration of sports for disabled into the international sports movement for able-bodied, always safeguarding its own identity'. In case there was any doubt, the constitution stated in Item 8: 'The IPC is the supreme authority of the international sports movement for the disabled'.

Membership of the International Paralympic Committee was to have three categories: full members, associate members and observers. Full members would include national organisations of sports for the disabled 'catering for one or more disability groups'; and international organisations of sports for the disabled. Associate members would be those national organisations not meeting the criteria for full membership (being a registered organisation for the disabled, or being certified by the national governing body for sports in the country). The status of observer would be accorded to national or international organisations not meeting the criteria for full membership or not participating in international competition. Funds would be raised from a membership fee, from hoped-for support from the International Fund Sport Disabled, and the expectation of gaining access to the financial support of the International Olympic Committee as the transfer of authority proceeded from ICC to IPC.

At the Duisberg meeting, elementary details had to be covered, such as who had to be formally notified that the IPC was in existence. It was agreed that the priorities lay in contacting the International Olympic Committee, the International Coordinating Committee, the International Fund Sport Disabled and the United Nations. Of course, some of these organisations had had individuals attending the meetings all along, including Arnhem and Düsseldorf. But the relationships had to be placed on to a formal footing to ensure that the correct posture was possible on each side. The IFSD had been waiting for this positive move to establish a new world organisation, since the time of strained relations with ICC. Hans Lindström suggested that, with IFSD backing, a Secretariat could be maintained in Brugge. Identity for IPC also had to be discussed immediately: the public image of such an organisation was crucial to credibility and good communication. Although the Seoul Paralympic Organising Committee had offered its 'five teardrop' logo to the ICC for use after the 1988 Summer Paralympics, the logo had not been brought into play before that time. Perhaps this was the ideal opportunity for the IPC to employ a very suitable symbol that was ready made.

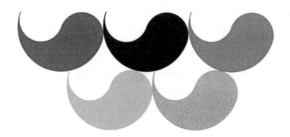

Of course, there was an urgent need to clarify exactly what the relationship between ICC and IPC was going to be in the immediate future and beyond. We have seen that prior to the Düsseldorf meeting, some of those involved with the International Coordinating Committee had expressed a strong preference for the ICC to reform itself into the new organisation that people seemed to be calling for. But this had not happened; the two discrete groups had visibly overlapping objectives and they needed to set out some sort of transitional programme – either to work towards the dissolution of the ICC or to agree a strategy that would enable both organisations to have a worthwhile function in the world of sports for athletes with a disability. The first meeting of the IPC Executive Committee acknowledged that the ICC had agreed that IPC would send observers to the ICC Executive and Technical Committee meetings. It was important to establish the exact legal position of the ICC with regard to identity and authority. Ongoing was the preparation for the Barcelona and Albertville-Tignes Summer and Winter Paralympic Games, and the IPC Executive assumed that there would be some sort of transfer of authority from the International Coordinating Committee to the International Paralympic Committee. But this final stage of the ICC's existence would be played out without changing the established patterns of communication and influence. The contracts had been signed between the respective Organising Committees and the International Coordinating Committee. In reality, many of the same people were involved in the practical management of these events; their expertise continued to be offered throughout the time of build-up for the Paralympic Games, regardless of whether the IPC or the ICC was at the helm.

Frustration and Slow Progress

The relationship of the International Paralympic Committee with the International Fund Sport Disabled was not yet cemented. André van Emden wrote to André Raes in Brugge on 16th November 1989, congratulating the IPC on its formation, but also expressing disappointment that the new organisation was so overtly catering for elite sports. He asked the IPC to 'reconsider this situation, as a true world organisation should cater for all aspects of sports'. Van Emden asked for more information about the constitution and structure of IPC before committing IFSD to financial support. He looked to the Assen meetings to confirm that the IPC was an organisation with sturdy enough credentials for the liking of the IFSD. When Bob Steadward met van Emden in March 1990, there was still no sign of progress towards sustained support for IPC. IFSD showed its support anyway, by declaring that it was offering to organise the General Assembly in Assen in July 1990, at the time of the World Games, and to provide a healthy subsidy towards administrational costs.

Classification Issues Raised by COOB'92

Meetings of members of the ICC and the Technical Committee took place with the Director of the Paralympic Division of COOB'92 (the Barcelona Olympics Organising Committee) and other members on 24th to 26th November 1989. The main topics for discussion were the Paralympic programme and functional classification for athletics and swimming. A classification study undertaken by COOB'92 Paralympics Division, in collaboration with the Polytechnic University of Catalonia, analysed results from Stoke Mandeville (1984–87), New York (1984), Brussels (1985), Rome (1985), Puerto Rico (1986), Paris (1987), Seoul (1988) and Nottingham (1989). Proposals were presented for discussion with ICC about the best 'grouping of classes' in competitions. The development of functional classification continued to be seriously researched, exploring the principles proposed by Birgetta Blomquist and her colleagues. The steady insistence of the Barcelona Olympic Organising Committee was that the Paralympic Games must be serious and that they must be only for elite athletes – distant from any notion of recreational sport. There was an obvious concern that there should be stringent limitations on the number of events admitted to the programme, and the negotiations were very even-tempered. It was reasonable that the hosts had no knowledge of the game of lawn bowls, and could not support the creation of facilities for an activity that would not be practised after the Games were concluded, for example.

Building Bridges, Not Walls

Hans Lindström put forward suggestions for the structure of the Sports Technical Department of the International Paralympic Committee, for the Executive Committee to discuss at its meeting in November 1989. There were to be annual General Sports Meetings for each of the sports involved in the Paralympic Games. Representatives would be elected by each country to discuss issues such as classification, rules and the sports programme for the Paralympic Games and multi-disciplinary World Championships. Each Sports Section would have authority over the conduct and administration of its sport; Lindström suggested that the technical authority of the Sports Sections should include: certification of referees; education of organisers; supervision of competitions; classification teams operating in conjunction with the Medical Committee; sanctioning of competitions in conjunction with the Technical Committee; ratification of records; and the establishment of minimum standards or criteria for qualification. These roles would require quite a lot of work initially in setting up procedures, but a strength of this structure was that most of the individuals who would become involved in the Sports Sections would be the same experts who were either already involved with sports disability organisations or with national federations. They would be operating within a different regime but using the same enthusiasm and dedication in serving sport for athletes with a disability.

Lindström then constructed an interlocking structure for a Sports Technical Committee, chaired by the Technical Officer. Annual meetings of a Sports Technical Assembly would be held, bringing together the chairpersons of the separate Sports Sections, with the chairpersons of the other sub-committees, and the Medical Officer. The Technical Assembly was to decide on issues such as:

> The general rules of IPC; the planning of sports programmes and calendar of sports; sports and disciplines for Paralympic Games and World Championships and Games; when possible, bids for World Championships and/or Championships with multi-sport programmes; give directives to the Sports Technical Committee, elect the members of the Technical Committee (every 4th year); and appoint a Records Committee.

The more detailed work of the Technical Committee was: to carry out specific commissions as directed by the Executive Committee and to present information back to the Executive for decisions; to run the Technical Assembly; to oversee the establishment and maintenance of appropriate rules for IPC sports programmes; to supervise and help the work of the Sports Sections; to 'co-ordinate international competition by sanctioning competitions and keeping the calendar of sports'; to take decisions on technical sports matters between Technical Assemblies; to appoint technical representatives of the IPC at competitions; to 'take initiative and promote research in sports for disabled'; to educate referees and trainers/coaches; and to work closely with the other IPC committees. A very important service factor for the new organisation was the encouragement of a coordinated approach to research.

The already-constituted groups of technical experts within the International Coordinating Committee were suggested by Lindström to help accelerate the establishment of the IPC Technical Committee. Hans Lindström contacted Colin Rains and Jean Stone, Chairman and Technical Secretary of the ICC Technical Committee to investigate an effective process for cooperation. With everyone sharing the same aims, this idea met with very little resistance. The next main task for Hans Lindström, as Technical Officer of the International Paralympic Committee, was to get the proposals for the sports sections through the Executive Committee in principle, and then to start working on the sports competition programme. The IPC Technical Committee started to work with one representative of each of the ICC federations to form an 'Interim Technical Committee', laying out a scheme for structure, by-laws and rules. The outcome of their deliberations was a configuration quite similar to the technical management of ISMGF and ISOD, which was reassuring to many of those who had been working within these structures for a number of years. The details had to be tidied up for the July 1990 General Assembly to approve in Groningen. The most remarkable departure from previous models was that the sports were being offered voting rights – not so far a feature of the international federations.

Michael Riding had been authorised to hold his position within ISMGF and also to be elected as Chairman of the IPC Medical Committee. This was an indication of the feeling of high regard for him by all those involved in the Paralympic Movement. Riding prepared a paper about the International Paralympic Committee as 'the view from the Medical Committee'. His words were both reassuring and provocative; they asked questions that had not been voiced before, but which were certainly concerns shared by many. He emphasised that everyone was really working towards the same goals but with different basic loyalties that created potential difficulties. The fact that the International Paralympic Committee had been created at this time 'would imply a dissatisfaction with the status quo' but a better understanding was needed of what the problems were before they could be resolved. Riding was tough on the IPC itself: 'I presume that the IPC's aspirations are Olympian. There is no doubt that the IOC represents excellence in the sports in its aegis and that the pinnacle of achievement for an athlete is an Olympic medal. Thus IPC must aspire to the excellence that IOC represents if we are to be credible in the sports community and the world at large'.

André Raes had indicated to the Executive Committee of ISMGF that he expected to stand down from its Executive once his role in the International Paralympic Committee was established. But when the handover of authority was delayed, Raes had to write twice in 1990 to John Grant, President of ISMGF, to emphasise that he had not in fact formally resigned yet. However, Raes's name had been removed from the list of members of the ISMGF Executive Committee, and he was unhappy about the treatment he was receiving. He stressed that he wished to be treated in the same way as Michael Riding in being permitted to hold posts in the two organisations, and that he wished 'to remain a member of the ISMGF Executive Committee until ICC transits its responsibilities to IPC'. Raes argued that the regulation made in the constitution of IPC that no post-holder in IPC could hold a position in any other organisation, was for the IPC to enforce if it wished. More than a hint of discontent is contained in Raes's statement: 'I wish to have the same status as Michael Riding until the situation ICC – IPC is cleared and decided, especially when so many ICC officers are questioning the (legal) existence of IPC'.

The Organising Committee of the Barcelona Olympic Games had put its concerns very plainly to the disabled sport community: to stop arguing among themselves and lift their effort to achieve a real parallel to the Olympic Ideal. Michael Riding used this rebuke from COOB'92 to urge the new world body to live up to its promises: 'The role of IPC then must be to build bridges not walls, to encourage but not bully, but to remember that we represent the elite competition in disabled sports. So what can we do to get there?' Riding went on to identify classification as an important current topic: integration across disabilities via combined classification Riding called 'the raison d'être of any disabled sport medical committee' up to the last few years. Although not everything had been settled, functional classification had been a way forward. Much more work would be needed on this. But Michael Riding identified the limitations of integration and functional classification, using the examples of wheelchair athletes and swimmers with cerebral palsy. In his view these athletes could be competitive in shorter distanced events with particularly appropriate training, but there would always be a shortfall in comparison with other athletes with a disability once longer distances were involved. Riding stated that the 'role of integration of classification rightly belongs to the IPC'.

With regard to the numbers of classes and the number of medals in Paralympic competition, Riding asked whether they were being realistic in the responsibilities now handed to IPC as the world coordinating organisation for elite sports for people with disabilities. Just as not everyone is equipped to compete in the Olympic Games, it is necessary for IPC to insist on strict constraints relating to the events that make up the ultimate sporting event for individuals with disabilities. Functional or integrated classification should not lead to a multiplication of events or individuals competing, nor should the process reduce the competitive or aesthetic impact of the Paralympic Games for the spectators. Riding stressed that the 'pursuit of excellence cannot always be fair, or equitable', and the IPC must take a firm lead in reducing the apparent contradictions of systems and attitudes that had emerged. The independence of the different disability groups was important, but there was a need to submit to the authority of IPC for those who wished to participate in the events under IPC's authority. Riding went on to say that the Medical Committee must bring together the disability groups and the sports sections 'to promote excellence through integration of disabilities and classes'. The work already done by particular disability sports organisations may not be transferable directly to others, and the IPC must be at the cutting edge of research to bring things together. As Riding so appositely put it, classification is both a philosophical issue and a technical issue at the same time. The different problems faced in classification of different disabilities would need research to rationalise classification procedures – combining them where possible. Research would have to feature as an important part of the IPC Medical Committee, and its hand would be outstretched for significant funding.

Control of doping was another area that IPC had to grasp firmly and show a lead in. The protocols and regimes for testing had been in place through the work of the ICC, with the International Olympic Committee being the reference point for comparison of procedures. Whereas classification might need sport-specific responses, doping should move towards a centralised coordination, and a unified reaction. Michael Riding also saw that there would be a need for the Medical Committee to look closely at sports injuries in the context of the very different needs according to sport and disability. As competition became still more intense and refined, much more would be needed in prevention and treatment of injuries. The International Paralympic Committee should see itself in a coordinating role: carrying out research and disseminating results to coaches, athletes and medical and technical officers at competitions. These were specific functions that the International Paralympic Committee could service.

Agreement with CISS Discussed

When the 2nd IPC Executive Committee Meeting took place in Brugge, Belgium, from 30th November to 1st December 1989, the members of the Executive Committee formally accepted the IPC Constitution, and it was ready to be placed before the General Assembly for final acceptance in July 1990. It was a great relief to the Executive Committee to have arrived at this point, although the resistance encountered both from ICC and IFSD, together with a certain hostility from the Barcelona

Paralympics Organising Committee, had dulled their euphoria. Bob Steadward's report reaffirmed IPC's aims as agreed in the founding General Assembly: 'The IPC is committed to the integration of athletes with a disability in all major world games besides the Olympic Games. This includes Pan American Games, Commonwealth Games, FESPIC Games, European Games, World Championships and other similar competitions.' He had been given the opportunity of addressing the Sport Committee and the Executive Committee of the Commonwealth Games Federation while visiting the 1990 Commonwealth Games in Auckland. There Steadward had received a positive response to the principle of integration, with the Commonwealth Games Federation going on to establish a commission to study the issue. Steadward also reported on his meeting with Jerald Jordan, President of the CISS, to work out an agreement between their two organisations. Steadward was aware that making exceptional arrangements with individual federations might appear to allow for dilution of the IPC's strength, and he urged the members to accept that 'CISS is a very unique organisation, and therefore, respect their past development'. The agreement was also to be put to the General Assembly in Assen.

Lindström met with the 'Assen Advisory Group' together with representatives of the ICC Technical Committee and the Assen Organising Committee, from 15th to 17th December 1989. The Director-General of the Assen Organising Committee, Major-General Kramer, hosted the meetings. Some late changes were of concern to representatives of the international federations: that an entry fee had been levied when there was originally none, and that limits were being placed on the number of competitors when there had been no earlier suggestion of there being any restrictions. There would be no national anthems or national flags at medal ceremonies – regretted by ICC members when this was discussed in their January meeting. Another source of concern was that the Assen Organising Committee appeared to be expecting the technical delegates to pay for their own expenses and costs, apart from 'local transport, and aperitif and buffet on the Saturday evening'. The ICC wrote to the Assen Organising Committee to insist that the proper payment of expenses be made under threat of having the ICC sanction withdrawn.

Steadward Addresses the ICC

Guillermo Cabezas welcomed the expectant delegates of the International Coordinating Committee to the Hotel Catalonia, Barcelona for their eighteenth meeting on 27th and 28th January 1990. While the morning of the first day was to be devoted to ICC matters, Cabezas informed the gathering that the President and Secretary General of the International Paralympic Committee had asked to be present as observers for the second part of the meeting.

Fernando Vicente outlined the request from INAS-FMH to hold separate Games under the Paralympic flag. Although there had been some disagreement about this happening in a Paralympic year, there was also a balance to be found considering the strongly expressed opposition to athletes with intellectual disability being accepted in the same arena as those with other disabilities. Vicente described the positive negotiations with the City of Madrid, where the Mayor had given his approval, and the Complutense University had also agreed to support the Games. The costs of the alternative Games would not be borne by ICC. As another positive demonstration of how this sector of sport for athletes with a disability had progressed, Fernando Vicente informed the meeting that INAS-FMH had met with Special Olympics Inc. half a dozen times in the past six months, and were maintaining very good relations. Vicente described Special Olympics Inc. as a 'private institution dealing with sport at a recreational level' and thereby not in direct competition for authority over elite sport for athletes with intellectual disability.

The delegates adjourned their deliberations temporarily, and enjoyed an extensive tour of the various sites for the Barcelona Olympic Games, a wholesome lunch being provided by COOB'92 after their excursion. On their return to the meetings, the representatives of the ICC were addressed by Bob Steadward, President of the International Paralympic Committee. He took the gathering through the progress of IPC meetings so far: preparation of the constitution for ratification, establishment of sub-committees, and introductory talks with a number of other organisations. As far as the assumption of responsibilities from the International Coordinating Committee was concerned, Steadward could not be precise. He explained that he had written to the organising committees of both Barcelona and Albertville to inform them of the establishment of IPC but to identify the intention to respect the contracts already signed with the International Coordinating Committee. Steadward admitted, in the first issue of the IPC Newsletter, that he and André Raes had travelled to Barcelona with the intention of persuading the International Coordinating Committee to hand over the reins as swiftly as possible, but he encountered strongly entrenched opposition from some ICC delegates. Delegates of IBSA were keen to provide continuity from the ICC to the IPC, and proposed that: 'There should be a permanent President, Medical Officer and Technical Officer of ICC and that these three officers should also be the officers of the IPC, and that this would be a way to show the world that a transfer was taking place'. The motion did not get any further.

The representatives of CP-ISRA raised the question of the autonomy of the international federations. The IPC's declaration that it would be the supreme authority of sport for the disabled was difficult for the federations to swallow. Each international organisation needed to feel that it could operate as a singular specialist in its field of disability. Without greater assurances it would be difficult to 'unequi-vocally approve a merger'. Bob Steadward tried hard to convince the members of ICC that the independence of the international federations would be respected at both national and international level. The IPC did not seek control over the federations. It is interesting to see that proposals to hand over all powers to IPC at the closing ceremony of the Barcelona Paralympic Games were ardently defeated at this ICC meeting. At least the ICC delegates agreed that the President and Secretary General of IPC should be invited as observers to ICC meetings. Steadward informed his IPC members that a temporary compromise was required, and that it would be necessary to wait until meetings in Assen in July 1990 'in order to complete the transfer of responsibilities'.

On the next day Juan Coll, Director of the Paralympics Division of COOB'92, spoke to the assembled ICC delegates. He presented a document that explained the organisation of the Games, and he also asked for regular dialogue as the time of the Games drew closer. A significant obstacle for Coll was the number of decisions still to be taken about the participation of athletes under the auspices of CP-ISRA. There were some complications caused by the functional classification of CP-ISRA athletes, and it had not yet been agreed which sports they would enter, apart from their exclusive sports (football seven-a-side, boccia and cycling). The problems seemed to arise in swimming and athletics. Jack Weinstein outlined the difficulties faced in classification of athletes with cerebral palsy using a combined classification system. Those athletes competing in wheelchairs would be at a distinct disadvantage if they were entered in the same event as wheelchair athletes without cerebral palsy. Michael Riding agreed that a degree of flexibility was essential in deciding the programme for athletes with cerebral palsy. The meeting headed into major disagreement until Joan Scruton quoted from the contract signed with the Barcelona organisers: 'For the sake of greater competitiveness, ICC shall supply COOB'92 with a system of functional medical classifications for as many sports as possible, and in particular for Athletics, Swimming and Table Tennis'.

Tensions and Resistance to Change

André Raes, Secretary General of the International Paralympic Committee, was quite outspoken about the barriers put in the way of the IPC's progress. Writing in the first IPC Newsletter in the Spring of

1990, Raes said: 'The great event in the last decades of sport for the disabled was the controversial, protested and exciting birth of the new world organisation in Düsseldorf'. He complained that it had not been allowed to grow according to expectation because the mandate given in the inaugural General Assembly was 'being contested by some of the international federations within ICC who desire to continue the control of sport activities until 1992'. He saw a conspiracy in the signing of the agreement between ICC and COOB'92 in July 1989, to organise the Paralympic Games in Barcelona. Raes attributed these actions to a 'strategic move completely in line with the aspirations and personal objectives of some members of the ICC Executive Committee'. André Raes was frustrated that the Secretary General of IPC was unable to have a clear steering hand on the pace of change towards the fully instituted new world body. The International Coordinating Committee seemed to have members who were clinging on to aspects of control, possibly in the vain hope that they might retain prominence as things inexorably changed.

Hans Lindström explained the differences in another way: that some members of ICC seemed to see the International Paralympic Committee as a 'tributary of ICC'. This implied that IPC could not take on its real work without receiving some sort of permission from ICC and other international federations. Of course the external view of such confusion was likely to have been detrimental to the Paralympic Movement more broadly, and Lindström, Raes and Steadward could see that firm but calm action was essential. Lindström was also capable of being provocative in pointing out that the essence of all their efforts was to provide opportunities for the very best sporting competition for athletes with a disability. He was clear that the IPC's emphasis, allowing for a national focus on sport representation, could see an eventual end to the dominance of the international federations. With the IPC taking charge of all multi-disability events, it would be for the nations to decide whether single-disability competitions remained – the federations would be irrelevant in that circumstance and, 'the member nations can decide to disband the international organisations. The decision is up to the members, not the executive boards'. But without a decision to pass full control over to IPC from ICC this would remain academic theory.

The caustic approach of André Raes could be seen in many of his letters. He wrote to Jack Weinstein in April 1990 to complain that the ICC had circulated its member nations to clarify matters that 'might be causing some confusion'. With characteristic directness Raes insisted that the information in the circular was 'NOT correct and tendentious, with the aim to turn the nations against the good intentions of IPC'. The letter related to the cancellation of a meeting between members of ICC and members of IPC relating to the future handover of control to IPC, and discussion of a draft constitution. Raes was furious that the ICC communication put the blame for the meeting firmly at the door of the IPC. Weinstein wrote back calmly to set the record straight (disagreeing with Raes in matters of fact), but also to reduce the temperature in their relations.

Cabezas Provides a Route Map for Transfer of Authority

The Second General Assembly of the International Paralympic Committee was judged to be a great success. At the meetings that took place in Groningen, the Netherlands, from 15th to 17th July 1990, Bob Steadward asked for the forbearance of the representatives as the new organisation found its way: there was a need to adapt and to accept compromise. Sponsorship had been welcomed from Air Canada for the IPC President's travel over a four-year period, as well as financial support from IFSD and the Belgian, Canadian and Scandinavian federations towards the IPC. There had also been contributions towards the costs of the General Assembly and Executive Committee meetings from the Rick Hansen Man-in-Motion Society. At this point in its existence the IPC had great need of this kind of support.

André Raes wrote to all member nations on 18th July to outline some of the most significant decisions taken. The members attending the General Assembly agreed that the constitution should be accepted.

An agreement was also formalised between CISS and IPC, straightening out some of the difficulties that had been present in the past. The agreement acknowledged that IPC recognised CISS as the supreme authority 'for sports for and of deaf people', and that IPC recognised the World Games for the Deaf as international events of equal status to the Paralympic Games. The International Paralympic Committee would encourage national and international bodies also to respect the autonomy and independence of national deaf sports federations. Included was an undertaking that IPC would not accept as a member a national federation claiming to represent deaf people unless it had been recognised by CISS. The particular nature of this relationship meant that the written agreement included automatic representation for CISS in any negotiations with representatives of international bodies such as the United Nations, the International Olympic Committee, the International Fund Sport Disabled or the General Association of International Sports Federations. CISS would also benefit from the establishment of a permanent secretariat: IPC would set aside office space for CISS, together with some financial provision for administrative costs. CISS would receive a portion of 'funds obtained in the name of sports for the disabled', shared in a proportional manner according to agreement with the IPC Executive Committee. This agreement was a substantial recognition by the International Paralympic Committee, a willingness to step well outside its relationship with the other international federations. With the lengthy history of CISS and the particular background to the relationship of CISS with the International Coordinating Committee, it was clear that CISS would not be willing to operate within the bounds of IPC as defined by its constitution. But it was also essential for IPC to have a relationship with CISS rather than encouraging CISS to remain utterly detached – IPC could not otherwise be fulfilling its mandate.

Prior to the General Assembly, several meetings of the IPC Technical Committee had taken place, as had gatherings of other sub-committees. Hans Lindström, Chairman of the IPC Technical Committee, had communicated with Stan Labanowich, as Chairman of the ICC Technical Committee, prudently exchanging information about aspects of their future relationship that would need sensitive treatment. They were careful to ensure that Labanowich was able to address the IPC General Assembly, asking for the floor to bring his views to the attention of the meeting. Their discussions included clarification of the position of existing recognised international bodies in particular sports, when IPC was suggesting the creation of Sport Committees. Labanowich was helpful in stressing the positive effect that would result from an insistence that an existing body for a specific sport would be recognised as the Sport Committee for the IPC-sanctioned event. The potential fragmentation of the separate sports within the movement into separate federations was also discussed between Labanowich and Lindström. The latter spelt out the desirability of IPC being given responsibility to pull the different groups together – but the national federations should determine this. What was obvious was the willingness of the two technical groups to communicate for the benefit of the future. Something else that was quite clear was the intention to make the Sports Committees much more a dynamic feature within IPC, with influence at the General Assembly, than had at first been considered. Hans Lindström explained his rationale in a motion to the General Assembly:

> It is essential that sports specialists are present with the right to speak and vote at the highest level of the IPC, the General Assembly. That would add to the joint knowledge of the Assemblies and serve to make the discussions livelier. More and more of the sports are reaching a level of independence of a kind that should be given the right to influence policy decisions. Simultaneously, an active participation in the Assemblies would serve to better enlighten the Sports Committees through their representatives on the . . . thinking behind policy development.

Just as wheelchair basketball in the United States had for many years insisted that the athletes must be full stakeholders in the administration and government of their national organisation, it appeared that the IPC could be moving to give a significant voice to the sports and athletes themselves.

A vital subject to be discussed was the transition from the International Coordinating Committee to the International Paralympic Committee. Guillermo Cabezas had put forward a route map for ICC and

IPC to reach agreement on transfer of responsibilities, and the General Assembly agreed to this process. Each sport was to become a standing committee within the International Paralympic Committee. Membership fees were set at US$50 per disability group within a country, and US$300 per international federation. Owing to the volume of work to be done, the next General Assembly was being planned for 1991, with a two-year interval after that. Each country was asked to help streamline the administration of the IPC by identifying a contact address to receive and deal with correspondence. This national federation would become the National Paralympic Committee (NPC) and would be seen by IPC as the national coordinator of national disability groups in relation to IPC. The initial tasks of the national federation would be to duplicate and distribute IPC material and to collect membership fees.

The transfer of responsibilities from ICC to IPC needed to be very visible, and within a reasonable time from the decision to establish the International Paralympic Committee. Otherwise the impact of the new organisation would be lessened, and its credibility would be damaged for the future. Jens Bromann spoke to the representatives in strong terms: 'The IPC is to be the supreme authority, which means that the only ICC task left is the practical carrying-out of the winter and summer Paralympics in Tignes and Barcelona because it (sic) is contracted by the ICC. IPC has to take over all other future events. We cannot wait for the IOC approval because there is already practical work to do'. He then proposed that the two bodies should meet to construct an agreement, using Cabezas' paper as a basis for discussion.

Signing an Orderly and Harmonious Transfer

The President of the International Olympic Committee, Juan Antonio Samaranch, maintained a suitably aloof posture with regard to the International Coordinating Committee. He had made it clear that he would not have a meeting with the ICC until a formal agreement had been reached between ICC and the International Paralympic Committee. The Executive Committee of the ICC was informed, when it met on 6th October 1990 at the Ludwig Guttmann Sports Centre, Aylesbury, that the International Olympic Committee had provided an advance of US$25 000, but this had not been followed up as yet with a full subvention. Unfortunately there had also been a setback in the arrangements for Winter Olympic Games exhibition events. The French Federation reported that there was no such event in the final programme of the IOC despite their efforts to meet with Walther Tröger. Bob Steadward spoke at this point, saying that he had a meeting scheduled with Samaranch for later in October. He would propose to make this a joint meeting with the ICC President pro tem, once there was an agreement in place between IPC and ICC. Steadward's suggestion was good politics, and served to give confidence to the ICC members.

The Presidents of IPC and ICC had met on 5th October to draw up a draft agreement. Time was spent perusing and debating the document and some changes were made. But the agreement was formally signed at 2.00 pm on 6th October 1990, by the President of IPC and ICC, together with the Presidents of the International Federations. Acknowledging the real triumph of this accord in very complex times, this agreement is worth looking at closely (Box 5.1).

The original agreement was signed with flourishes of ink by Jack Weinstein (President pro tem of ICC), Bob Steadward (President IPC), John Grant (President International Stoke Mandeville Wheelchair Sports Federation), Guillermo Cabezas (President ISOD), Jens Bromann (President IBSA), Jerald Jordan (President CISS) and Fernando Martin Vicente (President INAS-FMH). With this document firmly imprinted in the minds of all those involved in both the International Coordinating Committee and the International Paralympic Committee, there was finality to the result. There was no sense in the few ICC members holding tightly to the hope that there could still be a volte-face that would enable the situation to remain unchanged at the end of the year. Although there were still the dissenters, more people would positively embrace the changes to come.

Box 5.1 The IPC–ICC Agreement

IPC–ICC AGREEMENT: This agreement entered into by and between the ICC and the IPC this 6th day of October 1990, in Aylesbury, England, as follows:

WHEREAS, the ICC and the IPC are desirous of spelling out their working relationship between the date of this agreement and the conclusion of the 1992 Paralympics in Barcelona and Madrid, and

WHEREAS, the ICC is the contracting party with the Winter Paralympics in Albertville, and the Summer Paralympics in Barcelona and Madrid, and

WHEREAS, the IPC has formed and approved its constitution giving it authority over world multi-disability (more than one Federation) games from July, 1990 on, and the ICC has had authority over such games up to the date of this agreement, and

WHEREAS, the parties are desirous of spelling out the orderly and harmonious transfer of the control over world multi-disability (more than one Federation) games from the ICC to the IPC, it is

NOW THEREFORE, agreed by and between the parties as follows:

FIRST: That the ICC will continue its control over, and to handle and complete its contractual duties with respect to the Winter Paralympics in Albertville and the Summer Paralympics in Barcelona and Madrid; and

SECOND: That the IPC will assume immediate control over all other world multi-disability (more than one Federation) games, as spelled out in its constitution; and

THIRD: That in order to foster a harmonious working relationship and transition, the parties agree to the following:

a. The IPC will become full participating members in the ICC;
b. That the Presidents of the ICC and the IPC, upon the signing of this agreement, will jointly set up a meeting with the IOC to discuss the transition with the IOC between the signing of this agreement and the conclusion of the 1992 Paralympics;
c. The IPC as of the date of the agreement shall have full permission to the use of the logo of the ICC subject to the same terms and conditions as the ICC up to and including the 1992 Paralympics and shall have the sole and exclusive rights to the logo thereafter;
d. That upon completion of the Summer Paralympics in Barcelona, both organisations shall issue a joint communiqué spelling out the final transfer of power from the ICC to the IPC.

1990–1992: TIGNES AND BARCELONA

The 'Teardrops' or *Tae-Geuks*

When Juan Coll of COOB'92 reported to the ICC meeting on 6th October 1990, he informed the delegates that the IOC had requested that they should not use the 'five teardrop' logo because of confusion with the IOC's five rings emblem. Later in the meetings it was agreed that ICC representatives should strenuously insist that the logo approved by the IOC for Seoul should continue to be respected as representing the Paralympic Games. Even the published material of the IPC reinforces the parallels to the Olympic symbol of the five rings. On the front page of the IPC Newsletter of Spring 1991, the 'new IPC symbol' was proudly displayed and explained: five Korean *Tae-Geuks*, traditional decorative symbols, were arranged into a W-shaped pattern representing 'the five oceans and the five continents'. It was explained that the symbols formed the letter 'W' so as to show the initial letter of the word 'World', 'which represents the harmony and unity of the disabled all over the world through sports'. It was unfortunate for those trying to persuade the guardians of the Olympic symbols that the configuration of the *Tae-Geuks* – three placed horizontally above two more – was exactly the same as the configuration of the five Olympic rings (three horizontally aligned above two other rings). Additionally, the colours of the five *Tae-Geuks* also corresponded exactly to the colours of the five Olympic Rings. The text attributed further meaning to the IPC's adopted logo: 'The horizontal configuration of the *Tae-Geuks* represents equality and humanity, and the wave shape expresses the willingness and determination of the disabled to become fully active'. All member nations were encouraged to employ the logo in all possible appropriate uses. André Raes was to advise member nations on the exact dimensions of the logo so as to ensure accurate use of the new public image of IPC. Each country was to establish a National Paralympic Committee, and to incorporate the symbol, just as had been done by the International Olympic Committee. But this was not to be such a smooth process . . .

Coll further reported that there had been major arguments with INAS-FMH over the use of the word 'Paralympics' in conjunction with INAS-FMH's independent games being held in Madrid. In the end, Coll said, it had been decided to permit the use of the term so as to end the wrangling.

The Organising Committee for the 1992 Winter Paralympics in Tignes Albertville, France (COPTA), was represented at the ICC meeting by Mr M. H. Beguin, André Auberger having broken his leg. He reported that, with 500 days before the start of the Games in Tignes Albertville, there had been first indications of entries from over 460 athletes. Beguin hoped that this might reach the 500 mark, with more than 20 countries represented. Other development was going well, although in its early stages: the technical programme and facilities were starting to come together. The ski facilities were on target to be finished by the coming winter. Jean-Michel Folon, a renowned artist and the creator of the logo for the 1992 Winter Paralympic Games, would be responsible for preparation of an impressive cultural programme. Beguin was confident that the 1992 Winter Paralympic Games would cement a unique relationship between the Olympic Games and the Paralympic Games. He called the benefits to be derived 'reciprocal enrichment'.

Martin Mansell – Athletes' Representative

The Athletes' Committee was represented by Martin Mansell at the next Executive Committee meeting of the International Paralympic Committee. He asked that a report should be included as a matter of routine at future meetings, and this met with agreement. Mansell had immediately involved the other seven nominees for the Chair of the Athletes' Committee in the scrutiny of the major issues that might be covered in their Committee. This was an excellent use of the best resources. The Technical Committee and each of the Sports Committees would invite representation from members of the Athletes' Committee.

When the 4th IPC Executive Committee Meeting took place in Brugge, Belgium, on 16th and 17th November 1990, there was a feeling of quiet confidence and maturity in the air. Steadward had already been in contact with many key organisations that needed to be informed of the changes afoot in sport for people with disabilities. Integration of athletes with a disability into the framework of international sports federations had become a central concern. IPC had established a Commission on Integration, under the direction of Rick Hansen, and this was working vigorously. Anne Merklinger, who had worked with Bob Steadward before, was appointed Executive Director of the Commission. In Brugge, Jens Bromann insisted that the IPC's internal structure must be completely in place before launching new initiatives: 'An unprofessional start would work like a boomerang and lower our possibilities in the future. We need a powerful Integration Committee.' He was concerned that the group had not yet clearly defined its ground relating to integration. Hans Lindström agreed: 'Integration will be our most difficult task for the nineties'.

The work to establish National Paralympic Committees was inexorably slow, and in some countries it would be some time before existing structures would give way to this form of singular representation.

In line with the direction of the IPC structure, it was agreed at the meeting that the Technical Committee would be renamed the Sports Council Executive Committee, with the Sports Committee also being reassigned the name of Sports Assembly Executive Committee. Painstaking analysis of the regulations and by-laws of the International Paralympic Committee was made at the 4th Executive Committee meeting. As a result of small changes in the practical working arrangements already, several articles had to be deleted or amended immediately. This was a wholly constructive process; the IPC was clarifying its methodology through a redefinition of its first try at regulations. Some aspects could not be solved straightaway: regional representation was always going to be complicated by the separate international federations employing differing regional delineations. It was hoped that the unifying effect of the IPC could bring all definitions of regions into line with each other.

The contract for the 1994 Winter Paralympic Games was signed, with John Magdal, Technical Director of the Lillehammer Organising Committee, in attendance. Although there were a few details to be tidied up, there was confidence that this event would be a great success – in particular as for the first time, the Winter Paralympics would share the same organisational direction as the Winter Olympic Games. There was some disagreement on the big issue of whether sports for people with disability should be so closely tied to the Olympic Games, or whether the Paralympics should fight for an entirely separate identity. Martin Mansell and Jack Weinstein voiced the opinions that they did not wish the 'Paralympics to be accepted because of the bid of the Olympic Games'. They felt it would be better if the IPC could 'package the Games and bring it out as a strongly organised, separate event' with the IPC's governing regulations. In his typically practical manner, Michael Riding commented that accommodation alone would make being separate a limiting factor.

International Coordinating Committee Checks Preparation for Barcelona

The International Coordinating Committee met at the Hotel Catalonia, Barcelona on Saturday 16th February 1991. Before the discussions got underway, the Barcelona Olympic Organising Committee (COOB'92) led the delegates on a thorough tour of the Olympic Village and a number of sites for the Paralympic Games sports events. The hosts had prepared a booklet outlining the state of progress, and a brief address was made to expand on the information, covering: sports, services and operations; Paralympic Village; health care, technology and facilities; marketing; and volunteers. Questions relating to practical matters were effectively dealt with, and some further enquiries could only be answered when numbers of entries were more certain.

The ICC meeting proceeded with Fernando Martin Vicente informing the gathering about the Madrid Games, due to take place for INAS-FMH athletes. Although there had been consideration of a capitation fee to be charged to athletes, this was not going to be imposed – in fact, INAS-FMH would be paying an overall capitation fee of some US$10 000 to ICC, for which the ICC Treasurer was very grateful.

Stan Labanowich, as Chairman of the Technical Committee, reported that appropriate progress was being witnessed in each of the Paralympic projects, both Summer and Winter Paralympic Games. He informed the group that he had been present at the latest meeting of the Interim Technical Committee of the International Paralympic Committee, in Jackson Village, New Hampshire, USA. Labanowich explained that the aim of the meeting, and one to be held in Lillehammer, Norway, the next month was to produce 'a structure and policies related to the technical organisation of the IPC', to contribute towards refining the IPC Handbook.

When it was the turn of the Winter Paralympic Games Organising Committee, COPTA'92, to address the ICC, a sequence of setbacks was recounted. Heavy snowfall had slowed the rate of building of new facilities. Some sponsorship had been withdrawn as the Club Coubertin decided not to sustain its support. The Gulf War had made everyone's investment spiral downwards, and uncertainties over the future made things worse. It seemed to the Organising Committee that it needed to increase the entry fee in order to cope with the fall in value of the US dollar. Even acknowledging the particularly expensive nature of ski resorts, this was not a popular suggestion. Far more entries had been received in the initial posting than the committee could realistically manage. When the second entry form was sent in March it would also carry a specific entry fee – so far not published. Mr Garcia Soria of IBSA proposed that there should be a common level of entry fee for both Barcelona and Tignes. This received full approbation. Whereas the Barcelona Organising Committee had committed themselves to providing free medical care for all participants during the Summer Paralympic Games, COPTA'92 was insisting that all individuals had to have their own medical insurance.

As in each meeting of the International Coordinating Committee, there had to be some consideration of its standing with the International Olympic Committee. In this case, the ICC discussed the minutes of a recent meeting involving the IOC, the IPC and the ICC. As the debate warmed up it became clear that the record of the meeting produced by the International Olympic Committee differed in substance from the report of the meeting made by the Presidents of IPC and ICC. In the IOC account there appeared to be some expectation that the international federations would eventually disappear once the International Paralympic Committee took control. Some pains were taken in the ICC meeting to explain how this particular view may have been acquired. Bob Steadward spoke to the meeting to say that Samaranch had commented that he believed the IPC might not ever be successful as an international sport organisation for athletes with a disability. They discussed the difficulties to be faced in the future; particularly the complexity of a series of national structures that were inevitable, while 'the mandate that had been given to IPC was to recognise and support an umbrella organisation over a number of disability groups'. Although not entirely reassuring to all those at the Barcelona meeting, it was agreed that the ICC must indicate to the IOC that there was a discrepancy between their interpretations of the meeting, and this would need clarification. Other issues included the repetition of concern over the logo, and the refusal of IOC to permit demonstration events to involve athletes who were blind. Garcia felt ICC should insist that Samaranch change his attitude towards exhibition events for blind athletes, or ICC should withdraw from all exhibition events. Garcia considered that it was important to 'educate' the IOC. But any boycott would have a very negative effect on relationships and would penalise all other athletes.

IPC Supports Sledge Hockey and Dressage

The fast and demanding team sport of sledge hockey had been developed at the end of the 1960s in Norway and Sweden. By the later 1980s the Scandinavian countries were joined by the United Kingdom, Canada and the United States to arrange competitive opportunities. Canada lifted the title in the first World Cup in 1991, defeating Sweden by three goals to two. This was the sort of event that the International Paralympic Committee used to promote its new existence – while waiting for the full authority over the Paralympic Games after 1992 it was necessary to endorse other events. The next World Cup was already on the calendar, scheduled for Ottawa in March 1992.

The next opportunity for promotion of the International Paralympic Committee's objectives was through the 2nd World Dressage Championships, held in Denmark in August 1991. Dressage had featured in the 1984 New York Games for the Disabled, and it had been restricted then to athletes with cerebral palsy. It was natural for numerous other athletes to want access to this scale of event, when they saw the success of the New York competition. When the 1st World Championships were held in Sweden in 1987, the entries were opened to competitors from several disability groups: les Autres, amputees, blind athletes, athletes with intellectual disability and athletes with cerebral palsy. More than 70 riders represented 15 countries at these 2nd World Championships, held at Aarhus. The Danish National Riding Centre at Vilhemsborg was a perfect facility for the purpose. While the New York competition was organised within the framework of CP-ISRA, the IPC Sports Assembly agreed that equestrian sport should come under the multi-disability identity of IPC rather than remaining within CP-ISRA.

More Tears for the IPC Logo

The subject of the IPC logo continued to occupy the attention of the IPC Executive Committee, meeting in Lillehammer, Norway, on 9th and 10th May 1991. The ability of the International Paralympic Committee to market itself effectively, therefore its ability to sustain its existence, came from having an identity and appropriate symbols and emblems for use by sponsors. At this early stage very few membership fees had been received, and there was a feeling that the IPC should nurture the cooperation and confidence of member nations before pushing the financial 'button'. Only members with fees fully paid would be allowed to exercise democratic participation in the General Assemblies. Financial support from the International Fund Sport Disabled, certainly hoped for if not expected, had remained at the level of help for secretarial operation – not for the other activities of IPC.

Howard M. Stupp, the International Olympic Committee's Director of Legal Affairs, protested that unless the IPC was able to resolve the matter of the logo 'to the satisfaction of the IOC' there might be sanctions taken by the IOC against the International Paralympic Committee. For a young organisation hoping to secure significant financial subsidies from the IOC, the IPC could not afford to ignore this warning. The Executive authorized a search for a new logo, arriving at a circular pattern of six *Tae-Geuks*. The proposed new logo was displayed proudly in the IPC Newsletter of Fall 1991. An additional *Tae-Geuk* was in the logo – described as representing the six regions of IPC. The interlocking circular shape was to represent the harmony and unity of athletes with a disability through sports. The three colours (red, green and blue) were said to be the predominant colours in the flags of the world, and also were symbolic of sky, earth and water. But once this logo had been displayed, some countries were unhappy that IPC had turned away from the original one, democratically accepted as it had been. This then had to be another matter for discussion in Budapest, when the General Assembly convened in November 1991.

The IPC Secretary General continued to be dogged in his criticism of those post-holders in the Paralympic Movement who were obstructing progress. In the Fall 1991 Newsletter, André Raes slated some members of the international federations: 'It is frustrating to see that some persons are working solely for their personal glorification, and in the meantime, jeopardising the common interest of sport for the disabled. Creating possibilities for our athletes and setting up competitions should be our only objective.' Although it was commendable to be straightforward, Raes was managing to display remarkable insensitivity, especially considering the relationship the International Paralympic Committee would need to have with these organisations in future.

Progress towards the 4th Winter Paralympic Games in Lillehammer was excellent. Hans Lindström had visited the sites and considered the plans for accessibility to be excellent. Everything was positive: attitudes and facilities. This would be the first Winter Games with the Olympics and Paralympics using exactly the same facilities. 'Judging all this, the Technical Officer expects the 1994 Winter Paralympics to be the best ever organised.'

As for the planning of the Summer Paralympic Games of 1996, Atlanta had continued discussions, and was completing a feasibility study for hosting the Paralympic Games. In case it responded in the negative, Toronto and Melbourne were to be asked to consider activating their earlier expressions of interest in the

Paralympics. André Auberger, as IPC Treasurer, commented that he would be happier if the Paralympic Games employed the same facilities as the Olympic Games, and Eric Russell, representing the South Pacific Region, suggested that the media would be more likely to attend if the Paralympic Games preceded the Olympics: 'the media will lose interest if they take place after the Olympics'.

A testing time was to follow in the Executive Committee, when a proposal was made by James Neppl, representing the North American region, that the regulations of the international federations relating to the separate sports should be adopted, and not included in the IPC Handbook. Eric Russell and John Grant approved of this suggestion, inferring that the Sports Assembly Executive Committee would have to accept the rules as they stood from the international federations. Hans Lindström could not accept this proposal – he promised to resign if it was voted through. Neppl's proposal would, in Lindström's view, alter the basic principles of the International Paralympic Committee: 'It will then no longer be the organisation which I accepted to work for, but another ICC'. The voting in this motion was perverse: four in favour, six against, five abstentions. But this first major test of the integrity of the IPC's foundations was survived, just.

The rapidly changing situation of the former Soviet states was being felt in many international organisations, and the IPC had received a second request for membership from Lithuania. Earlier, the IPC had turned to the International Olympic Committee for guidance on the parallel application Lithuania was making to the IOC for membership. At this time the International Paralympic Committee looked for clarification of the basis on which the IOC had rejected Lithuania.

IOC Executive Discusses Disability, September 1991

The International Olympic Committee gathered its Executive Board together in Berlin over three days in September 1991. One item on the agenda was the relationship of the IOC with international organisations dealing with athletes with a disability. There had been progress within the IOC for the recognition of Special Olympics International, and this led to a broader discussion of leadership in the complex world of disability sport. Walther Tröger was emphatic about the need to only recognise one international umbrella organisation – as was the IOC policy. But recognising Special Olympics International would then make difficulties for IOC when the International Paralympic Committee formally replaced the International Coordinating Committee after the Barcelona Paralympic Games the following year. Rather than being an umbrella organisation, Special Olympics International was described by Tröger as: 'an individual, technical organisation, and should therefore not enjoy the same level of recognition as the IPC'. There was also the problem of the reluctance of organising committees to be involved with the Paralympics as well as the Olympic Games. Samaranch intimated that Lillehammer was not interested in hosting the Paralympics: 'Atlanta likewise did not want to host these Games, but were instead planning to stage a series of disabled sports exhibition events'. He went on to say: 'The IOC needs to decide whether it should be compulsory for OGOCs to organise the Paralympics in conjunction with the Olympic Games'. There was a regularly expressed view within the IOC Executive Board that the Paralympics would be better located in another city (and even country) from the city of the Olympic Games. Walther Tröger posited a solution to the venue: to offer the Paralympics to one of the unsuccessful bidding countries in the Olympic Games hosting competition.

CISS Withdraws from ICC

At the Bonnington Hotel in London, the next meeting of the International Coordinating Committee took place on Saturday 3rd August 1991. The first item for the committee to receive was the official withdrawal of the Comité International des Sports des Sourds from the International Coordinating Committee. Jerald Jordan had written to Joan Scruton on 18th March 1991 to tell her that it had been decided at the CISS Congress in Banff, Canada, that CISS should formally resign from membership of the ICC. With the signed agreement between ICC and IPC in place, clarification had been provided of the position of ICC in relation to the future – to fulfil its obligation to carry out its contract with the organisers of the Barcelona Paralympic Games. As Jordan wrote: 'Such matter is of no relevance to our organisation'. The decision of CISS to stand down from the International Coordinating Committee was not a surprise to the ICC members, and there was agreement that recognition should be accorded to CISS for its contribution to the work of the ICC in the past. Being objective about the precise impact of the elder statesman of organisations, CISS had gained very little benefit from its association with the ICC. The converse was true for ICC, however, with the more apparent global outreach of the umbrella organisation helping to persuade bodies like the International Olympic Committee that the International Coordinating Committee was the one to support in future.

John Grant, as the acting President of the ICC, had been surprised to learn while he was attending the meeting of the IPC in Lillehammer that the organising committee of the Winter Paralympics in Tignes was not happy with the dates of the Games. They had encountered some problems, and asked that the event be brought forward from March to January – this would cause a significant shift in preparation times. This also represented a major change in policy because the Paralympic Games would then be preceding the Olympic Games, rather than the other way around. Grant responsibly checked the feasibility of the suggestion with the Presidents of each of the participating international federations and, all having agreed, he wrote to the organising committee to say that ICC had reluctantly agreed to the change in arrangements. The next phase in this conundrum had two parts: the complaint of the athletes, and the action of the IOC. As the news of the proposed switch of dates from March to January spread around the Paralympic athletes, there was a general disapproval that January was not really the most suitable time for them to compete. A meeting was set up to discuss this. But at the same time the International Olympic Committee was gathering its own objections to the idea of the Paralympics being staged prior to the Olympics. It seems that it was this last influence that forced the arrangements to return to the original script: the Paralympics to follow the Olympic Games in March. André Auberger wrote to Jens Bromann expressing his frustration at the International Coordinating Committee's 'passive' behaviour in this, suggesting that greater assertiveness would have imbued the Paralympic movement with more self-assurance and stronger public standing. There would appear to have been little that the ICC could have done to impose its will on the Winter Paralympic Organising Committee (COPTA) in the face of the International Olympic Committee's insistence.

The status of the preparations for the Summer Paralympics had been discussed in a meeting with the Organising Committee, COOB'92. While there were some technical matters relating to the reallocation of spare places and the details of the second entry form, some important clarification was needed on aspects of classification. It was essential that the international federations should be able to handle the classification rules, rather than this being delegated outside the specialisms to general rulings. Michael Riding, Medical Officer, was full of praise for the arrangements in place for the Paralympic Summer Games. He had visited the facilities for medical treatment and found them to be of a very high quality. National teams were to have their own allocated provision for clinics in the Paralympic Village.

Relatively few overtly political issues affected the International Coordinating Committee or the Paralympic Games in this period, but there was a need for the Committee to discuss the re-admission of South Africa to the international sporting fraternity. The Barcelona organisers asked for clarification: the IOC had agreed to re-admit South Africa to the fold, as had the International Stoke Mandeville Games Federation. COOB'92 wished to know whether there was any intention of it being asked to provide places for South African Paralympic athletes. This clearly had not been something that the ICC had considered, and yet there were enough precedents already set for the ICC to agree that it would permit South Africa's participation in the Barcelona Paralympic Games if the IOC allowed its entry to the Olympic Games in 1992. This would have to be subject to the agreement of the international federations as well.

The ICC discussed some aspects of the structure of the IPC as it was taking shape. Hans Lindström described the different representation within the Interim Technical Committee of IPC, while Stan Labanowich said that the Technical Officers of the ICC federations were looking for a 'greater voice from a larger constituency' on the Sports Council of the IPC. The issue was that within ICC and the federations certain positions were *ex officio* and within IPC they were elected. The International Paralympic Committee would approve the admission of Technical Officers of each international federation as members of the Executive Committee of the Sports Council, at their next meeting in Hungary in November 1991.

At the February ICC meeting there had been an attempt to persuade the ICC to boycott the wheelchair demonstration events at the Olympic Games if the IOC did not change its attitude towards demonstration events for athletes who were blind. Jens Bromann revived the subject, and similar ground was covered: that everything that had been gained so far by the careful building up of trust between the IOC and the ICC would be lost if such a boycott happened. Bromann rejected the idea that ICC should treat the IOC as 'equal partners', but should rather prove that the different sportspeople in the different disability groups were treated equally. There was strong feeling that the integrity of the International Coordinating Committee was at stake. In the end Hugh Glynn proposed that it would be useful to mark the intention of ICC as 'trying to educate the IOC to include other disabilities in demonstration events'. Bromann insisted on voting on his original motion of boycotting the planned events 'if IOC still exclude the blind'. This was lost.

The members of the International Coordinating Committee reacted with dismay to information that the European Economic Community (EEC) was planning a seminar and the setting up of a European Committee on Sports for the Disabled. Jens Bromann wondered whether the ICC should take any action. Some members knew of this proposal, but those attending the ICC meeting had to acknowledge that there was little they could do: 'the EEC had power and money, we could not stop them only watch'. This was going to become something for the International Paralympic Committee's attention.

Athletes First, Disabled Second

Steadily through 1991 the problem of settling on a logo continued to take up time. There was no doubt about the reliance of the International Paralympic Committee on the International Olympic Committee, and as the IOC considered the Seoul 1988 Paralympics logo to impinge on its strategy of marketing and sponsorship, the IPC had to respond. Whatever wishes the member nations may have had for the IPC to make a stand and to retain what appeared to be rightfully its, there was also something to be said for a bold break with any approximation of the IOC's logo. This would mean the creation of something that the IPC could use to launch itself emphatically on the world. In the spring of 1992 this would eventually happen. The Executive Committee posed a number of vital questions: how reliant were they on the IOC grant?; was there such a thing as 'worldwide copyright'?; and even in which country the IOC might take the IPC to court if the IPC chose to defy it on the subject of the logo!

The 6th IPC Executive Committee Meeting and the 3rd General Assembly were held in Budapest, Hungary, between 1st and 3rd November 1991. Pal Nadas, President of the Hungarian Sports Association for the Disabled, and Deputy to the State Secretary of the Ministry of Sports and Education, welcomed the members.

Two of the elder statesmen of the international federations agreed in Budapest to draw more closely together. At the ICC Technical Committee meeting on 22nd November, Stan Labanowich (ISMWSF) told the representatives that the International Sports Organisation for the Disabled and the International

Stoke Mandeville Wheelchair Sports Federation (re-named to reflect its more clearly defined focus on wheelchair sports) had met to discuss bringing together more competitions under a common banner. It was thought that they would move towards combining the administration of the two organisations at some time soon. Filippo Dragotto (IBSA) voiced his hope that the motive behind the proposed amalgamation was not to make the joint organisation stronger than the others. In the Executive Committee of IPC there was concern voiced at the discussions the IPC President had had with ISMWSF examining a special agreement between the organisations. This would create yet another 'special relationship', as had been done with CISS. Although some members of the IPC Executive accepted the need for an arrangement with CISS, there was dissent from the view that the same recognition was sensible for ISMWSF. The IPC constitution should be enough, so thought some. Michael Riding emphasised that the problem arose from the multi-federational/multi-disability issue. Carl Wang and Hans Lindström proposed that constant liaison should be maintained with the international federations so as to ensure that 'all problems are resolved in a friendly and cooperative spirit'. This did not meet with the approval of everyone, but it was a compromise in the spirit of the International Paralympic Committee's mandate.

The delicate financial position of the IPC was made clear to the Executive Committee. In particular it was emphasised that quite a number of those attending the meetings in Hungary would be unsupported except by their own private funding. The IPC needed to establish the means to offer a greater base of support to the numbers of industrious members of the Executive Committee. Some national federations were helping with the costs of individuals attending meetings. Eric Russell asked whether it was really known what the true costs were of operating the International Paralympic Committee as an organisation – an impossible question at this time of establishing working patterns.

Michael Riding offered his Medical Committee's report, asking for approval of the position on doping control. He also informed the Executive that he was seeking assistance from Gudrun Doll-Tepper, of the Freie Universität Berlin, on exploring the best ways forward in sports science matters: 'this was a new thrust for the organisation and required innovative solutions'.

Rick Hansen and Anne Merklinger reported on the work of the International Committee on Integration. They were sensitive to the earlier criticisms of the Executive Committee relating to the all-Canadian membership, and the fundraising that had been done outside the parameters of the IPC Marketing Committee. Hansen described the frustration at the low response level to the questionnaire sent to nations, in the face of so many people identifying the importance of the subject of integration.

Membership numbers were rising, with the confirmation of admission of Brazil, Turkey and Zimbabwe. The three former Soviet states of Latvia, Lithuania and Estonia were judged eligible for membership. A decision on South Africa was questioned because, although the IOC had readmitted it, the Supreme Council of Sports in Africa had not. In the end South Africa was also accepted as a member of the International Paralympic Committee.

When Bob Steadward addressed the 3rd IPC General Assembly, the day after the Executive Committee meeting, he thanked Tamas Ajan, from the Hungarian Olympic Committee, for the welcome. Steadward spoke of his hope for positive meetings that would be conducted in an atmosphere of goodwill and friendship. The major issues identified by the IPC President were:

• support for the Sports Council and Sports Committees;
• more nations to bid to hold Games and meetings;
• to 'respect, support and work with CISS, as a lot of our work is absorbed by the other disabilities';
• large commitment to integration;
• growth of national Paralympic and regional committees;
• support for developing countries;
• that to develop 'an important and large image', finances and logo were needed.

In addition, Steadward specified that the two Executive Committee meetings in Belgium and Norway had thrown up issues of classification, minimum eligibility, multi-disability/multi-federational structure and demonstration events. The discussions were lively and fruitful at this General Assembly, attended by representatives from 43 countries and the six international federations. With South Africa admitted to IPC at this meeting, the number of bona fide votes was 239, of the 290 available within the membership.

Steadward announced that they had been successful in obtaining the agreement of the United Nations to a special recognition for the International Paralympic Committee. A 'Memorandum of Understanding' was signed with UNESCO, creating a formal relationship.

A very positive reception was given to André Auberger's announcement that a proposal for a Paralympic Solidarity Fund had been made: 'to cover the differences between rich and poor countries'. When Rick Hansen, Man in Motion, took the floor, he received a tremendous welcome from the General Assembly. Hansen described the work of the International Commission on Integration, stressing 'the importance of integration and sports for the disabled as a social issue'. He told the members that the inclusion of full medal events at major international competitions was 'a big step towards integration'. There had been some disquiet at the independence of action of this commission, and Hansen was keen to reassure participants that the International Commission on Integration was a part of the IPC, and would operate in close communication with the specific sports representatives to guarantee the greatest success. Bernard Atha commented that the present brief of the commission was too narrow: what would happen once they had achieved inclusion in the Olympic Games? Hans Lindström responded that Atha was quite right – there was a need for a broader policy on integration from the IPC as a whole. He took the opportunity of reassuring the General Assembly that integration into major championships would not threaten the future of the Paralympic Games.

The International Fund Sport Disabled had still not completed its realignment, but the General Assembly was able to appreciate that considerable support had been given to the secretarial work of the International Paralympic Committee.

Developing countries were to be aided through the energies of Horst Strohkendl, Peter Joon and Steffen Anderson. They had been instrumental in setting up the mechanism for helping developing countries through Stoke Mandeville before, and now they were asked to advise on the establishment of the IPC's own 'Development Committee'. The experience of the Project 001 work was shared, but the three put their minds to advising the IPC on what might be achievable. André Raes put a range of ideas to them: what to avoid, what to take on board, what scale of project, what content to plan and so on.

Winter Paralympic Games, Tignes 1992

The Games were in full swing. As the events were proceeding, members of the International Coordinating Committee were involved in the presentation of medals to athletes each day. The organising committee had generously supplied champagne and wine for the receptions held by ICC, and John Grant voted thanks to COPTA for its hospitality. As yet, however, there had been little opportunity to include the International Paralympic Committee officials in the proceedings – something that the ICC generously encouraged. André Raes asked for a greater involvement in the visible aspects of the Paralympic Opening and Closing Ceremonies, both in Tignes and in Barcelona. All agreed that this would be a good idea. The President of ICC and the President of IPC would discuss the best way of involving IPC in proceedings.

Michel Barnier and Jean-Claude Killy, Honorary Joint-Presidents of the Organising Committee (COPTA'92), declared: 'We attach great importance to the Paralympics, which, like the Olympic

Games, aim to highlight essential values: courage, perseverance, rigour, the desire to excel oneself' (Olympic Review 1992). 475 athletes representing 24 countries gathered at one of the venues just vacated by the Winter Olympic competitors. The rhythm of future Winter Paralympic Games was established at Tignes: use of the same venue as the Olympic Winter festival, and from these Games onwards to offset the dates of the Summer and Winter Games so as to have them in a different year from each other. The events at Tignes were limited to Alpine and Nordic competition, as there was no facility for ice-based sports. One of the outstanding athletes at Tignes was Katerina Tepla of the Czech Republic, who won three gold medals in Alpine events. She matched this again in Nagano. It was at Tignes that athletes with intellectual disability had the opportunity to participate in demonstration events in both downhill and cross-country. The biathlon joined the sporting programme for the first time in Tignes.

There would not be any exhibition events at the Winter Olympic Games this time, and there was some confusion about the cause. Walther Tröger had written to say that from the IOC's point of view the reason for the absence of exhibition events was the refusal of the French federation to permit them. But André Auberger, the federation's President, strenuously denied this claim. In a letter to Joan Scruton, Auberger pointed out that he had been the one to point out that there were no exhibition events in the preliminary programme produced for the Olympic Games when it appeared two years earlier. He put the blame squarely at the door of the International Coordinating Committee, saying that it was not for a national federation, or the Paralympic Organising Committee, to propose exhibition events to the IOC. Gilbert Felli, Director of Sport of the International Olympic Committee, had told Joan Scruton in a meeting that it was the Olympic Games Organising Committee (COJO), which had not been willing for the event to be held. He also stressed that the IOC did not have any influence as ICC had the contract rather than the IOC. From the year 2000 the contract with the International Olympic Committee for a country to organise the Olympic Games would include exhibition events as a requirement of the organisers. Because of the importance of public image, it was agreed that Joan Scruton would insert an article in the daily newsletter of the Winter Olympics to explain that neither the French Handisport Federation nor the ICC were responsible for the absence of exhibition events from the Tignes Winter Olympic Games. Unfortunately, although this article was written and submitted by Scruton, it was not published.

The exhibition events for the Summer Olympic Games in Barcelona were firmly cemented into the programme. There would be a selection event in New Orleans, and the Barcelona Organising Committee (COOB'92) was financing the travel costs, board and lodging for 16 athletes and seven delegates. Bob Wade and Chris Cohen would be the Technical Delegates. There was some disquiet from the Italian Federation that there had not been consultation about the location of the trials, as it had wanted to host a selection event in Italy. This was a case of the international federations not being involved in the decision making, and Stan Labanowich acknowledged that wider consultation should have taken place. The Presidents of IPC and ICC would be guests of COOB'92, along with John Grant as President of ISMWSF, from whose organisation most of the competitors in the exhibition events would be drawn.

The IOC had been asked for payment of the second part of the promised subvention. Joan Scruton explained to the gathered members of the ICC that the response from Walther Tröger had coupled the withholding of the money to the use of the *Tae-Geuk* logo. Scruton insisted that ICC was not using the symbol for any commercial purposes, but the IOC pointed to the continued use of the logo on ICC letterheads as unwillingness to act on the matter. Gilbert Felli had advised Joan Scruton the day before to write directly to Juan Antonio Samaranch to ask for the subvention to be paid. She should indicate that the International Coordinating Committee would be dissolved following the Barcelona Paralympic Games. When the final report of the Winter Paralympic Games was presented, it showed a very healthy surplus of some US$70 000 which the Organising Committee had proposed to donate to the Residence Handisport. This was agreed to be a very worthwhile cause.

IPC is Hot on the Heels of the ICC

Immediately following the meetings of the International Coordinating Committee, the IPC held its own meetings. The 7th IPC Executive Committee meeting was also held in Tignes, from 29th to 31st March 1992. André Auberger could only attend the third day of meetings due to his involvement in the organisation of the Winter Paralympics – as President of the French Handisport Federation.

The delegates attending the meetings were well aware of the importance of 1992 as the year in which the International Coordinating Committee would fulfil its final obligations by seeing the completion of the Tignes Albertville Winter Paralympics and then the Barcelona Summer Paralympics. The responsibilities would then fall to the International Paralympic Committee to help take the Paralympic Movement forward into the future.

Financially, things were not looking as desperate as before: relations with the International Fund Sport Disabled appeared to be improving, especially as discussions were heading along the lines of promoting a single fundraising body for sport for athletes with a disability in the world – a possible future role for IFSD? There was a meeting pending with the International Olympic Committee that would help clarify the next subvention. Meanwhile, progress had been made with IBM, which was looking into support in practical provision of equipment, and Crédit Lyonnais, which was on the point of making a significant subvention.

The bid progress from Atlanta was reviewed. Things were better advanced than at the last IPC Executive Meeting, and a formal bid had been submitted. Harald Hansen, Chairman of the Atlanta Paralympic Organising Committee (APOC) told the Committee that its bid had the full support of the US Government 'at the highest level', and that its umbrella organisation (CSOD) and the Atlanta Olympic Committee endorsed the bid for the Paralympic Games, with financial support promised. It was agreed that the Atlanta bid should be accepted, subject to a suitable contract being constructed. The Tignes meeting also gave the opportunity for an introduction to the bid from Nagano, Japan, to host the 1998 Winter Paralympic Games. Mr Ite, from the Nagano Bid Committee, was introduced at the meeting. Although the gathered IPC members were impressed with the Nagano bid, they had a little bit of time until the deadline for bids arrived, and wished to wait before making a final decision. Meanwhile the Sport Technical Committee could study the details of the bid and advise the Executive for its next meeting.

Michael Riding raised the subject of drug testing for athletes with intellectual disabilities at the Executive Committee meeting. At the present juncture these athletes were not being tested. But Riding felt this could not continue for long without outcry from other athletes: 'there would be no justice at all if all other athletes could be dope tested and the Mentally Handicapped not'. Riding then proposed a motion that the participation of any athletes with intellectual disability in the 1994 World Championships must be on the condition that the Legal Committee had clarified the status of their testing. This was strongly supported in the vote. As there had been bids from Berlin and Sweden to host the 1994 World Championships in athletics and table tennis respectively, including events for athletes with intellectual disability, this was an important problem to sort out.

The plans for an international congress to be held in Canada in May 1993 were presented. The Vista '93 International Symposium was to be a milestone in the extension of sport science into the subject of sport for people with disabilities. Bob Steadward was acting as Chairman of Vista '93, and it would be held at the Rick Hansen Centre, University of Alberta.

Rick Hansen himself gave a presentation on the work of the International Commission on Integration. The Commission had circulated some proposals for the inclusion of full-medal status events at the Atlanta Games, with three possible plans. Unfortunately the plans were criticised because all three precluded blind athletes from participation, and appeared to give the impression that all sport for persons with a disability was wheelchair-based. It was agreed that something must be taken to the negotiating table with the International Olympic Committee, and that the IPC President should use 'Option 3' (wheelchair marathon for male T54 athletes, wheelchair basketball for male IWBF athletes, 100 m freestyle swimming for female S9 athletes, and standing table tennis for male class 6–10 athletes) as a guideline for negotiations with the International Olympic Committee.

During the planning stages for the 1993 IPC General Assembly Bob Steadward suggested that a congress should be held in Sydney during the time that everyone was gathered. He thought that the focal points should be: minimum disability; functional classification; integration; and developing countries. The venue for the meeting later had to be changed to Berlin.

Sports without Limits: Barcelona Paralympic Games

The Barcelona 1992 Paralympic Games provided the opportunity for the 22nd Meeting of the Executive Committee of the International Coordinating Committee, held at the Mapfre Hotel on 30th August 1992. Jose Maria Villa, representing COOB'92, welcomed the ICC delegates to the Games and offered his help in solving any problems members might have. He described some of the ways in which awareness was being raised among members of the public. Specially adapted buses were being used for the first time in Spain. Alberto Jofre was directing affairs from the Coordination Centre, located together with the main organisation of COOB. Accreditation was running smoothly, and the schedule was being kept up in classification. Minor adjustments were needed at the venues for shooting and powerlifting, but these were in progress. Media attention was very strong, with 42 television channels represented in Barcelona, and requests from 1300 members of the press for accreditation.

Even in the earliest stages of preparation there were a few problems being encountered by the ICC members. Hugh Glynn voiced his concern that there were countries present at the Games that were not members of ISOD: the same was thought to be true of ISMWSF, according to Joan Scruton. Some concern was noted about the amount of promotional material appearing on some competitors' clothing. Jofre insisted that the same principles as for the Olympic Games were being applied at the Paralympic Games – although he acknowledged the severe financial difficulties of some countries in getting their teams to the Games. Individual countries should contact COOB'92 'who might be able to waive some of these rules'. Once the Barcelona Organising Committee representatives had left the meeting, Jens Bromann voiced his concern that COOB'92 had only sent out the detail of the regulation on advertising one month before the Paralympics were due to begin. It had been relatively normal for competitors to bear promotional material on clothing other than sports clothing, and some teams felt compelled to buy new outfits just before leaving for the Games because of the regulations – an unwelcome expenditure, and one that could have had a longer period of notice. Guillermo Cabezas suggested that this important subject would have to be one for the International Paralympic Committee to pick up.

The great success of the Paralympics in Seoul had been slightly marred by the lack of effectiveness of communication between essential members of the ICC and the Organising Committee. Pagers were issued to many of these key people in Barcelona in order to improve their accessibility. For a little while some difficulties followed the issue of the pagers, as they gave their information in Spanish, but a short tutorial was all that was needed to permit those carrying the pagers to switch them to English usage. During the Games the ICC representatives were provided with a car and driver, as well as a personal assistant. COOB'92 was proving to be highly efficient.

The exhibition wheelchair demonstration races in the Olympic Games were a great success. The spectators were highly appreciative and a high level of excitement was evident in the stadium. In the evening a dinner was hosted by ICC for participants and officials. The Barcelona Olympic Games were just spectacular in every way: a Paralympic archer, Antonio Rebollo, lighting the Olympic Flame at the Opening Ceremony in front of 100 000 spectators; the astonishing success of Vitaly Scherbo (Unified

Team) winning six golds in gymnastics, the unbeatable US basketball 'Dream Team' of NBA professionals; the return of South Africa to the Olympic Games; a unified Germany; and Linford Christie (UK) a surprise winner in the 100 m sprint event.

While the Barcelona Paralympics were underway, final preparations were being made for the competitions for athletes with intellectual disabilities, which were being hosted in Madrid. This was the first such venture: both events were under ICC purview, but the Madrid Games were to be completely funded by INAS-FMH. Fernando Vicente responded to questions from François Terranova (ICC Technical Officer) on the organisation of the competitions in Madrid. Athletes had qualified according to qualifying standards set in advance. The competitions were entirely parallel to the events of the corresponding international federation without any adaptation for particular disability. The competition was 'open' – no classification was taking place. Vicente responded to the question of whether they hoped to participate in the Paralympic Games in Atlanta by insisting that 'they were going to demand the right to be able to take part'. Elizabeth Dendy asked how the organisers managed the complication of bringing together athletes from different countries where there were differing principles used for defining mental handicap. The contemporary definition of mental handicap maintained by the World Health Organization related to individuals with an IQ below 70. The issue was one being examined closely by INAS-FMH, with a common definition being drawn up that might be proposed for use by every country.

Practical difficulties encountered in Barcelona by the athletes with cerebral palsy were the first topic for the meeting on 3rd September 1992 between the Barcelona Organising Committee and Guillermo Cabezas, Joan Scruton and Francois Terranova. The escalator in the dining room was of such a speed as to cause problems for some athletes, and Cabezas asked for a few volunteers to be on hand to assist individuals to carry food trays on the escalator. Other wrinkles in the otherwise smooth-running Games included a need for clearer and more numerous signs and notices to offices and rooms where meetings were to take place. The international federations were not finding the ICC Secretariat easily, and this needed the attention of the organisers. Always the epitome of tact and diplomacy, Joan Scruton praised the organisers for their efficiency and support for the work of ICC. She emphasised the need for excellent communication, and the wide distribution of daily bulletins giving details of changes in venues and of meetings taking place. One particular inconvenience was that the transport for officials of ICC could not drive into the Village because the appropriate accreditation had not been allocated to the drivers. The convenience of such a facility was rendered much less effective when the officials themselves had difficulties with mobility. The Organising Committee gave statistics to the ICC representatives: 3029 athletes had been accredited with 1046 accompanying officials, giving a total of 4175 in total for the national delegations. From the perspective of officials, 251 referees had been welcomed, along with 56 classifiers, 24 technical officials and 21 sports technicians.

An irregularity had arisen with regard to the Unified Team. Their Chef de Mission was invited to the breakfast meeting of ICC and COOB to explain how substitutions had been made to enable athletes not originally entered to compete in the Paralympics. The prevalent political situation in former Eastern Bloc countries was complex and not altogether stable. At first only Russian athletes had entered for the Paralympics in Barcelona, but COOB'92 later specified that a Unified Team would be encouraged. Entry forms were then sent out to Byelorussia and the Ukraine, although the Russian entry form had already been received. So as to be seen to embrace the competitors from the other states, the organising committee permitted substitutions to be made for existing named Russian competitors. To make this possible COOB extended the entry deadline for the Unified Team. Oleg Scheppel, from Byelorussia, legitimately replaced Temir Bulatov of Russia for the 400 m. However, Scheppel indicated on his arrival at the Paralympic Village in Barcelona that he also wanted to be able to compete in the long jump and the high jump events. Similarly Kolmykov of the Ukraine provided a conundrum for the assembled representatives of ICC and COOB. He had, in fact, never been entered at all but arrived on 5th September with his request to be permitted to compete in the high jump, long jump and relay events.

While COOB suggested leniency, the ICC officials felt that the competitors had not used earlier opportunities to bring their requests forward, and the precedent set in this case would prejudice the other 98 requests they had received for late entries to be considered. As a result of this consultation the two athletes were prevented from entering the events – with the exception of Scheppel's legitimate entry in the 400 m race.

Returning to the Mapfre Tower Hotel on 13th September, the Executive Committee of the International Coordinating Committee ran through the various subjects that had been covered in the regular breakfast meetings. Guillermo Cabezas was only just managing to be heard, not due to the rowdiness of the members of the Executive Committee, but because he had steadily been losing his voice as the Games had progressed.

The two athletes involved in doping offences, and their sanctions, were discussed. A Hungarian athlete and a South African athlete had been separately detected as having contravened the regulations and the Medical Committee had investigated their cases. Testing programmes had been present for many years, but the problems were growing in both Paralympic and Olympic Games. The Hungarian was found to have a steroid present in his urine, and he later admitted taking a performance-enhancing substance that was on the banned list. He was stripped of his medal and sent home. He would be banned from international competition for four years. The case of the South African was quite different because it was judged by the Medical Committee that he had not been advised by the South African Sports Association for the Disabled that the medication he was taking contained a banned substance – it was also judged that he was not intending to enhance his performance by taking the substance. The Medical Committee recommended that the South African athlete, who had already withdrawn from further competition, should be allowed to keep his medal. Guillermo Cabezas, as President of ICC pro tem, had approved the recommendations of the Medical Committee but the Executive Committee needed to ratify the decisions. Unfortunately, this was not to be the end of the doping problems relating to the Barcelona Paralympic Games.

As the members of the ICC Executive Committee were leaving Barcelona and heading for Madrid on 15th September, the B sample of an American wheelchair basketball athlete, David Kiley, was announced to be positive for dextropropoxyphene, a banned painkiller found in the prescription pharmaceutical Darvocet. As the athlete concerned had already left the country before the B sample was tested he was not in a position to make an appeal at the time. The recommendation of the Doping Commission in Barcelona was that Kiley was found to have tested positive for a banned substance, and should be 'suspended for a minor doping offence. The suspension is recommended as three calendar months.' When Michael Riding communicated this recommendation to ICC President Guillermo Cabezas, the latter sought the views of the Presidents of the international federations in membership of ICC, together with Bob Steadward as President of IPC. Their consensus was that the matter was to be treated more seriously, with the US team to forfeit the final match, and the medals awarded to the American team to be returned and reallocated (involving the Netherlands, Germany and France). Further sanction of David Kiley would fall to the sport's governing body. This was entirely in keeping with the ICC guidelines. The United States Disabled Sports Team requested a hearing, and was invited to attend the Larnaca meeting of the International Coordinating Committee in March 1993.

Another drug infringement was announced after the close of the Games: Vladimir Kazakov, a gold medallist in the judo (over 95 kg category), was found to have taken a performance-enhancing drug, norandolone. Kazakov, a member of the Unified Team, was stripped of his medal and banned for life.

A strange outburst had visited one of the medal ceremonies at the Paralympic Games. When Jack Weinstein had presented the bronze medals to the Korean athletes following the boccia event, the Koreans immediately removed their medals and threw them to the ground together with the bouquet of flowers. The boccia competition, appearing for the first time in the Paralympic Games, had been very hard fought with the Koreans being placed third behind the Danish and Spanish teams. The interest shown in this new event meant that the world's news media and television crews were well represented at the competition and the medal ceremony. The Koreans' protest related to a sport-specific rule regarding the reporting time prior to competition. After very lengthy debate between the Executive Committee members, Jack Weinstein proposed that the seriousness of the Korean team's actions warranted banning them from competition for life. Jens Bromann pleaded that people who were very severely disabled had few opportunities for participation in competitive sport, and boccia was a godsend. But it was thought important to maintain the same outlook as the International Olympic Committee in dealing with difficulties of this sort, just as the International Coordinating Committee had taken the IOC's lead in approaching drug abuse. Bromann recounted how journalists had commented to him that the Paralympic Games were quite different from the Olympic Games; they were 'elite games with a human image'. To prevent these athletes from competing for the rest of their lives was less humane than the Paralympic Movement professed to be. Bromann implored the Committee to consider the discrepancy when: 'a person who is banned for four years for taking drugs, be allowed to take part next time in Paralympic Games, while some Koreans who have made an emotional protest ... are banned from taking part in Paralympic Games for life'. At the vote there were five in favour of a life ban, one vote against the motion, with one abstention. The Irish team, having finished fourth in the boccia competition, were awarded the bronze medal in place of the disqualified Korean team. Following the conclusion of the Paralympic Games there was further thought on this matter and it was considered that the enforcement of the sanction on the Korean athletes would be a matter for the International Paralympic Committee, and a letter was sent to the Korean Paralympic Committee saying that the competitors were to be banned from the next Paralympics. This was clearly not in keeping with the decision taken by the Executive Committee in Barcelona, and the matter would surface again at the final meeting of the ICC in Larnaca. Eventually the ban was lifted for these Korean athletes from the end of the Atlanta 1996 Paralympic Games.

In a less notable demonstration, a Canadian athlete was disciplined by his team for being aggressive towards two Spanish athletes. The Canadian wished to run a lap of honour following his victory but the Spaniards, who had placed 2nd and 3rd, ran in front of him, spoiling the Canadian's moment. He became abusive towards the other two athletes and officials prevented him from running a lap of honour.

As the Paralympic Games closed it was traditional for the flag to be handed over to the president of the organising committee for the next Paralympic Games. This part of the Closing Ceremony was particularly poignant for the members of the International Coordinating Committee, who would also be seeing the demise of their organisation soon afterwards. The Executive Committee was not happy with the proposal of COOB'92 that the protocol was to be that 'the flag would be passed from the President of ICC to the President of ONCE to the Mayor then to Mr Fleming of APOC'. There were all sorts of complications to iron out: Jack Weinstein felt that the protocol should be for the flag to go from the Mayor of Barcelona to the Mayor of Atlanta, but Jens Bromann pointed out that the Mayor of Atlanta was not in Barcelona. Joan Scruton also commented that the President of the Barcelona Olympic Organising Committee and the Mayor of Barcelona were one and the same person. Weinstein emphasised that the International Paralympic Committee had to be very visible in this process as well. François Terranova suggested that the same procedure could be adopted as at Tignes for the Winter Paralympic Games: the flag was handed from the President of ICC to the President of IPC, then from the President of COPTA to the President of the Atlanta Organising Committee. This looked like the right protocol, and the next day's breakfast meeting with COOB'92 would confirm it. Some sort of statement was also going to be needed to announce that the International Coordinating Committee would be concluding its work and closing down business, handing on all responsibilities to the International Paralympic Committee. This would be announced to provide a respectable period following the Madrid Games. Elizabeth Dendy stressed that the ICC should make more effort to show recognition of the Madrid Games.

The financial position following the winding up of ICC was clarified. Once the expenses of the meeting in Barcelona had been cleared, it was proposed by Jens Bromann and seconded by Bob Steadward that any remaining funds be transferred to the International Paralympic Committee. This was not to the liking of all those present, the vote being tied with three votes for and three against. This meant the motion was lost. Bob Steadward then proposed that the US$10 000 should be made over to each of IBSA, ISMWSF, CP-ISRA and ISOD. Because the INAS-FMH still owed the same amount to ICC for the agreed capitation payments from the Madrid Games this seemed a fair outcome.

The International Paralympic Committee's newsletter, *The Paralympian*, looked back at the Barcelona 1992 Paralympic Games ten years on, from the perspective of 2002. The perspective of time has not dulled the effect of the Barcelona Games on some of the most significant members of the Paralympic Movement:

> The Paralympic Games in Barcelona were the first of their kind, crowned with success, which highlighted to the world the human quest for great sporting achievements. They were a collective undertaking which . . . make all those involved very proud. We should however, once again pledge to continue supporting the development of sport for athletes with a disability. (Juan Antonio Samaranch)

> The Barcelona Games were my first as a technical delegate and not as an athlete . . . On the second evening, 12,500 spectators packed the Badalona basketball arena for Spain versus USA and 4,000 potential spectators were turned away. Barcelona '92 turned Paralympic sport into elite spectator sport. Thank you Barcelona! (Phil Craven, IPC President, Technical Delegate for Wheelchair Basketball in 1992)

> I have now been to three Paralympics and I belong to a very special group of athletes. Barcelona was the beginning of it all. I will never forget my first Paralympic gold medal and the feeling of having it around my neck with the anthem being played and the Australian flag raised up high because I was the best in the world. Barcelona gave me the taste and I wanted more. (Louise Sauvage, Athletics, Australia)

> When the ISOD President Guillermo Cabezas informed me that Barcelona would take the Paralympic Games with the condition that classification would be by sport and not by disability, I hugged him. When I accompanied Her Majesty Queen Silvia of Sweden to a Swimming event at the Barcelona Games, we both saw how perfectly everything was set up. I had to explain the tears in my eyes to Her Majesty, saying that I had never expected to see this true recognition of athletes with a disability in my lifetime. (Hans Lindström, Secretary General of ISOD and IPC Technical Officer 1989 to 1997)

> Barcelona was, together with the Paralympic Games in Seoul in 1988, a turning point for the Paralympics, with a single triad for the first time: Same country, same city, same facilities as the Olympic Games. This seems very regular now, but it was a huge victory at the time. (François Terranova, IPC Vice President, ICC Technical Officer for Barcelona Games)

> If asked for the greatest experience in my 20 year-long wheelchair sports career, then Barcelona and Sydney are always mentioned in first place. Barcelona gave a completely new dimension to the Paralympic Games, provoked by the pride and sports enthusiasm of the Catalan people. We stayed in the best Olympic and Paralympic Village that I have ever seen. (Heinz Frei, Athletics, Switzerland)

> In Barcelona the Paralympics came of age. I have many happy memories: the professionalism and commitment of the organisers, the excellent facilities in a beautiful and friendly city and the enthusiastic support of the crowds. What more could athletes ask for? (Elizabeth Dendy, President CP-ISRA in 1992)

> The Barcelona 1992 Paralympic Games were a magnificent opportunity to use sport as a vehicle to get across our message of integration and normalisation for the disabled, an aim we have been striving to achieve for more than 64 years now. I honestly believe that the major achievement of Barcelona '92 was to bring dignity to disabled sportsmen and women and, as a result, to all persons with a disability. (José María Arroyo Zarzosa, President ONCE)

> Every day throughout the Games, we noticed long queues of people who were excited about catching every event. It was the first time we experienced such overwhelming public support. As well, the

Paralympic Summer Games in Barcelona represented a historic milestone for the IPC with the official handover of the Games from the ICC to the IPC. (Bob Steadward, IPC President in 1992)

The city took a whole-hearted interest in the competition, previously of a secondary character, setting these games in the limelight. In addition to the city's physical transformation, the legacy of the Barcelona 1992 Olympics and Paralympics included the civilities and participation of the people of Barcelona and the confidence we showed as a city. (Joan Clos, Mayor of Barcelona)

I believe the most powerful impact was standing on the podium and hearing the American Anthem for the first time being played during the award ceremony. This was a very emotional and monumental moment for all athletes who were able to hear their national anthem after winning a gold medal. This huge step could not be made without the help and commitment of the Organising Committee of the Barcelona Games. (Trischa Zorn, Swimming, USA)

The *Paralympian*, no. 4, 2002

Paralympic Congress in Barcelona, September 1992

Scientific meetings had long been associated with major sporting events. A conference had been held in 1980 at Ustaoset, Norway, coinciding with the 2nd Winter Paralympics at Geilo. This had been called the 'First Medical Congress on Sports for the Disabled' and featured 30 papers, mostly presented by speakers from Scandinavian countries. However, two papers were presented by Bob Steadward, then of the Canadian Paralympic Sports Association. The Congress at the Barcelona Paralympics was being called the First Paralympic Congress, held from 31st August to 3rd September. Manuel CaJudo Pinillos, President of the Organising Committee, recorded that the Congress had welcomed over 800 participants, representing 86 countries. He recognised the impact the Congress and the Paralympic Games were to have on the people of Spain: spreading awareness of the great opportunities for athletes with a disability, and encouraging governmental support for projects in his country in future. The First Paralympic Congress was made possible through the cooperation of three organisations: Organisatión Nacional de Ciegos Españoles (ONCE), Federación Española de Asociaciones de atención a las Personas con Minusvalía (ASPACE), and Federación Española de Deportes de Minusválidos Físicos (FEDMF). Financial support had been forthcoming from the Fundación ONCE, International Fund Sport Disabled, Coca Cola and various municipal and regional offices of government.

The conclusion of the Congress led to a number of plenary recommendations. The spirit of the few days' meetings is shown in the unified and dynamic expression of the recommendations. The vision of the founder of the modern celebration of the Olympic Games, Pierre de Coubertin, was invoked in the very first recommendation: just as de Coubertin was convinced of the social value of competitive sport, the Congress called for Paralympic sports: 'to be integrated into the Olympic framework in order to combat the lack of importance that society places on any forms of competition taking place outside the Olympic framework. This "relegation to a second division" takes place irrespective of how important these events are.' Although cautious, there were calls for international governing bodies of sport to include events for athletes with a disability in their world and regional championships. This had been steadily on the increase already, partly due to the weighty influence of the International Olympic Committee and the work of the ICC in past years. Grass roots development was needed on a long-term basis in order to encourage normalised attitudes towards integrated participation. This could be enabled by the widespread adoption of appropriate strategies for adapted physical activity in educational settings. Governments were called upon to legislate for the security of financial support for national programmes and organisations for athletes with a disability. The work done over the past ten years by the International Coordinating Committee was recognised by the Congress, while the participants expressed their 'unwavering adherence to the International Paralympic Committee', and respect for the international federations. Developing countries needed greater levels of practical assistance in order to bring on their programmes, and the Congress endorsed all support to those countries that could be embraced by others.

The high levels of media presence in Barcelona made it clear to all participants at the Congress that here was the start of a much higher profile for their activities. The Congress recommended that all participants should be mindful of the potential for greater positive exposure, while also calling on the world's media to 'approach the sports movement of the physically handicapped with the highest degree of sensitivity and objectivity'. Democratic representation within international federations was recommended by the Congress, including active encouragement for the participation of athletes in the government of their own organisations. Research in the specific fields relevant to sports for athletes with a disability had to be better coordinated and more widely recognised. The separate meetings at the Congress afforded the opportunity for numerous technical examinations of particular sports regulations, bringing together the many officials, scientists and coaches who worked hard to enable the athletes to perform at their best. There were recommendations for amendments to rules and structures of separate sports events, and there was further progress in the classification debate.

The conclusion of the First Paralympic Congress was heartened by the words of the President of the International Olympic Committee on the rostrum. Juan Antonio Samaranch spoke with great feeling about his personal connection in the development of relations with the Paralympic Movement: he was in charge of sport in Barcelona in 1968 when Guillermo Cabezas was elected President of the newly formed Spanish national federation of sport for athletes with a disability. Here they were again, one President of IOC and the other President pro tem of the International Coordinating Committee. When Samaranch was elected to his position as President of the IOC in 1980 he began to encourage a single international umbrella organisation to speak on behalf of sports for athletes with a disability. This permitted IOC funding to be released, and other influence could be brought to bear by the IOC. Samaranch recounted the gradual appearance of demonstration events in the Olympic Games, beginning with Sarajevo in 1984 and followed closely in Los Angeles. He identified that there was still a need to persuade the Organising Committee of the Atlanta Olympic Games to agree to host the Paralympics as well. He was hopeful and promised to do his best to succeed, but he acknowledged that it was dissatisfying for those passionate about the Paralympic Movement to have to wait for a 'yes' or 'no' from Atlanta. Finally, Samaranch tantalised the delegates at the First Paralympic Congress by telling them that he was just finishing the draft contracts for the organisers of the 2000 Olympic Games, and that he believed there was still time to write into these contracts: 'that the city that has the luck and the honour to be chosen for the Games of the year 2000 will also be obliged to organise the Paralympics (in this case the XI Games) a few weeks later'. What could be a more positive message for the gathered delegates to hear from the President of the International Olympic Committee?

FAREWELL TO THE ICC

Our Origins are not Nearly as Important as our Destination

Just before delegates packed up and headed home, the International Paralympic Committee Executive met informally for what it called a 'business meeting'. On 7th and 10th September, discussions ranged over a number of very practical matters. The budget was high on the priority list: the IOC had been helpful, but wanted a four-year plan, with fewer details. Also the IOC wanted the IPC to acknowledge that some income should be derived from marketing. The marketing aspect was also raised with Andy Fleming of the Atlanta Paralympic Organising Committee (APOC) in attendance. A businessman from Atlanta, Mr Bevilaqua, was able to advise on approaches that could be made to those corporate sponsors who had not been successful in gaining recognition from the Olympic Games programme as official sponsors. Bevilaqua had been helping the Bidding Committee for Atlanta, and had applied to be retained by the Atlanta Paralympic Organising Committee. He suggested that these sponsors might be interested in taking up significant stances in the funding of the Atlanta Paralympic Games. The figures being talked about were in the range of US$6 million for Official Sponsors, with a $500 000 contribution to a Paralympic Sports Foundation. Bevilaqua International would stand to gain 17.5% commission. The logo again became a contentious subject: Bevilaqua had been in touch with Copeland Design to come up with some ideas, with the approval of the IPC President. The future involvement of the IPC with Bevilaqua International would be dependent on the company gaining the marketing concession with the Atlanta Paralympic Organising Committee – the decision would be on 5th March, when APOC was to meet.

Anne Merklinger gave a brief report on the work of the former Commission on Integration – the name had been changed now to reflect the mandates of the group: the 'Commission for the Inclusion of Athletes with a Disability' (CIAD). Bob Steadward had submitted a formal proposal to the IOC for the inclusion of full medal events in the 1996 Summer Olympics. Meanwhile the Commission had been successful in having events included in the 1994 Commonwealth Games in Victoria. The agreement made included the development of distinctive medals, accommodation within the Athletes' Village, full accreditation and inclusion in Opening and Closing Ceremonies. The athletes would be entered for: men's open wheelchair marathon, men's open 800 m wheelchair, women's 100 m freestyle swimming (S9), women's lawn bowls singles (visually impaired), and men's lawn bowls singles (visually impaired). Although the work of the Commission was appreciated, Martin Mansell, the Chairman of the Athletes' Commission, voiced the concern shared by athletes that the inclusion of events in the Olympic Games could divide the sportsmen and sports women into 'privileged and non-privileged athletes'. A greater value could be accorded to the participation in the Olympic Games than in the Paralympic Games. The Athletes' Commission needed to give direction on this subject. But the work of the CIAD must go forward.

Although the next General Assembly had been planned for Sydney, the Secretary General had received a letter to say that Sydney had withdrawn the invitation for financial reasons. This prompted the decision to build in a number of obligations on the host city of the Paralympic Games at the contractual stage, including the hosting of a General Assembly three years before the Paralympic Games and an Executive Committee meeting one year before. Effectively this would give a pattern of meetings that was clear and predictable in future: 1993 Executive Committee meeting in Lillehammer, 1995 General Assembly in Nagano, 1995 Executive Meeting in Atlanta, 1997 General Assembly in the city to host the 2000 Paralympic Games, 1997 Executive Committee meeting in Nagano, 1999 Executive Committee meeting in the city to host the 2002 Paralympic Games. It remained to find a host for the forthcoming General Assembly.

Alberto Jofre of the ONCE Foundation was introduced to the meeting. The foundation was enormously influential and financially supportive of the Barcelona Olympic Games. It had given US$8 million for the preparation of the Games, and was also very much involved with the Paralympic Games Organising Committee.[1] Jofre had met with Samaranch after the Paralympic Congress had closed. In that meeting, several subjects were covered that really should have been matters for the International Paralympic Committee. Jofre explained that the meeting had originally been for another purpose but had meandered in the direction of the inclusion of events in the Olympic Games. Apparently they discussed the acceptance of between seven and nine full medal events at the 1996 Olympic Games and the agreement that the IOC would try to 'convince Atlanta to involve the Deaf Paralympic Games'. The

---

[1] Miguel Sagarra, Secretary General of IPC, has confirmed that the budget for the Paralympic Games in Barcelona was 9500 million pesetas, the contribution from ONCE Foundation being 3800 million pesetas. With an average exchange rate of 1US$ = 120 pesetas, the contribution of ONCE Foundation would have been US$31.6 million in total.

reaction among the IPC Executive members was dismay that another organisation could have this level of discussion on matters so fundamental to the dealings between the IOC and the IPC. Of course neither IOC nor IPC could ignore the financial input of ONCE, and no one wished to give offence to a potential or actual donor. Jofre apologised for the fact that the discussion with Samaranch had headed on to IPC territory; it was 'a mistake', and he asked that ONCE should work cooperatively with IPC. When Jofre had left the meeting, the IPC representatives agreed that they needed to meet with and listen to the ONCE people, preferably before having another meeting with Samaranch. Jens Bromann emphasised that everyone must get the clear message that IPC represented sport for people with disability, and that the IOC should not have dealings with others – even if one tolerated its relationship with Special Olympics. Bromann went on to inform members that ONCE had, in fact, been one of the organisations 'against the establishment of the IPC. ONCE was strictly against having one strong unified disabled sports organisation.' But ONCE was a member of the International Blind Sports Association, and IBSA was represented in IPC. The best idea would be to encourage a relationship with ONCE as a sponsor, as André Auberger emphasised: 'sponsors will never be allowed to dominate the IPC'. It was considered that the national representation of the IPC would prove to be the strength in the end, and this would reduce the threat of any impact from an aggressive organisation – if this was what they were experiencing.

Steadward and some other IPC Executive Committee members met with Jofre, Duran and Sanz of ONCE on 10th September. The meeting was positive, and calmed several misgivings of the IPC. ONCE had no wish to take over at all. Steadward stressed that the different organisations working in the same field needed to operate together. ONCE was working to integrate blind people into society, and sport had an obvious place in this process. Duran wished to ensure that ONCE helped the IPC to achieve its own goals, but he was also keen to clear up any misunderstandings. Enrique Sanz and Alberto Jofre were nominated to meet with IPC representatives to explore ways that ONCE could help in future.

Manchester Welcomes the International Paralympic Committee

A very full agenda was planned for the interim meeting of the IPC Executive Committee when delegates met in Manchester, UK on 5th and 6th December 1992. Congratulations were extended to Elizabeth Dendy on her election to the Presidency of CP-ISRA.

Bob Steadward had met Juan Antonio Samaranch earlier in the year, and discussed the status of negotiations about the IPC logo. The Lillehammer Organising Committee would continue to use the five *Tae-Geuk* logo, as any changes at this stage would affect the position with sponsors. Carl Wang considered that 'the LPOC got the impression that President Samaranch let go the logo problem for Lillehammer in 1994'. Steadward confirmed that this was already in place for 1994. While talking to the IOC President, Steadward had taken the opportunity of raising the subject of inclusion of events in the Olympic Games.

The Manchester meeting once again welcomed Rick Hansen to talk about progress in the Inclusion Commission. There was a concern that the inclusion of athletes with intellectual disability at the Atlanta Olympic Games might lead to the incongruous position of these athletes being permitted to compete in the arguably higher profile event, when they were still being prevented from entering the Paralympic Games because the Legal Committee still had to clarify the position of drug testing of athletes with intellectual disability. Another problem would arise if athletes competing in the Olympic Games did not then also compete in the Paralympic Games: the very highest tier of competitors would have been filtered towards the Olympics. At the other end of the spectrum was the question of the rights of the severely disabled to be involved in the Olympic Games as well. For them the public perception of what constitutes elite athletics would be the issue. Finally, a straightforward question was put to Anne Merklinger: had the athletes themselves been involved in the consultations about the ideal programme to take forward to the IOC? Merklinger explained that they had not been consulted. Martin Mansell, the

Chairman of the Athletes' Commission, emphasised that the athletes were vital in this process because they needed to understand the principles behind the policies. They were supportive of demonstration events, but had still to be convinced that full medal status events were valuable to the Paralympic Movement. The real ideal was most clearly stated by Eric Russell (Australia), describing the Olympic Games demonstration events as an opportunity to 'promote sports for people with a disability through a window that the world is looking at'. Having demonstration events within the Olympics and keeping the integrity of the Paralympic Games served the Paralympic Movement best.

New sports to the Paralympic Movement were evolving as more and more people with disabilities found expression and enjoyment through physical activities. The Executive Committee enjoyed an animated debate about 'what constitutes a sport'. This was sparked off by the announcement that wheelchair dance was becoming more formalised, and approaches had been made to include it as a sport of the International Paralympic Committee. Elizabeth Dendy was sceptical about wheelchair dance being a sport. Hans Lindström confirmed that ISOD had wheelchair dance under its umbrella. He considered that half of the world thought it constituted a sport and the other half disagreed – he believed the same was true of chess. Elizabeth Dendy also threw lawn bowls into the melting pot; the sport had only limited regional participation, and she was 'anxious that we do lose it from the Paralympic programme'. Carl Wang joined the debate, emphasising that wheelchair dance had already held two European Championships, with the third taking place the next year. Wang supported the inclusion of wheelchair dance in the IPC programme. As neatly as possible, Hans Lindström turned the discussion towards the sports calendar, and the arrangements for World Championships in 1994. Most sports had venues for their championships, with a few more under discussion. Only swimming and lawn bowls still needed venues and willing organisers.

With the arrival of Andy Fleming to the meeting came the disappointing news that there was a difficulty between the Atlanta Paralympic Organising Committee (APOC) and the Atlanta Olympic Organising Committee (ACOG). The Olympic Organisers would not include the Paralympics in their bid to host the Olympic Games. ACOG said that it had 'never considered taking the Paralympics on board'. Extensive discussion between the two Atlanta groups still had the same outcome. The gesture that had been made by ACOG was to pledge US$10 million towards the budget identified by APOC as $50 million. Andy Fleming also told the IPC Executive Committee that a marketing agreement had been signed with ACOG to 'eliminate any confusion between Olympic and Paralympic sponsors'. The agreement compelled APOC to only approach Olympic sponsors, still talking about 'big money'. Companies like Coca Cola had shown interest in the worldwide opportunities (at $8 million), but they wanted to be confident that the input would find appropriately genuine targets: the IPC and the Paralympic Movement more broadly. Fleming advised the IPC to 'develop a very clear explanation as to how these funds are going to be spent'. One critical issue that received attention in the public domain later was the restrictive management of the marketing practices by the two Organising Committees and the United States Olympic Committee (USOC). An aspect of the agreement on marketing was that no approaches could be made by APOC or IPC to competitors of Olympic sponsors, without the permission of the Olympic sponsor. Andy Fleming explained that his committee had considered trying to go it alone, but the control in the hands of the Olympic Games Organising Committee meant that the Paralympic organisers could possibly be 'locked out of the Olympic venues, because ACOG has contracts to control the venues far beyond the closure of the Olympic Games'. In fact the criticism of the marketing agreement was heightened when, according to Andrew Jennings: 'The US Olympic Committee . . . demanded a share of the royalties raised by the Paralympics' mascot, a lively bird named Blaze. They didn't just want them during the Games – they wanted a cut long after the event was over' (Jennings 1996). This dispute was settled in favour of APOC, rejecting the USOC's demands.

Delicately, Bernard Atha took the Executive Committee through a paper on the participation of athletes with intellectual disabilities. He demonstrated that he was aware of all the pitfalls and misgivings already made clear by people recently, but Atha was very coherent in his purpose. His premise was that it was appropriate to have a very limited programme of events at the Atlanta Paralympic Games. He suggested that these competitors should have minimum standards stringently applied, and that people with learning difficulties should not be admitted to the Paralympic Games. Only the very highest standards would be acceptable. In the opinion of Atha the 'more severely handicapped and the multiple handicapped are taken care of in other games and other activities'. André Auberger called for a very gradual progress. He stressed that the press would be watching very closely, and 'we cannot permit the Games to be discredited'. According to Martin Mansell, the athletes' assembly in Barcelona had not really understood the differences between the purposes of INAS-FMH and Special Olympics; most had only heard of Special Olympics anyway. Ever practical, Hans Lindström put the technical perspective. In his view the area was more complicated because of the relatively early stages of development of sport for people with intellectual disabilities in some countries. He felt that the leadership in those nations was still one of: 'don't send athletes but rather patients to participate'. Because of the diversity of interpretation it was only possible, at the moment, to subject the athletes to minimum standards. With a sign of greater openness, the Executive Committee voted to include athletes with intellectual disabilities in the Atlanta Games, with the details of the programme to be worked out between INAS-FMH and the IPC Technical Committee.

The Paralympic Programme Committee had arrived at a list of sports to be included in the Paralympic Games: archery, athletics, boccia, cycling, equestrianism, fencing, goalball, lawn bowls, powerlifting, shooting, soccer, swimming, table tennis, wheelchair basketball, wheelchair tennis and volleyball. Snooker and billiards were being removed from the list, and it was recommended that judo, wrestling and wheelchair handball should be removed as well because there had not been any entries received. The Programme Committee recommended that sailing should be included in the Atlanta Paralympics, and that racquetball should be admitted as a demonstration sport. The Executive Committee wanted more work to be done on sailing before including it even as a demonstration sport. Wheelchair dance was going to be referred to the winter sports programme. After an appeal by Elizabeth Dendy, the status of judo in the Atlanta Paralympic Games was discussed again, and led to a decision to keep it under consideration for the moment.

Lengthy reports had to be received on the ever-more complicated subject of finances: as the IPC was in line for more subventions and donations, the accounting became more intricate. Although no contract had yet been signed by Bevilaqua International and the Atlanta Paralympic Games Organising Committee, Bob Steadward and André Auberger had met with representatives of the ONCE Foundation. ONCE had agreed to donate to IPC the computer software developed and used in Barcelona at a cost of US$6 million. For this the International Paralympic Committee had to agree to make it available to other organising committees free of charge. Beyond this, Steadward had informed ONCE of IPC's suggestion that ONCE should contribute $10 million for four years. André Auberger concluded that he thought they would receive at least $1 million once the ONCE Board had met in February 1993.

The burden of sorting out the IPC logo seemed to be reducing. The recommendations from the Copeland Company public relations experts was that a three *Tae-Geuk* symbol, in red, green and blue, associated with the words 'Mind, Body, Spirit' was the best representation of the image and philosophy of the International Paralympic Committee. Further discussion among key members of IPC took this suggestion forward, and the IPC Executive approved the idea with some relief.

The International Federation for Adapted Physical Activity (IFAPA) had contacted the IPC with a view to becoming involved in IPC activities. IFAPA was a sport science oriented organisation with a broad remit, including elite sport, recreation and physical education. It would certainly have a positive input to make in the Sport Science Sub-Committee. Michael Riding offered to look at the possibilities together with some of the Medical Committee members, and present some views at the Lillehammer meeting. Bob Steadward thought there could be a benefit in IFAPA becoming involved in work on the Paralympic Conference Committee.

One more topic found its way into the forward-looking discussions in Manchester. Steadward informed the Executive Committee members that he had been in consultation with the International Olympic Committee about helping to support the redevelopment of sporting structures in Eastern Europe. The IPC obviously needed to promote a growth of stability and ease of communication in the former Soviet states, and Steadward had offered the assistance of the IPC in an area that was definitely going to benefit the operation of the IPC itself. Gilbert Felli (IOC) had been in touch with Jacques Rogge (Belgium), in his role as President of the European Olympic Committee, asking for assistance in the process of supporting the establishment of National Olympic Committees in these countries. There was even a possibility that National Paralympic Committees could be integrated within the National Olympic Committees in the Eastern European countries – especially as some countries would be starting from scratch.

Larnaca Send-Off to the International Coordinating Committee

The International Coordinating Committee met for the very last time in Larnaca, Cyprus, on 24th and 25th March 1993. The Sandy Beach Hotel, about seven kilometres outside Larnaca, provided an appropriately relaxing location for the saying of farewells as the ICC was wound up. Jack Weinstein should have been present as President pro tem, but he had been forced to withdraw from re-election as President of CP-ISRA because his member organisation could not support him in office financially. As a result he could not preside over this final meeting of ICC. The representatives at this historic meeting were:

Elizabeth Dendy, President pro tem (CP-ISRA)
Jaap Brouwer (CP-ISRA)
Colin Rains (CP-ISRA)
Jens Bromann (IBSA)
Bjorn Eklund (IBSA)
John Grant (ISMWSF)
Claude Sugny (ISMWSF)
Donald Royer (ISMWSF)
Guillermo Cabezas (ISOD)
Hugh Glynn (ISOD)
Bengt Nirje (INAS-FMH)
Bob Steadward (IPC)
Hans Lindström (IPC)
Carl Wang (IPC)
Michael Riding (IPC)
Joan Scruton (Secretary General)
Kate Lambrechts (Minutes Secretary)
Sergio Blanco (Interpreter)

Even with the winding up of the ICC at this meeting, there was still important business to do. The inconsistency of the action taken over the Korean boccia competitors featured early in the Larnaca discussions. While the ICC could be seen to have questions about the legitimacy of a life ban, it was certainly guilty of being muddled in its messages: the letter sent to the Korean Paralympic Committee did not convey the true severity of the sanction decided by the ICC. In the end it was agreed that the Boccia Committee would have the problem placed in its lap 'bearing in mind the discrepancy between the motion made (in Barcelona) and the letter sent to the Koreans'. A statement was added to the Barcelona minutes of 13th September: 'This meeting regrets the confusion that has occurred as the result of the letter sent to the Koreans. We accept the motion that has been recorded in the minutes but regret that the letter sent to the Koreans did not reflect this. Further development to be left to IPC.'

Representatives of the United States Disabled Sports Team attended the Larnaca meeting to present their appeal on behalf of David Kiley, who had failed a drugs test after the victory of the US team in the wheelchair basketball final. Paul de Pace, Chef de Mission at Barcelona, read out a statement from the team coach, Harry Vines, who could not be present in Cyprus: Kiley had been in notable pain very late at night on 8th September, resulting from an injury to his toe while training in France prior to the Games, and had been unable to rest recently or get any sleep, so he had been offered Darvocet as a painkiller by his coach. Harry Vines' deposition categorically stated that he had checked 'the pamphlet' on banned drugs and did not find Darvocet listed there. De Pace asked that the circumstances under which the banned substance had been taken should be considered when deciding finally on whether to confirm the proposed sanctions. Evidence was heard from David Kiley and Dr Gregory Pelutsis, team physician, before the US delegation withdrew. Phil Craven, who had been the ICC Technical Delegate at the Barcelona Games, and President of the International Wheelchair Basketball Federation, asked to attend the meeting in Cyprus. Craven stated that the IWBF wholeheartedly supported the ICC policies, and wanted an opportunity to hear the full story, and to wish for: 'a fair outcome in the best interest of Paralympic sport'. He had contacted numerous people connected with the case immediately following the end of the Barcelona Paralympic Games, and he had squarely accused the ICC of overreacting to the infraction. In Craven's view, wheelchair basketball had made great progress as a result of the Games, and the publicity surrounding a scandal of this sort would be highly damaging for the future of the sport. It would be a pity to allow the incident to 'gain proportions way above the actuality of what happened'. There had been some concern among the Executive Committee involved in the immediate discussions that Phil Craven's obvious interest in the case could lead to the perception that he was leading the USDST appeal, rather than appearing in his impartial international leadership role on behalf of ISMWSF and IWBF. At one point at the end of January Joan Scruton wrote to Paul De Pace to say that as all documents appeared to have been widely circulated, including correspondence with Phil Craven, Elizabeth Dendy, ICC President pro tem believed 'no purpose could be served by Phil Craven's coming to Larnaca'. Craven had expressed considerable anger to Jack Weinstein late in September 1992 at the way the case had been handled by the ICC Executive: the announcement of a positive test had been made by Michael Riding in Barcelona before the subject had been discussed by the ICC Executive Committee, and Riding informed Mike Mushett, Deputy Chef de Mission of the US Team, of the proposed action to be taken. Kiley was a spectacularly successful athlete: a multiple gold medal winner in different Paralympic events in previous Summer and Winter Paralympic Games. Phil Craven was given an opportunity to comment further. The sanctions were out of proportion to the seriousness of the transgression, said Craven. As Michael Riding had confirmed, the amount of the banned substance found in the sample was a trace, suggesting that this was not a major infraction. Craven emphasised that Kiley having taken the Darvocet did not affect the outcome of the final in any way. The Executive Committee of ICC then discussed the case in great detail. Michael Riding wrote to Joan Scruton on Christmas Eve 1992, giving his opinion of the case for the benefit of the hearing: the drug dextropropoxyphen was clearly listed on the IOC banned list under Schedule B; the athlete did not disclose that he had taken the drug although he had opportunity to do so at the testing stage; as a prescribed drug the distribution of it to another party could be considered an illegal act in USA and in Spain. The hearing discussed the details further before confirming the decision that the US team would be disqualified from the event, with medals being returned and redistributed. A two-year ban was levied on Kiley for his infringement of the doping regulations.

The finishing touches were still being put to the report from the Barcelona Paralympics, and the ICC meeting was informed by Juan Coll that the Games had suffered a very significant deficit. The costs were covered by the Organising Committee and the ONCE Foundation.

The official report of the Madrid Games organised by INAS-FMH was presented in Larnaca. Bengt Nirje told of the gathering of athletes and officials from more than 70 countries, numbering some 2500 in total. He explained that this number was more than had been originally planned, and there was strain caused to the systems of organisation by this overload. Transportation had been the worst affected. The sporting events had been very good, with the basketball particularly successful. Standards of officiating were variable in several areas, but things got better as the competitions progressed. Nirje expressed his assessment that many nations would have drawn meaningful motivation from their participation in this world event.

The Larnaca get-together was a celebration as well as a farewell to ICC as an organisation. Of those who could attend the meeting, four people had also attended the very first ICC meeting on 11th March 1982 at the Second World Championships in Winter Sports for the Disabled at Leysin, Switzerland. They were Hans Lindström, Claude Sugny, Jens Bromann and Joan Scruton. These last two had actually attended each and every meeting of the International Coordinating Committee – on more than 20 occasions altogether. A gala dinner was held to celebrate the completion of the work of the International Coordinating Committee, and the handing over of the reins to the International Paralympic Committee. This was a festive and light-hearted occasion, recorded on celluloid by Bengt Nirje.

Almost two months later, Joan Scruton accompanied the circulation of the minutes of the Larnaca meeting with a letter dated 18th May 1993. In sending it she carried out the last duties as Secretary General of the International Coordinating Committee. She informed the Presidents of the international federations that she had written to the United States Disabled Sports Team asking for the return of the gold medals for the wheelchair basketball event at Barcelona. She had also written to the relevant organisations in the Netherlands, Germany and France to inform them of the action taken. Scruton confirmed that she had arranged the transfer to the four federations of the funds agreed at the last meeting. And with that the International Coordinating Committee's role was complete.

CONCLUSION

The magnificence of the Barcelona 1992 Paralympic Games was a fitting tribute to the work of the International Coordinating Committee. Its role in supporting the Organising Committee exhibited the very best cooperation and communication that was possible in the preparation of such a splendid sporting festival. The same was true of the 1992 Paralympic Winter Games in Tignes, with the subtle differences that have always distinguished the Summer from the Winter Paralympic Games. The final gatherings of the ICC served to tidy up loose ends, handing over a healthy Paralympic Movement to the new guardians, the International Paralympic Committee.

Blending the work for the future with a sensibly paced handover from the ICC, the International Paralympic Committee continued to bolt together the machinery for a permanent, modern world organisation. Very few problems were created by the waning influence of the International Coordinating Committee; everyone now accepted that the principles of representation had shifted to a structure with a national voice rather than dominance from disability sports organisations. But the same people who had been so heavily involved in the former days of the Paralympic Movement willingly offered their experience and expertise to the good health of the International Paralympic Committee.

Some different problems were going to face the International Paralympic Committee in the next stage, but these were going to serve to build the character of the new organisation, rather than threaten it. The future was faced with hope, and with great appreciation for the work of the ICC.

CHAPTER 6

Spirit in Motion: 1992 to 1996

OVERVIEW

The Paralympic Movement had completely redefined itself in the period from 1982 to 1992. While businesslike negotiations had to continue for the Paralympic Games, and each spectacle seemed to add more and more superlatives to our vocabulary, the guardians of the trust and hopes of the athletes had been working towards the establishment of the International Paralympic Committee (IPC).

As the IPC grew in confidence as an organisation, aspects of its operation became routine – although no less important for their regularity. The calendar of sporting events was balanced over a four-year cycle, and provided a steady schedule of work in progress. This was a very specialised and dedicated international organisation emerging from the 1980s into the 1990s. The structure of the International Paralympic Committee was to be closely analysed by all stakeholders: they wanted to invest still more energy in fine-tuning the organisation. The Paralympic Movement had matured in its demands, and needed such a mechanism as the International Paralympic Committee to keep the Movement's ideals foremost, and to service the needs of a more focused, specialised and knowledgeable group of athletes.

The next period in the history of the Paralympic Movement can be explored more thematically, dividing the time into convenient phases. The periodisation follows the cycle of Paralympic Games: from Barcelona to Atlanta, via the Lillehammer Winter Games (1992–1996); from Atlanta to Sydney, via the Nagano Winter Games (1996–2000); and from Sydney to Athens, via the Salt Lake City Winter Games (2000–2004). Using these phases we can see certain themes reappearing consistently as the main concerns of those involved in the Paralympic Movement: the relationship with the International Olympic Committee; finances; inclusion and integration; preparation for Paralympic Winter and Summer Games; technical issues; doping; minimum disability; athletes with intellectual disability and so on. Some themes would have prominence for a while but would not be of equal concern throughout all phases.

Prominent in this decade of the Paralympic Movement was the willingness of the International Paralympic Committee to delve into its soul and interrogate its effectiveness. This was exactly how the IPC was created: from the International Coordinating Committee looking to restructure its operation and the 1987 Arnhem Conference determining that an altogether different format was most relevant to the contemporary situation. The Düsseldorf meetings in 1989 brought the IPC into being. In this section we will see that the effects of speedy expansion of the International Paralympic Committee led in 1995 to the formation of a Task Force to propose a revised structure. This was presented to the 1996 Extraordinary General Assembly in Atlanta. Not every interest group was satisfied with the process or the results, but the IPC moved on to work with its renewed mandate.

Athlete First: A History of the Paralympic Movement   Steve Bailey
© 2008 John Wiley & Sons, Ltd

'THE FUTURE OF IPC – WHAT DO YOU WANT?' – FROM BARCELONA TO LILLEHAMMER

In preparation for the General Assembly in September 1993 an Ad Hoc Committee produced some statements relating to the future of the International Paralympic Committee for members to consider. Members had an opportunity to comment on the paper. The IPC was wanting to acknowledge that it was ending its first four years in existence: from the meeting in Düsseldorf in September 1989 to the 4th General Assembly in Berlin in September 1993. The consultative document was entitled: *The Future of IPC – What Do You Want?* As the Paralympic Movement faced its first independent years, it is valuable to see how the 'insiders' assessed their movement. The content of the document helps identify how the organisation perceived its own position in relation to its membership and its purpose:

> The International Paralympic Committee promotes and develops the Paralympic Movement through a united voice for athletes with a disability around the world. The IPC is:
>
> - The recognised world leader and resource for persons with a disability within the sport community
> - An organisation comprised of national member organisations of sport for athletes with a disability
> - An international multi-sports federation that promotes and supports the ideals of the Paralympic Movement
> - An organisation that provides athletes with a disability with their choice of a range of quality sport opportunities in the environment of their choice at the level of their choice.

The document then asked the members to review the statement and make additions, deletions and clarifications. Values important to the International Paralympic Committee and its operation were then declared:

> The values of the IPC are:
>
> - It will not discriminate or tolerate discrimination of any form (including racial, faith, political, gender, disability or age)
> - Mutual respect and understanding for all involved in sport
> - Sport should be athlete centred i.e. organisational decisions should be made such that they are in the best interest of the athletes and athletes should be involved in the decision making process
> - Honesty, integrity and fairness.

The member nations were asked to indicate whether these values 'reflect the kind of behaviour you would like to see in the IPC?'

The Ad Hoc Committee identified issues that would need particular attention from the IPC and its membership. The members were asked to prioritise these and also to indicate any additional topics, or suggest that a topic should be deleted. The fact that these themes were highlighted at this time allows analysis of the contemporary concerns of the participants in the Paralympic Movement and in the administration of the International Paralympic Committee. It also permits a consideration of the similarities between the issues of the present day and those of the 1990s. Many of the fundamental issues that were central to providing the very best opportunities for athletes with a disability would remain the same years later. Conversely, certain topics had only a temporary episode under the spotlight; they were specific concerns that were assessed and resolved or tolerated.

The topics listed by the Committee were, in order:

- Involvement of athletes with mental handicap in the Paralympic Games
- Roles, responsibility and relationships between IPC, IOC and the International Federations (e.g. FINA, IAAF)
- Sport specific development and autonomy

- Classification
- Minimum disability
- Revenue generation or financing
- Research training and education priorities
- Including events in able bodied competitions – strategies and priorities
- Place of recreation in IPC and sport specific development models
- Integration with able bodied sport

Finally, this worthwhile exercise concluded with statements of the International Paralympic Committee's goals. They were introduced as defining the organisation's 'major areas of emphasis':

- To promote, support and develop the Paralympic Movement worldwide
- To facilitate communication and liaison amongst member federations and sport commissions of IPC
- To develop and maintain ongoing communication with international sport and multi-sport organisations
- To promote and support sport specific development and to promote the autonomy of sports through inclusion into the relevant able bodied international sports federation
- To facilitate the organisation of Winter and Summer Paralympic Games
- To include events for athletes with a disability in major international competitions
- To seek the integration of sports for athletes with a disability whilst safeguarding and preserving the identity of sports for athletes with a disability.

In his Presidential Report to the 4th General Assembly, Bob Steadward made it clear that he had no magic formulas for the challenges and issues the Movement would face. The delegates were located at the Hotel Radisson Plaza, Berlin, where Friedrich Ruth, the Vice President of the Berlin 2000 Olympic Bid Committee, had warmly welcomed the Executive Committee the evening before. The IPC President expressed his willingness to bring all his energy, enthusiasm and commitment to the development of the Paralympic Movement over the next quadrennium, 1993 to 1997. He articulated his attitude in the following words: 'Coming together is a beginning; staying together is progress; working together is success'.

Administration

The process of opening up contacts between the IPC and other sports organisations was enhanced by its acceptance into membership of the General Association of International Sports Federations (GAISF) at a meeting on 24th October 1992. Admission as an associate member was agreed unanimously by the GAISF General Assembly.

National Paralympic Committees (NPCs) were a big feature of the period from Barcelona to Lillehammer, with the IPC writing to all National Olympic Committees to seek their help in establishing NPCs in their country. If a country had already gathered all disabilities together in one representative body, as rarely happened, then a National Paralympic Committee was unnecessary.

The role and effectiveness of regional representatives and committees would take some time to clarify, but it was entirely logical for Elizabeth Dendy and John Grant to propose, in March 1993, that the Far East and South Pacific Games for the Disabled (FESPIC) be recognised as the official representative body for the South Pacific and East Asia areas, encouraging the election of a regional representative to attend IPC meetings. Bob Steadward had attended the meeting of the FESPIC Board of Directors in March 1992 in Guangzhou, China. Carl Wang would energise the European membership into forming an effective regional body as well. This subject had remained a passion of Wang's; he had first suggested to Ludwig Guttmann at the ISOD General Assembly in 1979 that the cause of sport for athletes with a disability would be stronger for the establishment of regional committees.

Elizabeth Dendy addressed the 1993 IPC General Assembly in Berlin on the official winding up of the International Coordinating Committee. The final ICC meeting in Larnaca, Cyprus, in March 1993 had bittersweet memories, but Elizabeth Dendy reminded the assembled IPC delegates that they owed much to the international federations, and that the Paralympic Movement would still need to look to these organisations as a central part of the family. Dendy presented the President of the IPC with a cheque for US$40 000, representing the agreed sharing out of ICC monies (US$10 000 for each of IBSA, ISMWSF, CP-ISRA and ISOD). In response Bob Steadward thanked all the Presidents and Secretary Generals of the international federations for their dedication during the twelve year period of the ICC. In particular Steadward paid tribute to Joan Scruton for her 'great support, her integrity, leadership and commitment to sports for disabled, to which she devoted her life'.

The Berlin General Assembly saw representatives from 47 countries meeting together, with 6 international federations bringing the total number of votes to 247. New voting members included the Czech Republic, Guinea, Moldavia, Croatia, Slovenia and Slovakia, after their membership was ratified. Armenia had applied for membership and received observer status at the General Assembly – its application would need scrutiny to ensure that it met with all IPC conditions. Applications pending were: Honduras, Kazakhstan, Uganda, Belarus, Ukraine and the United Arab Emirates. The restructuring of Europe was certainly extending the membership of IPC, along with a natural process of expansion due to the maturity of the Paralympic Movement.

The IPC Constitution could never be seen as a perfect document set in stone, and the General Assembly immediately faced complications as a result of the technicalities of the voting arrangements. The international federation representing deaf sports, CISS, objected to the proxy voting that enabled some delegates who were not deaf to vote on behalf of the deaf sports organisation in their own country. This was contrary to the constitution of CISS, which had its own special relationship and agreement with the International Paralympic Committee. Only people who were deaf could represent them. But in six countries the mandate had been given to the representative who could attend the General Assembly, who happened not to be deaf. In another complication, CISS also objected to the refusal of the voting system to permit the deaf representatives from one country to represent the deaf from another country. Bernard Atha recommended that it would be even-handed to insist on the IPC Constitution being upheld at this meeting, but for the Executive Committee to discuss the specific requirements of CISS, putting a proposal before the next General Assembly. So, for the Berlin voting, those countries with membership of CISS would be allowed to vote for the deaf athletes of their country.

CISS expressed its discontent at the communication system within the IPC structure: the IPC Secretariat would send correspondence to the 'national contact address' for a member country, but the effectiveness of distribution of materials or information would be totally dependent on that body's actions. In some cases the national contact address was a newly established National Paralympic Committee, in others it was an existing disability sports organisation or a government department.

The Sports Council Executive Committees felt that their work was fundamental to the purpose of the International Paralympic Committee – as it obviously was. However, the constitution of IPC failed to give them an automatic voice in the General Assembly. Hans Lindström presented a statement to the General Assembly requesting the establishment of the principle that the Sports Council Executive Committee Chairpersons could speak at General Assemblies. Voting rights had already been denied to these Committees when voted on the day before, but the General Assembly did agree to permit these crucial representatives to speak on the issues of great concern to them.

While the senior officers of the IPC (President, Secretary General, Treasurer, Technical Officer and Medical Officer) were returned unopposed to their positions, the 4th General Assembly held a secret ballot to determine the other people to take the IPC Executive Committee on for the next four years.

Jens Bromann defeated Carl Wang, Reiner Krippner, Miguel Sagarra and York Chow for First Vice President; Nabil Salem was elected Second Vice President over Miguel Sagarra, Carl Wang and James Neppl; Members at Large were to be Marie Little, York Chow and Colin Rains.

The CISS had made an independent agreement with the International Paralympic Committee that it would cooperate within the umbrella of the IPC, but that it wished to retain its own major sporting events and not be involved in the Paralympics. In 1993 the CISS Congress gave serious consideration to participating in the Paralympic Games. When the Executive Committee of the IPC considered the letter from CISS, the immediate concern was the implications for the size of the Games of adding deaf athletes – the World Games for the Deaf in Sofia had seen 1700 competitors. To be able to respond properly, the CISS letter had to be circulated to national members and international federations for comment, and a report constructed that could be considered by the Executive Committee. The Paralympic Movement had managed so far with the exceptional appendage of CISS to its normal activities, but the impact of total involvement would be significant, albeit a welcome fulfilment of the aims of uniting all disabilities. The subject was brought into discussion at the 1994 Lillehammer Executive Committee meeting of the IPC, and the representatives were very welcoming. Up to this point there had been reluctance on the part of CISS to fully involve itself in the activities of IPC, except to attend meetings. There had always been the understanding that the International Paralympic Committee benefited from CISS's willingness to be part of it, because the IPC could be acknowledged to be truly representative of all disability groups. Now Jens Bromann and André Raes proposed that CISS should be admitted to full membership of the Paralympic Movement if it asked. Should this request be made it would make redundant the agreement in place, and put CISS into the same relationship as the other international organisations for sport for persons with a disability. Any eventual participation in the Paralympic Games would have to be determined by the Sports Technical Department. A very important feature of the Lillehammer discussion was the agreement that CISS should be asked not to withdraw from the agreement already in place with IPC, should it decide not to seek the altered status of membership with IPC.

At the Lillehammer Executive Committee meeting, Bob Steadward recommended four individuals who had served the Paralympic Movement outstandingly in management of the Lillehammer Winter Paralympic Games. The Gold Order was awarded to Gerhard Heiberg, President of the Lillehammer Paralympic Organising Committee (LPOC); Silver Order went to John Magdall, Managing Director of LPOC; Bronze Orders were presented to Lill-Unni Ostern and Rolf Jenssen, Venue Consultants.

One international competition that broke new ground during this period was the 1993 Mediterranean Games, held in Languedoc-Rousillon, France. André Auberger had maintained close contacts with the organisers, who were willing to include athletes with a disability in a manner not so far experienced. As was reported to the IPC Executive Committee in Berlin in September that year: 'For the first time in an international able-bodied event, disabled athletes were fully integrated, receiving full medals, participated in the parades of Opening and Closing Ceremony and the number of medals of disabled athletes were added to the number of medals per nation'. This was great progress in the acceptance of sport for athletes with a disability.

International Olympic Committee

In a summary of the meetings between the IPC and the IOC over the first four years, André Raes noted that they covered a relatively narrow range of topics: financial support, integration of IPC (competition, administration and marketing), the logo and the relations between both headquarters. Juan Antonio Samaranch had boosted the prestige of the International Paralympic Committee when he wrote in December 1992 to announce that the IOC Executive Board had voted to grant the IPC 'official recognition'. The International Paralympic Committee had now become a 'Recognised Organisation'. For his part, Walther Tröger also wrote to the IPC President in February 1993: 'From the beginning of this important year you and your committee have obtained full responsibility for the coordination of Sports for the Handicapped worldwide, as well as the future of the Paralympics'. As the IOC Delegate for the Disabled (and President of his National Olympic Committee) Tröger offered his 'continued assistance and advice in matters of mutual concern'. A useful meeting had taken place in May 1992 between Dick Pound and Bob Steadward, with a number of IPC and IOC representatives present. This was a straight-talking meeting in which Pound made the problems relating to the IPC logo very plain: the IPC five *Tae-Geuk* logo was 'confusingly similar' to the Olympic Rings. The agreement was reached for IPC to launch a new logo and therefore release more funds through IOC subvention and income derived from marketing. Somehow, while being told how the IPC had behaved badly over this subject, Steadward still managed to ask insistently for further funding from IOC to help produce a new logo. The three *Tae-Geuks* emblem was launched. The IPC emblem was being protected in the Benelux countries: the name 'Paralympics' and the motto 'Mind, Body, Spirit'. In 20 other countries, the IPC undertook to protect the trademark for a fee of US$250 for each country.[1]

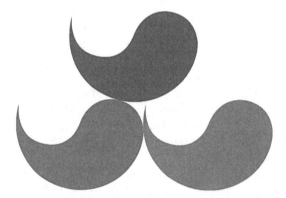

Identity is fundamental to any organisation, particularly in its infancy. So the International Paralympic Committee needed to pave a clear path for itself that would serve to mark the identity of the organisation it wished to be. Carl Wang voiced the elementary, but indispensable question to the Executive Committee: 'What is the exact relationship between the International Olympic Committee and the International Paralympic Committee?' This question would most likely produce a different reading of 'temperature' at different times during the life of the Paralympic Movement, but in March 1993 the question was aimed at the connection between the cities bidding for Olympic Games and the staging of the Paralympic Games. André Raes told Wang, and the other members gathered in Lillehammer, that those cities bidding for the Olympic Games were asked whether they intended also to bid for the Paralympic Games. Raes went so far as to add that 'the next step will be to include it in the Olympic Charter. If not included, IPC will establish its own Charter.' Of course, the hypothetical IPC Charter would not carry any weight unless the influence of the International Olympic Committee was applied, to suggest that bidding for both Games would improve their standing in the competition to be awarded the Olympic Games.

Bob Steadward and André Raes had the opportunity of meeting with the IOC President on the occasion of the World Athletics Championships in Stuttgart in August 1993. In the company also of Walther Tröger

---

[1] The Benelux registration was extended to 18 countries in 1994 and was renewed in 2004.

and Gilbert Felli, the meeting with Juan Antonio Samaranch covered important updates. The inclusion of full medal events for athletes with a disability in the Olympic Games was discussed. Some concerns were raised about the effect on the marketing programme of the Atlanta Paralympic Organising Committee of the restrictive marketing agreement between USOC, ACOG and APOC. Although Samaranch would not be drawn, he indicated that he was in favour of a single organising committee for both Paralympic and Olympic Games, and he would encourage the two Atlanta committees to greater cooperation. Some restraint was evident from the International Olympic Committee, however, not wanting to make the IPC manual for bidding cities an integral part of the IOC manual. The IPC's bidding manual had been put together, and served to ensure a direct overlap. An important recognition of closer relationship came in the invitation of the IOC President for André Raes to attend the 101st Session of the IOC in Monaco on 23rd September, at which the decision for the host city for the 2000 Olympic Games would be announced. Samaranch agreed that the contract for the Paralympic Games would be signed soon afterwards.

The IOC support for the Paralympic Movement was reaffirmed in a very practical sense by Samaranch agreeing that the IOC would make a subvention of US$250 000 per year for 1993, 1994 and 1995. He wrote to Steadward in October 1992 to also tell him that the Vista '93 Conference in Jasper, Canada would be supported to the tune of US$45 500. These were welcome gestures of genuine help.

Finances

The promising connection with ONCE (Organisatión Nacional de Ciegos Españoles) was to have a disappointing start: André Auberger had to inform the IPC Executive that some restructuring within ONCE, following its elections in September 1992, had shifted the people the IPC had been dealing with. The economic downturn had also caused ONCE to step back a bit from its initial position. The IPC Executive Committee meeting in Lillehammer in March 1993 was told that the original assurance to the value of US$10 million would still result in the computer software used in Barcelona being given to the International Paralympic Committee, but the remaining US$4 million was very much in doubt. The Management Committee[2] had then submitted a proposal for a subvention of US$100 000, and was awaiting a response. The other type of support being considered by ONCE was practical help in printing the IPC Newsletter and the Handbook. It was heartening that ONCE was prepared to help the IPC establish a promotional and marketing system, and it would offer advice and expertise to complete this task. The computer software was available immediately, but as the manuals were only available in Spanish at that time, there was a delay while they were being translated.

Further information was available about the situation within the ONCE Foundation when the Executive Committee of IPC met in Berlin in September 1993. The Berlin meeting heard from André Raes that the smooth flow of the relationship between the two organisations was totally conditional on Miguel Sagarra being elected as Vice President of the IPC. As the Executive Committee Minutes state, André Raes explained that: 'The promised financial support as well as the printing of the IPC Handbook and Newsletter are subject to the election of Mr Miguel Sagarra as Vice President of IPC. In case of non-election, negotiations would have to start all over again' (IPC EC V/10/2 Item 5.2). This suggestion of pressure was not unique, but it makes international organisations vulnerable to particular influence, in exchange for support being proffered. Sagarra was not voted in. Although this may have been reported to IPC. it is not accepted as the accurate account of events.

---

[2] The Management Committee had been established in 1991 at the suggestion of Carl Wang that the IPC needed a means of managing the day-to-day business in between the biennial meetings of the Executive Committee.

Miguel Sagarra was named by the Spanish Paralympic Committee as its nominee for the position of Secretary General in 1997.

The IPC had not quite worked out the best way to address the wide differences between countries in membership. Developing countries were difficult to define, and more traditional criteria did not apply wholesale to the organisation. The General Assembly led to some limited discussion, but rejected the proposal that there should be distinctive membership fees charged to developing countries. André Auberger considered that all countries should have the same obligations and therefore the same rights; any difficulties a country might experience in paying fees could be adjusted using the Paralympic Solidarity system. Each country would be judged on an individual basis. The Executive Committee would need to formalise the principles that would allow this to function effectively.

Inclusion and Integration

Having united the nations, sports and international sports federations for different disabilities under one 'roof', the International Paralympic Committee needed to work to ensure that the phenomenon of the Paralympic Games was manageable. The Games initially had too many events and too many medals. Sport-specific functional classification was the effective way to progress, but problems followed this path as well. Integration of different disability groups in the same event meant that it was difficult to identify the concept of the 'elite' in sport. Also the range within the continuum meant that definition of minimum levels of disability was needed. Athletes with a severe disability were entitled to access to high-level competitive sport, and their inclusion tended to raise more complex reactions in the uneducated among the general public. As well as integration of disabilities with each other, there was an agreed objective to seek opportunities for athletes with a disability to compete in the programmes of international sports federations for mainstream sport. This tended to be referred to as 'inclusion'.

The regular updates on progress by Anne Merklinger or Rick Hansen are an indication of the importance of the subject of inclusion at this time in the Paralympic Movement. When the IPC Executive Committee met in Lillehammer in March 1993, Merklinger described the list of sports that had been reviewed by the Commission for the Inclusion of Athletes with a Disability (CIAD). The Executive Committee had provided some input, as had the international federations and the Sports Council. Now a proposal had to be put to the International Olympic Committee of a package of events that might be accepted as having full medal status within the Atlanta Olympic Games in 1996. The list put together for the IPC President, Bob Steadward, to present to the IOC comprised:

- two wheelchair track events;
- two wheelchair basketball events;
- two swimming events;
- two table tennis events (one sitting and one standing);
- two track events for blind athletes;
- two swimming events for athletes with intellectual disability;
- two track events (one for athletes with cerebral palsy, one for amputees).

At the same time, the Commission was looking for clear direction from the Executive Committee, and posed certain questions: What are the final objectives for CIAD in respect of the inclusion of full medal events for athletes with a disability in the Olympic Games and other major international competitions? What are the assessments of IPC on the impact of inclusion of full medal events in the Olympics on those same events in the Paralympics? And what are the assessments on the impact of the inclusion of full medal events on the Paralympics in general? These were fundamental questions, really asking the Executive Committee to be mindful of how far the subject should be taken.

Jens Bromann underscored the democratic intent of IPC by asking that no decision on the inclusion of the proposed events or agreements with the IOC should be made without discussion in the forum of the General Assembly, and without a mandate from that body. Hans Lindström emphasised that the General Assembly needed to work with concrete proposals, and Elizabeth Dendy agreed that preparatory work by a small group should establish specific recommendations for the September 1993 meeting of the General Assembly in Berlin. As had been noted before, the Athletes' Committee wished to be involved in these matters, and Martin Mansell indicated that extensive debate had been seen at the most recent meeting. The athletes asked for a presentation at their meeting from CIAD, and they wanted an input at the General Assembly. The earlier deficit of consultation of athletes had still not been attended to. This seemed very short-sighted in the context of 'ownership' of the Paralympic Movement: who were the beneficiaries of the principle of inclusion supposed to be?

In an attempt to establish something definite to take to the General Assembly, Hans Lindström and Michael Riding proposed to accept the list of events as presented by Anne Merklinger. The votes made it obvious that they would have to take a longer route to a solution: six in favour, four against, seven abstentions. Discussion followed, and another vote underscored the stalemate: seven in favour, seven against and three abstentions. Hans Lindström, Elizabeth Dendy, Colin Rains, Anne Merklinger and Martin Mansell would form an Ad Hoc Committee and draw up a background paper. Before sending it to the nations in the package for the General Assembly it would be circulated to the Executive Committee members to enable some feedback.

The ongoing disagreements over integration and inclusion became more vocal at the Berlin General Assembly of the IPC in September 1993. While the work done by Rick Hansen and his group relating to the inclusion of full medal events in the Olympic Games remained well received by the Executive Committee, the General Assembly was less welcoming. Similarly, Elizabeth Dendy's Ad Hoc Committee was to receive quite a grilling in the larger forum of the membership. But it was made clear to the 4th General Assembly that the work of Rick Hansen's Commission for the Inclusion of Athletes with Disability was part of the broader picture of integration. This also served to put the CIAD's status within IPC in a clearer light.

The main issues identified in discussion were the following.

- The priority of the IPC is the uninterrupted progress of the Paralympics, not integration.
- There is a lack of knowledge about the impact on the Paralympic Games, if some full medal events are included in the Olympic Games.
- That full medal status in the Olympic Games could encourage a split in the Paralympic Movement, creating two tiers of athletes and a less clear identity.
- That integration should ideally begin at the national level and work upwards.
- If suitably administered, full medal events in the Olympic Games 'could be a stimulus to enhance the events of the Paralympics'.
- Media coverage at the Olympic Games would advance public awareness.
- Integration would probably improve access to sports science research and training programmes.
- The process of integration must be evolutionary: gradual and adaptable.
- The IPC will be flexible enough when the time comes to make decisions about integration.

The report of the Commission for the Inclusion of Athletes with a Disability for the 4th General Assembly did emphatically identify the potential benefits of inclusion of full medal events in the Olympic Games. The report first explained what 'inclusion' means: 'that events have full medal status and are equal to other events on the competition programme; athletes with a disability enjoy the same privileges as all other athletes; athletes reside in the Games Village; athletes participate in the Opening and Closing Ceremonies; and athletes are full members of their national teams'. To try to explain the importance of including events in major international competitions, the report suggested that this would:

> mean full and equal participation for athletes with a disability; send a powerful social and educational message and generate positive social change; have a powerful impact at all levels of sport; help promote full inclusion in society for people with a disability; enhance the profile of the Paralympic Games; provide valuable linkages with potential corporate and media partners; enhance the profile of sport for athletes with a disability; increase understanding of the high level skills displayed by athletes with a disability; extend sport's ability to unify, preserve identity, redress inequities and abolish discrimination; mature attitudes in all aspects of community living by minimising social, attitudinal, environmental and physical barriers; provide inspiration for people around the world to overcome adversity; and extend opportunities for athletes with a disability to compete in world class competition.

Rick Hansen's commission saw inclusion in the Olympic Games as just one of a list of opportunities for athletes with a disability. The other components available to participants might include: Paralympic Games, multi-disability, multi-sport world games and championships, single-sport world championships, single-disability world championships, regional championships, national championships, events with full medal status for athletes with a disability in major able-bodied competitions. It was clearly the intention of the Commission to reduce the claim that opportunities would be lessened by pursuit of inclusion in the Olympic Games. According to the CIAD, all disabilities and all existing sports on the Paralympic Games programme would be eligible for consideration.

The list of events for submission to the IOC, agreed at the Lillehammer meeting, was revised after it became obvious that some aspects of the IPC charter were not being followed in relation to equality of opportunity. Gender equity was also an issue that needed to be addressed. So an extended plan of events for inclusion was generated, leading to a total of 536 competitors and 242 officials. The events were listed as: 1500 m wheelchair track (male, open), 800 m wheelchair track (female, open), wheelchair basketball (male and female, IWBF), 100 m freestyle swimming (male and female, S9), 100 m freestyle swimming (male and female, mentally handicapped), standing singles table tennis (male, open class 6–10), sitting singles table tennis (female, open class 1–5), 200 m track (male, B2 and female, B1), 100 m track (male, leg amputees and female, cerebral palsy class 5, 6, 7, 8). This was a monumental proposal.

A questionnaire was circulated at the Lillehammer Winter Paralympics, asking athletes for their detailed views on the inclusion of full medal events in the Olympic Games. The Executive Committee, meeting in Lillehammer, considered that most information would be gained if the same procedure were carried out at each of the 1994 world championships of the summer sports as well.

Paralympic Games Preparation

The Paralympic Programme Committee had proposed the inclusion of sailing in the Atlanta 1996 Paralympic Games, but this had met with the opposition of the Sports Council Executive Committee. At recent national championships, the competition had permitted five different types of craft to be used, with four different combinations of crews, combining different locomotor disabilities. While this might be laudable flexibility and integration, it did not comply with the IPC's usual requirements for Paralympic sports. It was essential to pin down the variables in planning Paralympic sports so that true elite competition could be engaged. The Sports Council Executive Committee persuaded the IPC Executive of its preference that sailing should be included as a demonstration event only in Atlanta, and then it could enter the 2000 Paralympic Games as a full status event.

The vote in Barcelona to exclude weightlifting from the Atlanta programme was strongly criticised by George Dunstan. The heated disagreements about the safety of the bench press had clouded the judgement of people at that meeting, so Dunstan claimed, and the vote (40 to 33) should not be allowed to stand. Hans Lindström and George Dunstan worked out a delaying position, where a Sports Assembly would be held at the forthcoming Powerlifting World Championships in Uppsala, Sweden. The Assembly should be managed so that the issue could be calmly raised for further exploration.

The Lillehammer Paralympic Winter Games were in a harmonious state of preparedness. John Magdall, Director of the Lillehammer Paralympic Organising Committee (LPOC), reported in March 1993 that the funding from sponsors was well under control, and the venture was on target with its budget schedule. The Executive Committee had the opportunity of seeing many aspects of the preparation for the Games, and the detailed information made available served to give great confidence that all was secure. Carl Wang gave an account of the planning for the 2nd Paralympic Congress, which was to be held in conjunction with the Lillehammer Winter Paralympics, in the afternoons of 12th to 17th March. Participants would be free in the mornings to enjoy the spectacle of the Games. The topics selected for the programme were: winter sports, classification, medicine, sports for the mentally handicapped, integration, and 'towards the year 2000'. A visit was also planned to the health and sports centre at Beitostølen.

When Andy Fleming addressed the Executive Committee on the preparations for the Atlanta 1996 Paralympic Games he also gave an upbeat position statement. He suggested that they even found themselves ahead of schedule. Fleming had to tell the Committee that owners of the facilities to be used for the Games had insisted that the dates of the Games were shifted to operate from 16th to 27th August. This gave 12 days between the ending of the Olympic Games and the Opening Ceremony of the Paralympic Games. The marketing report was promising: Coca Cola was eager to be named as the first sponsor, and it was hoped that something would be agreed very soon. Television rights could only be negotiated in train with the process completed by the Atlanta Olympic Games Organising Committee, so the Paralympic Organising Committee had to wait for the 'go ahead' from its counterparts. The next phase could then begin. The principle that the Atlanta Olympic Games Organising Committee had established was that it needed to market the Olympics first, and then to promote the Paralympics subsequently.

André Raes asked for comment on the current status of the use of the term 'Paralympics', particularly whether the United States Olympic Committee had expressed a view. James Neppl, Regional Representative for America, explained that the use of the term 'Paralympics' was permitted until the year 1996. Andy Fleming indicated that he hoped to have a 'political and legal solution in the near future'.

The sports programme for Atlanta had not included lawn bowls, and Hans Lindström wished to hear why a sport identified by the IPC as one of the 'family' of Paralympic sports was not on the Atlanta list as: 'only the IPC has the authority to make such a decision'. Fleming countered that lawn bowls was not a commonly practised sport, and in any case it had not been included in the contract. Of course, it had been omitted accidentally from the contract with the Organising Committee, and Bob Steadward calmly insisted that lawn bowling must be on the programme for the Paralympic Games in 1996. Fleming agreed to take the matter back to the APOC Board for discussion at its next meeting.

The Winter Paralympic Games to be held in Nagano in 1998 were considered at the Lillehammer meeting of March 1993. Hans Lindström, André Raes and Michael Riding had made a visit in December 1992, and their report was very positive about the site and the planning. A further progress update was given in a slide show at the Lillehammer meeting by Masanori Miyatsu. This gave a good idea of the layout to those who had not been able to see the venues for themselves.

In this very positive spirit, the Executive Committee received 30-minute presentations from each city bidding for the 2000 Paralympic Games: Berlin, Beijing, Manchester and Sydney. Large piles of documents supported the bids, and highly professional audio-visual material illustrated the talks of the four bidding cities. Tashkent, Brasilia, Milan and Istanbul did not show any inclination towards hosting the Paralympics, and did not enter a bid. It would be interesting to obtain an official view of whether this fact actually affected the success or failure of bidding cities for the Olympic Games at this time.

On the 2nd March Tony Sainsbury, Vice Chairman of the British Paralympic Association, faxed a letter to the IPC Secretary General expressing concern about rumours they had heard. Sainsbury suggested that the IPC intended to confidentially indicate to the IOC President the single city that would be preferred as the hosts of the Paralympic Games. André Raes replied to Sainsbury to say that the Chairmen of the Bidding Cities had received letters in December 1992 that made clear that: 'After the presentation in Berlin a letter of approval and evaluation of the ability to host the Paralympics will be communicated to the IOC'. Raes stressed that the British Paralympic Association chose to read too much into the letter, and that it was the intention of the IPC only to indicate to the IOC 'which cities are capable to host the Paralympics and ensure good conduct of the Games'. However, Raes did tantalisingly close by saying: 'It is obvious that cities like Istanbul, Brasilia and Tashkent, will not be recommended to the IOC, as they have not introduced their bid to the IPC before the deadline (neither did Manchester – there is only a letter of intent)'. Bob Steadward added his degree of disapproval to this communication from the British Paralympic Association by telling the IPC Executive Committee that he wholeheartedly disapproved of any bidding city telling the IPC what it could and could not do: 'It is entirely up to the Executive Committee to decide on the number of cities they want to recommend to the IOC'.

When the Berlin meetings came, the site inspections and the presentations of the bids by the cities were considered carefully. Care was also taken over the manner of expressing the IPC Executive Committee's views on suitability. They agreed to recommend that Beijing, Berlin, Manchester and Sydney were all capable of delivering a Paralympic Games fulfilling the standards and philosophy of the Paralympic Movement. The members of IPC and the IOC would be sent a 'factual summary of the IPC's enquiries'. Highlighted by the concerns already expressed by the British Paralympic Association, the IPC needed to tread a careful line in dealing with the politically delicate area of bidding cities. Having acknowledged that all four of these cities would be able to host the Games, the Executive Committee agreed that its evaluation would be sent to the IOC without expressing preferences: 'it would place IPC in a very bad position if our No 1 choice would not be elected'. The members of the Executive were concerned that the credibility of the IPC would be damaged if bidding cities came to believe that the IPC had no importance in this matter. So the International Paralympic Committee wanted to give the impression of being centrally influential, while not wanting to express any partiality. As a rider to this, it was suggested that the IPC President might wish to prepare his own report for the eyes of the IOC President and the IPC Executive Committee members only.

At the Berlin General Assembly the Nagano bid to host the 1998 Paralympic Winter Games was officially accepted by the IPC. It was also agreed in Berlin that future Paralympic Games would have a requirement placed upon the organising committee to include the organisation of an International Youth Camp during the Paralympic Games. With all the agreements already being in place with the Lillehammer and Atlanta Organising Committees, this would come into effect for the Nagano Games onwards.

Wheelchair rugby was to be proposed to the Atlanta Paralympic Organising Committee for inclusion as a demonstration event. This received much support from the IPC Executive Committee. Women's Powerlifting received a negative response when put to the Executive for inclusion on the Atlanta programme. Exhibition events in shooting for the visually impaired would be reassessed after the Shooting World Championships in Austria. If this were thought suitable, the Sports Assembly

Executive Committee would recommend the event for inclusion in the Paralympic programme to replace racquetball, which no longer met the criteria.

There was some uncertainty about the motives of the Atlanta Paralympic Organising Committee, when it proposed the acceptance of a 'Paralympic Philosophy' specifically for the Atlanta Games. The IPC Executive Committee acknowledged that the Sports Council had approved the adoption of the statement from APOC:

- The Paralympic Games are the highest-level multisports competition for athletes with disabilities
- The Paralympic Games are a defined competition where only elite athletes participate
- The Paralympic Games must be governed by similar criteria as those in the Olympic Games
- Therefore, the Paralympic Games must be managed with the utmost discipline in the programming of sports and events.

The purpose and timing of this 'philosophy' are reminiscent of the Barcelona Paralympic Games Organising Committee's emphasis on the elite nature of the Games.

Minimum Disability

The Sports Committees were the obvious forum for discussion and decisions about the eligibility criteria for the highest level of international competition. The IPC Executive Committee agreed that as much work should be done as possible to provide the Sports Committees with a rationale to work from, then they should provide the sport-specific benchmarks for acceptance. Clarification would come from the Sports Science and Medical Committee, together with the Sports Technical Committee so as to arrive at a definition of 'minimum disability'. In Lillehammer in March 1993, Jens Bromann proposed that a definition should be circulated to the nations and the Athletes' Committee before being put before the Executive again. To this proposal Michael Riding added that there should be very active encouragement for more inclusion of athletes with severe disabilities, through the sports classification systems for the separate sports. This subject would remain central to the qualifying criteria for athletes participating in Paralympic Games.

Intellectual Disability

Bernard Atha had been elected President of INAS-FMH in 1993, so he joined the Lillehammer Executive Committee meeting of the IPC in March representing the highest level of authority for his members. The inclusion of athletes with intellectual disability was almost to be a test case of the credibility of the IPC's declared aims. The progress report on the Atlanta Paralympic Games preparations given by Andy Fleming caused concern. Fleming emphasised that there was no provision in the plans for athletes with intellectual disability, on the following grounds: no minimum standards were in place; there was no classification system; there remained a political problem between INAS-FMH and Special Olympics that could put at risk the successful marketing and financing of the Paralympics; Atlanta had not included 'the hosting of the mentally handicapped athletes' in its bid; and the United States Athlete's Advisory Committee was not in favour of athletes with intellectual disability being included in the 1996 Paralympic Games. This position reflected the concerns in differentiating the Paralympic Games from Special Olympics – the latter being well recognised in the United States. In the opinion of many at Lillehammer, the decisions taken by the IPC Executive Committee in Manchester were taken in good faith, but Fleming suggested that the concerns of the Atlanta Organising Committee had not been considered. Elizabeth Dendy pointed out that back in the Tignes meeting, the potential problems between INAS-FMH and Special Olympics had been discussed, and Fleming had given assurances that APOC would carry out the wishes of the IPC.

There was a need for the IPC to be sensitive to the needs and problems of the Atlanta Organising Committee, and John Grant and Carl Wang felt that such an important principle as this could only be decided in the forum of the General Assembly. For information, Michael Riding told the Executive Committee meeting that the problem of doping control had been satisfactorily resolved. He emphasised that athletes with intellectual disability would have as rigorous a system of testing as any other athletes. Classification proposals had also been formalised, and Bernard Atha described the most recent General Assembly of INAS-FMH, when the particular classification system was agreed upon. This allowed eligibility criteria to be more firmly established. But there was a basic difference from other athletes with a disability, because those with intellectual disability, once registered with INAS-FMH, did not need reclassification. This particular procedure would turn out to be a weakness in years to come. Bernard Atha reassured the members that there were no difficulties encountered with Special Olympics on a national level, but more needed to be done with International Special Olympics to resolve differences. He wanted to stress the showcase that Atlanta would be for the Paralympic Movement: 'the Paralympics belong to the athletes of all disability groups ... the media worldwide would be very negative if Atlanta excluded the participation of the mentally handicapped athletes'. As predicted by Atha, by July 1994 national newspapers would be decrying the stance of the Atlanta Organising Committee.

Bob Steadward returned to the comments of the APOC presentation, in particular to the potential for marketing of the Paralympic Games to be negatively affected by athletes with intellectual disability being included. He strongly felt that the marketing of the Paralympic Games should be concentrated on the image of a sporting festival, rather than focusing on disability. With regard to the relationship between INAS-FMH and Special Olympics, Steadward was happy to offer any influence he could. Hugh Glynn felt that it would be most appropriate for the IPC President to be fully involved with this matter, but also that the overt support of the International Paralympic Committee would 'give INAS-FMH more credibility'.

The Stuttgart Athletics World Championships in 1993 gave rise to a letter signed by 15 athletes and four coaches expressing their disagreement with the possible inclusion of athletes with intellectual disabilities in such competitions in future. When this was reported at the Berlin meetings of the IPC Executive Committee and the General Assembly later in the year, it was felt suitable to acknowledge the opinions expressed but to continue to encourage the debate. There was no question about the IPC's position regarding protecting the rights of all athletes with a disability to participation in appropriate events.

The Atlanta Paralympic Organising Committee had agreed to reconsider its initial position in relation to including 'a special programme' for athletes with intellectual disability. It informed the Executive Committee in September 1993 that it would thoroughly evaluate the participation of INAS-FMH athletes at the 1994 World Championships in Swimming and Athletics. The Athletes' Committee would undertake a survey of opinions of athletes worldwide. In some sort of concerted action, Martin Mansell also wrote on the same day to raise the same two points. The International Paralympic Committee could only respond positively to these suggestions, as it was taking two reluctant groups towards a better understanding of the position of athletes with intellectual disability. It might also lead to provision in the Atlanta programme for these athletes – an important milestone if reached.

When the IPC Executive Committee met during the Winter Paralympics in Lillehammer, there was agreement that there would be events for athletes with intellectual disability at the Berlin Athletics World Championships. Competitors must be members of INAS-FMH in order to be allowed to participate. This was quite a different circumstance from other athletes, because of the need for classification of intellectual disability through INAS-FMH registration.

The Athletes' Committee helped to construct a questionnaire for distribution at the Lillehammer Games on the inclusion of athletes with intellectual disability in the Paralympics. Although this had been done at the request of the Committee for the Inclusion of Athletes with a Disability and INAS-FMH, the Executive Committee felt that it should approve any questionnaire first. Bernard Atha gained the agreement of the meetings in Lillehammer, when he suggested that it would be more useful to obtain opinions of participants after the Berlin World Athletics Championships, when they would have had an opportunity to reflect on their experience and observations, rather than asking them to comment before actually encountering athletes with intellectual disability. He stressed that prejudice was more likely to be expressed than a fair opinion based on knowledge. The questionnaire was deferred until Berlin.

Technical Matters

Additions to the list of recognised Paralympic sports were requested at the 4th IPC General Assembly, held in Berlin in September 1993. Applications had been received from the sports of water skiing and surfing for Paralympic status. Wheelchair dance applied for recognition as both a sport of the IPC and for Paralympic status. One level of recognition would lead to sanctioning of sport-specific championships by the IPC, and the other would mean the inclusion of the sport in the Paralympic Games.

The list of sports that were termed 'IPC sports' had expanded. These were sports in which the IPC had responsibility for organising world championships:

- Alpine
- Archery
- Athletics
- Cycling
- Equestrian
- Ice sports
- Lawn bowls
- Nordic sports
- Powerlifting
- Shooting
- Swimming
- Table tennis

Representatives from each of these sports, together with the non-IPC sports that had Paralympic status, made up the Sports Council of the IPC. Also on the Sports Council were the Technical and Medical Officers, the international federations' Technical Officers, and the elected members of the Sports Council Executive Committee. The Chairman of the Athletes' Committee was also invited to be a member of the Sports Council. Jean Stone was appointed Technical Secretary. The non-IPC sports that would have Paralympic status for the 1996 Atlanta Paralympic Games were:

- Boccia
- Fencing
- Goalball
- Judo
- Soccer
- Wheelchair basketball

- Wheelchair tennis
- Volleyball.

A task that was nearing completion was the construction of the IPC Handbook, with the rules of all the international organisations of sport for persons with a disability in one manageable tome, including all applicable disability groups. The sports each had a different rate of progress in this venture, and each was affected by the response to functional classification and some elements of joint rules. As Hans Lindström admitted in explaining the time taken to achieve the goal: 'After all we have started from scratch to achieve a concept which was totally new for a great many people involved'.

The lack of constraint over inclusion of sports and events in the Paralympic programme before the existence of the IPC had led to a chaotic expansion of the Games. The Sports Council Executive Committee recommended to Bob Steadward that a Paralympic Programme Committee should be formed, establishing criteria that could be applied when considering sports, disciplines and events in the Paralympic Games. The Committee would also evaluate the extent to which the existing sports met the criteria – possibly removing sports that failed. The Committee was a small and effective threesome: Anne Merklinger, Horst Kosel and Guy Princivalle. The Paralympic Programme Committee was later to be dissolved during the meeting of the Executive Board in Lillehammer, in March 1994. This was effectively a sign that the separate sports had established firm rules, and principles were cemented in place for the inclusion of new sports and the removal of obsolete sports from the Paralympic Games. The debate centred over the need for a committee to decide which sports were viable – at this point the parameters precluded the necessity for a separate group to meet to decide. Hans Lindström pointed out that the Paralympic Games should not be the place for decisions about viability. Only events with appropriate standing and proven status should be included. The Technical Department would embrace the work formerly done by the Paralympic Programme Committee.

Hans Lindström, the workhorse of technical matters, was feeling frustration that there was still a lack of commitment to embrace unity among some factions, as the first four years of IPC were closing: 'It is quite clear that some international leaders still today in words and deeds advocate an international sports system for disabled athletes as segregated as possible in different international organisations, rather than have it organised per sport as is the intention of IPC'. Lindström was clear that the sports technical side was largely free of the problem, but he decried the divisive attitude that slowed progress: 'in some cases this has taken the form of creating problems where there actually were none, with unnecessary mistrust as a result'. The advantage of the IPC technical structure that had been the inspiration of Birgetta Blomquist and André Deville, but which had been breathed to life by Hans Lindström, was that the IPC Sports Assemblies' Executive Committees possessed a large degree of autonomy and self-determination. Their national influence guaranteed this autonomy, but there was a need for the Assemblies to recognise their implicit position within the umbrella of the International Paralympic Committee – as one international sports organisation.

US Wheelchair Basketball Team Still Had Not Returned Gold Medals

The United States Wheelchair Basketball team had still not returned their gold medals from Barcelona, and the IPC Executive Committee made it clear, at its meeting during the Lillehammer Paralympic Games, that the US team would not be allowed to participate in Atlanta unless they did return the medals. The sanction related to the doping offence of David Kiley in Barcelona in 1992. As the team that was moved into first place as a result of the ban, the Netherlands, had not received their gold medals, the Barcelona Organising Committee were to be approached about the provision of further gold medals.

Sport Science and Medicine

With the amount of underpinning work that was necessary in the first four years of the IPC's operation, the Sport Science and Medical Committee considered its primary role as one of supporting the establishment of the Sports Council Executive Committee. Michael Riding was able to be confident that the people involved in his committee were largely active in sports medicine already and had been active in the International Coordinating Committee's programmes anyway. As he looked to the period beyond the first four years, Riding saw that he must encourage a plan to consolidate doping control and the care and management of athletes.

The protocols and regulations of able-bodied sport were being employed as the model for the IPC's procedures for doping control. With the specific application to sport for athletes with a disability there was the regular return to the question of whether the banned drugs list should be the same as the one for able-bodied sport. Riding was adamant that it should, particularly in that the evidence showed that very few Paralympic athletes were taking any of the banned drugs for medical reasons. Rather than trying to create an unnecessary distinctive list for athletes with a disability, Riding thought it more important to draw the IOC Medical Commission and the IPC Medical Committee closer together. He had written to the Chairman of the IOC Medical Commission, Prince Alexandre de Mérode, but had so far not had a response. The delay was starting to cause problems, however, because changes to the IOC procedures were only reaching the IPC via the national members in Australia and Canada. The International Paralympic Committee was constantly altering its protocols to match those of the International Olympic Committee, as was deemed desirable, but the time lag was now a significant problem.

Whereas in the earliest days of sport for athletes with a disability, classification was a central medical issue, it had now moved into the arena of the sports themselves. Functional classification had simplified and demythologised the method by which athletes were organised into appropriate groups for competition. Classification had shifted into the technical department now that it was not based on a medical model of disability. While he applauded functional classification and the reduction in number of events, Riding identified a fine balance between having too few and too many classes in individual sports.

The connection between the International Paralympic Committee and the International Federation for Adapted Physical Activity (IFAPA) was confirmed at the Lillehammer meeting in March 1993. Michael Riding was asked to continue to negotiate future cooperation, and the possibility of IPC contributing to the journal *Palaestra*. At the Vista Conference in Jasper, Canada, an Ad Hoc committee was put together under the leadership of Gudrun Doll-Tepper, to identify a position statement and formulate a strategy for sport science applicable to athletes with a disability. The Sport Science Sub-Committee of IPC had its first meeting in Berlin, beginning on 5th April 1994, at the German Olympic Institute. This was a natural direction for the Paralympic Movement; once the practical administration of the IPC was in place there must be a launch of high-level research into the fast-expanding area of sport for athletes with a disability. Michael Riding felt that his own preference was for practical research that directly impacted on the lives and performance of the athletes, rather than purely academic, publication-motivated sports science that was removed from the applied environment. He was hopeful that both goals, of publication and spreading the products of the research, would be achieved through appropriate attention to effective communication. The fortunate delegates attending the Vista '93 Conference enjoyed Alberta's stunning scenery while being stimulated by the impressive speakers and debate. Located at Jasper, in the Rocky Mountain range, Vista '93 collected together 163 scientists from 18 countries over the period from 14th to 20th May 1993. Gathering first at the Royal West Inn, Edmonton, participants registered and booked into rooms for one night. The evening's entertainment was in the form of a reception, with native Canadian dancers giving a taste of traditional cultural heritage. The following morning delegates were transferred to the Jasper Park Lodge for the main conference events. On the Tuesday (18th May) participants were encouraged to get out into the countryside and to get active: horse riding, white water rafting, cycling, golf were on offer for those who did not just wish to walk and talk with new friends or old adversaries.

The schedule of plenary sessions followed the current themes relevant to the Paralympic Movement, as well as serving to pose and answer some questions important to the International Paralympic Committee:

- sport performance:
  a. exercise physiology
  b. advances in training techniques
  c. technical developments
  d. sports medicine;
- classification;
- integration;
- ethics;
- organisation and administration.

Important information was shared during these meetings that had immediate and dynamic impact on the athletes with a disability. On sports injuries and boosting, presentations by Kathleen Curtis, Mike Ferrara, Robert Burnham and Duane Messner were highly significant. 'Boosting', or the intentional induction of autonomic dysreflexia, was of concern because of its increase among quadriplegics. Physiological characteristics of higher spinal cord injury (usually above T6) can mean that autonomic dysreflexia will stimulate venous return, and encourage the redistribution of blood flow, among other effects. Autonomic dysreflexia can be brought on by athletes over-tightening leg straps, over-consuming water, clamping the catheter prior to competition to hyper-distend the bladder, or harming themselves with a sharp object. Research demonstrated that significant risks to the health of athletes were created by boosting, particularly increases in blood pressure, and moderate to severe hypertension. There were implications for body temperature issues that needed further investigation, but risks of hyperthermia were realistic. Boosting by quadriplegic athletes had become a problem of substantial proportions for the Sport Science and Medical Committee. The stance taken focused on the responsibility of the IPC to protect its athletes' own health. It is revealing that Riding acknowledged that the seriousness of commitment of athletes with a disability had now reached a point where: 'most athletes ... would jeopardise their present and future health for victory. It is our duty, therefore, to protect them from themselves.' There was a known effect on performance through autonomic dysreflexia, and the practice sat squarely alongside doping as cheating in elite sport for persons with a disability.

Another sign of change in the Paralympic Movement was that attention turned towards management of health care for athletes with a disability at Paralympic events. This was a natural shift once classification was no longer based on medical and disability categorisation. Also, as the Paralympic Movement gained in momentum, the commitment and dedication of the athletes meant that much more time was spent on training, and a much more extensive competitive season was on offer. Athletes with a disability might experience quite a different range of injuries from other athletes, and patterns of injuries could also be entirely different dependent on the disability of the athlete. Sports medicine needed to be intensified in prevention and management of injuries for athletes with a disability.

Doping control was constantly reviewed, and Michael Riding submitted a written motion to the Executive Committee at the Lillehammer 1994 Winter Paralympics encouraging that all member nations should 'enrol their athletes in national out of competition unannounced drug testing programmes'.[3]

---

[3] Minutes of 11th IPC Executive Committee Meeting. 7th–10th March 1994, Lillehammer, Norway.

This had become a feature of elite sport, and needed to apply visibly to the Paralympic Movement in order to sustain the progress of the philosophy.

'No Limits': 5th Paralympic Winter Games, Lillehammer, Norway 1994

Before the Paralympic Winter Games, the splendour of the 17th Olympic Winter Games had produced an exceptional sporting gathering, with some 1750 athletes competing. The image remains of the Olympic Flame arriving in the hand of a ski jumper at the Opening Ceremony. Particularly of note was the presence of 11 former Soviet republics, all of which had been admitted to membership of the Olympic Movement as independent states. The most prominent athletes at the Olympic Games were Johan Olav Koss of Norway, the speed skater who won three Olympic medals, taking his country's total to 26 medals; Manuela Di Centa of Italy, who was awarded five medals in cross-country skiing; and Lyubov Egorova, representing Russia, who won three golds and a silver medal. Later in the year Koss was named Sportsperson of the year by *Sports Illustrated* magazine. Grinkov and Gordeeva repeated their gold medal winning performance in the ice dance competition. It was a deep disappointment that no demonstration event could be arranged within the Olympic Games programme. Bob Steadward expressed his frustration at this, but said: 'we shall put it behind us and work towards the future'.

Ten days after the Olympic Games Closing Ceremony, Queen Sonja of Norway officially declared the Paralympic Winter Games open. The Lillehammer Paralympic Organising Committee chose as its motto for the Games: 'No Limits', expressing that potential of the athletes and the potential of the phenomenon of the Paralympic Movement. Particularly of note was the fact that this was the first Paralympic Games completely organised under the banner of the International Paralympic Committee.

As the athletes and supporting staff worked their way through the majestic celebration of the Opening Ceremony, the venues were in their best state of preparedness: Hjafell for Alpine events, Birkebiner Stadium for Nordic skiing events, the Hamar Olympic Vikingship Hall for ice sledge racing, and the Kristin Hall for the ice sledge hockey competition. The celebrations at the Opening Ceremony were fittingly brought to a peak with wheelchair dance sport and traditional Norwegian folk dancing.

Cato Zahl Pedersen lit the flame at the Opening Ceremony of the Paralympic Winter Games, and then promptly won three medals: two golds and a silver in Alpine events. Ice sledge hockey emerged as a dynamic and dramatic sport, much enjoyed by the supportive spectators. The final had to be decided in a penalty shoot-out, with Sweden eventually beating Norway to take the gold medal. There were many disappointed people who could not get tickets to see the last rounds of the ice sledge hockey; a black market even sprang up, miraculously producing the scarce means of entry, but at a high price. The women's biathlon was won by Marjorie Yvette Van de Bunt (Netherlands) in the amputee class, with Anne-Mette Bredahl-Christiansen (Denmark) winning the gold in the visually impaired group. Hakon's Hall was brimming with people and noise as the Closing Ceremony colourfully peaked everyone's high spirits. The Organising Committee, presided over by Gerhard Heiberg, who had also been President of the Olympic Games Organising Committee, with John Magdall as Executive Director, received much-deserved praise for their magnificent efforts. At the Closing Ceremony, Juan Antonio Samaranch presented Gerhard Heiberg with the Gold Medal of the International Olympic Committee.

In an unusual move towards solidarity of all people with a disability, the United Nations encouraged all medal winners to sign an appeal 'for the world community to spare no efforts to help the disabled all over the world'. The spectacular setting for the Winter Games was a great success, particularly because the same facilities and the same organising committee were used for both Olympic and Paralympic Winter Games in Lillehammer. The Paralympic athletes numbered 491 in all, representing 31 countries. Another feature of the welcoming atmosphere of the Lillehammer Paralympic Games was the close proximity of everyone involved: the Paralympic Village was temporary home to officials, athletes, escorts, volunteers and organising staff.

Socially, the Lillehammer Paralympic Games were exceptional. The programme of events beyond the athletic competition was very extensive. Films were shown in the Village Cinema every night, and the disco next door seemed to be buzzing – no matter what was happening the next day.

The lasting effects of the Lillehammer Paralympic Games on the people of Norway were soon evident. The financial base of the Games was strong, with the donation by the Norwegian Storting (National Assembly) of US$15 million, and another US$3 million from the excellent sponsors being more than enough to run the Paralympic Games and leave a significant surplus for national initiatives.

Second Paralympic Congress in Lillehammer

During the ten days of the Winter Paralympic Games, each of the Winter Sport Committees held meetings, as did the Athletes' Committee. As had become customary, a most successful Paralympic Congress took place between 12th and 17th March, drawing together scientists, coaches and technicians from the winter sports world. The IPC Executive Committee met for the 11th time from 7th–10th March. Having been involved in hosting a medical conference at the time of the Geilo Winter Paralympic Games in 1980, Norway had been very positive about the IPC's idea of attaching such conferences permanently to the obligation of organising committees. The Lillehammer Congress drew participants from 35 countries, about 180 individuals in total. Features of the Congress were the uniform wish to look forward to the year 2000; to address the issue of integration/inclusion; to discuss the situation of the intellectually disabled; and to focus, as expected, on winter sports for people with a disability. The Second Paralympic Congress took place under the direction of the Royal Norwegian Ministry of Cultural Affairs. Organised to operate directly in parallel to the Paralympic Winter Games, half of each day was left free for delegates to take advantage of the spectacle of the Games – some delegates were centrally involved in the participation of their national teams anyway. The Secretary of State for Cultural Affairs, Ole Jørgen Johannessen, welcomed guests and delegates to the Quality Hotel, Øyer, on 12th March, with the encouragement to participate so as to find ways for greater 'normalisation' through research and sharing of ideas: 'no unnecessary dividing lines should be drawn between disabled and able-bodied people with regard to medical and social treatment, conditions for growing up, education, employment and welfare. A society adapted to the needs of persons with a disability will benefit us all.'

Carl Wang, stressing that his paper was born out of his personal observations and studies and not representing any faction, insisted that we must all look at sport in its social and political context. It is a phenomenon that cannot be examined in isolation from the real world. He said sport relates to: general politics/conflicting interests; human affairs/fundamental human rights; economics/relationship between the affluent world and the developing world; and social affairs/culture. In a liberating paper, Wang employed the works of popular 'futurologists' such as Toffler and Nasbitt to explain recent changes in society, and described trends for future development that might prove useful in appraising a phenomenon like the Paralympic Movement. He condensed the influential factors as: increased knowledge of human development (health now meaning more than absence of illness), able-bodied and disabled; safeguarding of the underlying principles of human rights; and the maintenance of the principle of 'normalisation'. Wang went on to decry the situation in developing countries, where millions of persons with a disability were being denied even the simplest trimmings of civilised society: often families were disgraced to have a person with a disability among them. These individuals were disenfranchised; they had no position in society that enabled them to affect their own situation. There would be a significant increase in the numbers of persons with a disability over time because of increased life expectancy, and better medical systems aiding the support of the newborn as well. The demands on society would multiply phenomenally. Sport is, by definition, rehabilitation, but at the same time it is tied closely with culture and society. Wang stressed that for persons with a disability and those without, sport 'has to do with the care of the environment, well being, humour, enthusiasm and excitement connected to events and experiences that fill your mind and emotions. Sports enrich life. Sports are engagement. Sports bring people together in a friendly atmosphere.' Carl Wang led the delegates to accept that 'sport is necessary to the individual and to the society as a whole'.

Classification, as a subject, received a comprehensive airing at the Congress. The detailed analysis of the separate disability groups, and the evolution of the systems of classification currently employed, was tremendous. Harald Natvig, former Medical Officer of the International Sports Organisation for the Disabled, presented a provocative paper on minimum disability. Of particular note were excellent contributions on aspects of intellectual disability by Årstein Skiftun, Kristjana Kristiansen and Adri Vermeer. Three presentations from Norwegian speakers launched the topic of integration, always emotive within the context of the Paralympic Movement. Six 'free papers' then extended the discussion, before Hans Lindström posed his thoughts for the future of integration in international sport for people with a disability.

The strength of the Lillehammer Paralympic Congress lay in the passion of the speakers, and their commitment to the work they were engaged in. Whether in agreement or not, the participants were left in no doubt that they were among the most dedicated and well-informed scientists, administrators and coaches in the world.

TRIUMPH OF THE HUMAN SPIRIT: FROM LILLEHAMMER TO ATLANTA

Open-mindedness, discipline and integrity were the characteristics called for by Bob Steadward as he welcomed delegates to the 12th meeting of the IPC Executive Committee in Paris, 18th to 20th November 1994. This was a very strong period for the organisation; the Winter Paralympics had been a great success, and everyone could now work with renewed enthusiasm towards the Atlanta Paralympic Games of 1996. But there was growing discontent within the Paralympic Movement about the diversity of systems of management and organisations that member nations and athletes had to deal with. The multiplicity of memberships and allegiances that were encouraged – all supposedly coming under the IPC umbrella – was draining to the participants. It was also a drain on their resources: countries had to be members of several organisations in order to retain legitimacy of their standing. There was obvious duplication of administration as the international federations held on to their secretariats; the IPC tried to encourage a centrality itself and from the nations, and the sport-specific organisations needed their own means of communicating and operating. Committees seemed to bring the same people together over and over, all 'wearing different hats' as they managed to represent disability groups while holding national influence and so on.

An outcome of the period in question was the withdrawal of the Comité International des Sports des Sourds (CISS) from involvement with the International Paralympic Committee. There had been a lengthy process of steady decline in commitment from CISS, and it might be considered to have hung on well beyond the time others had expected it to. CISS did not gain enormously from its involvement in the International Paralympic Committee, and its continued willingness to listen to proposals to keep it under the umbrella of IPC was largely attributable to the personality of Jerald Jordan. He could see that there was an inherent desirability to having all international sports organisations for persons with a disability together in one forum. But once his organisation was plugged in directly to the International Olympic Committee, and things were going well, the last real reason for holding on to the coat-tails of IPC was gone. The oldest organisation of its kind had respectfully come along as the newer bodies were finding their feet, but in the end CISS did not need IPC in order to continue its already significant successes. The 34th Congress of the Comité International des Sports des Sourds, meeting in 1995, would vote to withdraw from membership of the International Paralympic Committee. Both Walther Tröger and Hans Lindström addressed the Congress prior to the vote to withdraw from membership of the International Paralympic Committee.

The Brighton Declaration on Women and Sport was adopted by the Tokyo 1995 General Assembly of the IPC. The involvement of women in sport for people with a disability had been flagged up by the IPC prior to the Barcelona Paralympic Games as a subject that would need particular consideration. The world's attention was drawn to the subject by this powerful conference that concluded with the Declaration. The IPC General Assembly adopted the 'scope and the aims' of the Brighton Declaration: 'The overriding aim of the Declaration is to develop a sporting culture that enables and values the full involvement of women in every aspect of sport'.

A feature of the importance of elite level sport to the individual and the public was the increase in litigation relating to management of and performance in competition. When Steadward reported to the 1995 IPC General Assembly, he sounded almost exhausted by the two lawsuits dragging themselves through their necessary processes. One was the ongoing difficulty of concluding the US Basketball Team's return of the gold medals from the Barcelona Paralympics, when David Kiley tested positive for dextropropoxyphene, a banned substance. The other was associated with a claim of discrimination from Wayne Washington, a powerlifter who believed that the 20° armlock rule was not applicable to him because of the physical restrictions of his disability. These issues focused the minds of the Executive Committee on the personal liability they risked in the course of their duties on behalf of IPC. Washington had brought a lawsuit that sought indemnification of US$20.5 million because 'the loss of his arm extension is higher than allowed according to IPC Powerlifting regulations' and this would not permit his participation in the Atlanta Paralympic Games. The President agreed to explore world-wide insurance cover for all IPC officials. Both suits eventually went in favour of the International Paralympic Committee, but the time and attention they required put strain on everyone involved.

Administration

The status of observers at IPC meetings had not been officially established until the Paris meetings of the Executive Committee, and the Legal Committee had been asked to come up with a policy. It was agreed that at all meetings, with the exception of the General Assembly, only members of the committee should be present except when the chairperson invited someone to attend for a specific part of a meeting. Then the individual should have the right to speak but not to vote. The implications of this decision led the representatives of the Atlanta Paralympic Organising Committee to walk out of the Paris meetings of the Executive Committee: 'and to return to Atlanta, where time and energy could be better spent directly on the organisation of the 1996 Paralympic Games'. The IPC Executive Committee had clearly insulted one of its partners. André Raes wrote to Andy Fleming on 22nd November 1994 to apologise for 'the surprising decision of some members of the Executive Committee' (the vote had been carried with only two abstentions). Raes explained that the reason for wishing to exclude people was due to embarrassing situations that had arisen in the past, and because delegates felt inhibited when people other than elected members were present. Raes also acknowledged that the communication between the Executive Committee of IPC and the Atlanta Paralympic Organising Committee was vital, and could only be maintained by attendance at each other's meetings. The decision was to be reconsidered so as to permit two observers from the Paralympic Organising Committee to each meeting of IPC, but with the requirement of withdrawing if confidential matters were being discussed.

Day-to-day running of the International Paralympic Committee had quickly become a very demand-ing operation. The volume of communications and production of materials was overloading the limited numbers of staff. Many essential jobs were carried out by people outside the Headquarters in Belgium, by officers of the IPC who had considerate and flexible employers willing to tolerate the shared attention of secretarial staff. But even this voluntary support was being overwhelmed by the fast growth of the organisation. The facilities used by the IPC Secretariat until 1995 were to become more expensive as the Flemish League for Sports for the Disabled moved out of the offices. The IPC had to undertake the total costs. In a show of further support the International Olympic Committee produced a generous promise of additional support, but for one year only. It was now time for a permanent Headquarters to be planned, with all departments centred under one roof. Bob Steadward informed the Executive Committee, at its meeting in Atlanta in April 1995, that his unofficial contacts with potential host cities had not led to a formal proposal. York Chow pointed to questions that would have to be considered: the effect of moving to another country when the IPC was registered in Belgium; the financial package for office rent and staffing; the quality of communication afforded by the country; the language of the country related to the language skills of the office staff; the support of the government; and the ability of the country to support the image of the International Paralympic Committee rather than affecting the IPC's image politically. This subject needed more formal proposals, and the President agreed to bring it back to the Executive Committee.

There had been regular returns to discussion about how membership fees were being collected, and how complex the situation had become in some countries. The nations themselves had wanted regularity over how many sets of fees they were obliged to pay – to the National Paralympic Committee, to IPC or to the international federations for people with a disability. It was decided that a single membership fee was desirable. A knock-on effect was a need for some technical adjustments to the voting procedures, notably in Tokyo for the 1995 General Assembly, where there was an appeal for 'honesty and integrity' in identifying the entitlement of the number of votes. The General Assembly brought together representatives of 45 nations and five international federations. Representatives from Nepal attended as observers, together with the Chairpersons of some sports: Alpine skiing, archery, athletics, boccia, cycling, ice sports, judo, lawn bowls, powerlifting, soccer, shooting, swimming, wheelchair basketball and wheelchair fencing. These observers from the sports had no voting rights, but they did have the right to speak.

Over the previous two years, a number of countries had applied for membership. These were ratified at the Tokyo General Assembly in 1995, bringing another 12 into the IPC: Kazakstan, Bermuda, Ukraine, Ivory Coast, Former Yugoslavia, the Kyrghz Republic, Qatar, Macedonia, United Arab Emirates, Saudi Arabia, Angola and Bosnia Herzegovina. The International Paralympic Committee was fast becoming an essential organisation for all countries to join. There were limitations that related to the local management of sports for people with a disability, but the world stage provided by the Paralympic Games was very meaningful – especially to smaller nations and newly emerging former Soviet states. The Secretary General told the General Assembly that there were still applications from another 22 countries pending. The representation of countries within the International Paralympic Committee was now up to 143.

EUROCOM, the European Regional Committee of IPC, had issued a Technical Handbook of its own. This was proving to be a help in the preparation of national and European events. Tony Sainsbury undertook to update this handbook when necessary, and the closer monitoring of the activities in the European countries had a very positive effect on the level of interaction and cooperation within the region. Athletes with intellectual disabilities took part in the European Swimming Championships in France, a major step along the right route. EUROCOM was also highly involved in preparing structured assistance for countries of the former Eastern Bloc. They were being steered towards regular involvement and membership in the International Paralympic Committee.

The East Asian Region had much of its successes through participation in the FESPIC Games and related activities. While 40 countries took part in the FESPIC Games of 1994 in Beijing, China, only

16 countries were members of the East Asian region of IPC. Yasuhiro Hatsuyama, chairing the Regional Committee, was concerned that there were another 13 nations with good levels of participation that were not members of the Regional Committee.

As the Lillehammer Winter Paralympics had permitted the Athletes' Committee to elect three representatives of winter sports, the total membership on the Committee stood at ten. The surveys that had been conducted by the Athletes' Committee at the Athletics and Swimming World Championships were certainly inconclusive. The questions related to the inclusion of full medal status events at the Olympic Games, and the inclusion of athletes with intellectual disabilities in the Paralympic Games. Unfortunately the response rate from these surveys was so low as to be embarrassing: at the Athletics World Championships 1100 questionnaires were sent out, but only 12 were completed and returned; at the Swimming Championships, 600 were distributed and a meagre two responses were received! However there were meetings held for athletes at both competitions, and the same questions were put to them by the Athletes' Committee. In answer to the question about full medal events in the Olympic Games, the athletes voted to cease the work of the Commission for Inclusion of Athletes with a Disability towards full medal events in the Olympics. To the other question of the inclusion of athletes with intellectual disabilities, the gathering voted to encourage the participation of these athletes in the 1996 World Championships in both athletics and swimming.

International Federations Attempt to Take Control of Finances

Some indication that the international federations were feeling a need to gain more control came when the regular meeting of IPC representatives took place with the International Olympic Committee on 13th June 1994. The President of IOC had been called away (to meet with the Director General of the United Nations and Nelson Mandela), but the IOC ensured that the next most important people were there to face the IPC: Walther Tröger (IOC Delegate for the disabled), François Carrard (Director General of IOC), Gilbert Felli (Sports Director) and P Miró (Deputy Sports Director). The international federations presented the IOC with a letter they had signed proposing an alteration in the financial arrangements between the IOC and the IPC. The suggestion was that 25% of any subvention from the IOC would go to the IPC, while 75% would go directly to the international federations. They specified that the IPC money would go towards 'the development and organisation of Paralympic Games, IPC Regional Games and World Championships involving more than two disability groups'. The money for the international federations was 'for expenditure on development of sport by the ISODs with the intention of achieving an equitable share for each organisation'. Although all six international federations had signed the document, the explanation seemed to exclude the CISS from the arrangement for dividing up the money. Gilbert Felli sought clarification from the meeting and was informed that CISS would not be involved in the 25%–75% split, but would pursue its own arrangements. The fact that CISS was involved in the negotiations at all was remarkable, especially as Bob Steadward had informed the Executive Committee of IPC that the CISS had formally withdrawn from membership at the April meeting in Atlanta. The organisation for deaf sports already had its own agreement with the IOC, and monies were pledged, but it is likely that each side wanted to ensure that there was a fair distribution of IOC generosity. The International Olympic Committee still seemed to be insisting on the authority of the IPC in distributing the total subvention. The IOC delegates agreed that the IPC must decide how to divide the funds given to it by the IOC, but the international federations' proposal 'changed the financial report fundamentally'. The IOC made its subvention on the basis that 100% went to the IPC. If the allocation of funding were to be changed, all the projections presented by the IPC for the next budget would need clarification in terms of receiving only 25% of the subvention. Bob Steadward, who had been virtually silent on this matter, responded meekly that the IPC 'were working on this, and that details would be given in US dollars'. He appeared to have been 'Shanghaied' by the action of the international federations. Interestingly, the June 1994 minutes of the International Olympic Committee Executive Committee meeting in Lausanne describe this major affront to the IPC President in a much more tame manner: 'It seems there has been a slight misunderstanding between the IPC and the international organisations as far as the separation of duties is concerned, and in relation to certain financial aspects'.

Signs of the IOC's willingness to work hard on behalf of the International Paralympic Committee were evident in Gilbert Felli's writing to Jean-Marie Weber, Chairman of the Board of ISL Marketing AG on 5th January 1995. This marketing company was conducting the International Olympic Committee's programme, and had been approached by the IPC with a view to employing ISL as well. The response of ISL had been to request a fee of approximately US$65 000 to conduct a preliminary test analysis of the market for IPC. Felli wrote to convey the view of Juan Antonio Samaranch, that ISL should conduct this first level analysis without charge to IPC.

Increasingly evident during the period between the Barcelona Paralympic Games and the Atlanta Paralympic Games were world championships in IPC sports, and also opportunities for demonstration events in other competitions. One such example was the World Track and Field Championships in Gothenberg, Sweden, from 9th to 13th August 1995. Among the top athletes in the world were the competitors in the men's 1500 metre and women's 800 metre wheelchair events. As with so many other such occasions, the sporting spectacle offered another opportunity for meetings between Bob Steadward and Juan Antonio Samaranch. Steadward was sure that the increasing regularity of their meetings was helping the two organisations move closer together: 'I am discovering that the more frequently he and I meet, the more at ease we are in our discourse and consequently the better he can understand and appreciate our issues and our goals'. Also while they were in Gothenberg, John Grant and Bob Steadward signed the contract for the Sydney 2000 Paralympics.

Finances

After a lengthy period of questionable security for the finances of IPC, there was optimism that things were getting better. With the release of some funds from the International Olympic Committee, and the possibilities of income from commercial sponsorship, the IPC was more confident of riding the variable waves of the near future. The work to establish a new logo had received a subvention from the IOC of US$40 000, and this led to a revised budget being prepared by the Management Committee for 1994. Unfortunately, as we have seen, the promising position with ONCE did not produce further tangible financial support for the IPC.

Advertising had to be well controlled, and proposals for regulations were discussed at the meeting of the Executive Committee in November 1994. This Paris meeting set up a framework to be adapted once there was a marketing programme in place, but the nations needed something to base their principles on, as fundraising was absolutely crucial to ensure the viability of participation. The International Olympic Committee had provided details of its own guidelines and regulations.

André Auberger was keen that the membership fees should be increased to US$1000, with the approval of the 1995 General Assembly. This would serve to bring all members into the same level of payment, with those nations with specific financial problems being supported through the Paralympic Solidarity plan. The meeting did not accept this idea, and preferred a sliding scale within agreed limits. Some other possibilities were discussed, such as basing fees on the Gross National Product of member countries, or on the level of participation in the activities of the Paralympic Movement. But the motion passed was for the Executive Committee to establish a sliding scale with three or four categories of fees, ready for 1996–97. This was a complication for the Treasurer, who had prepared the next budget on the basis of the expected income from fees.

Subventions from the International Olympic Committee had helped buoy up the IPC finances. In addition to a supplementary grant of US$100 000 – for the 'initial stages of administration settlement', the IPC President's request for a separate subvention for his travel was not granted – the IOC's subvention of US$250 000 annually was considered adequate to cover these expenses. In fact, Air Canada was to provide a number of complimentary flights per year for the IPC President throughout his period of office.

The Treasurer's report to the General Assembly was very positive. In the period from 1992 to 1995 the income of the International Paralympic Committee had been increased from US$108 000 to US$632 000 – a six-fold multiplication. A beneficiary of this welcome increase was the Technical Committee, having its budget increased during the four-year period from US$28 000 to US$187 000. But there was still a difficulty in persuading member nations to pay their membership fees in good time. By mid-August 1995 only 80 out of 143 countries had paid up. They would need to settle their fees before having voting rights in the General Assembly, or taking part in any IPC competitions.

The Paralympic Solidarity programme was fully operational, developing countries could be helped with membership fees, courses and athlete support. This initiative of André Auberger had received warm support from the President of the IOC, and funds were forthcoming on top of the subventions already received by the IPC. Regional courses and projects were also able to receive additional funding from Samaranch, who had been enthusiastic about the influence of the IPC on countries seldom in the front line of support for persons with a disability. The current project was for the IOC to directly finance the travel and subsistence of two athletes and a coach from developing countries to compete in the Atlanta Paralympic Games.

Inclusion and Integration

Inclusion and integration had received a great amount of attention in the past few years, and Bob Steadward gave the 1995 General Assembly an account of the chronology of decisions and progress. The success of the IPC's Commission for Inclusion of Athletes with a Disability (CIAD) was appreciated, and the General Assembly agreed with the Executive Committee's decision to include the women's 800 m and men's 1500 m wheelchair races in the Sydney 2000 Olympic Games.

Steadward acknowledged that there was still concern over 'the selection process of the events proposed, fear of losing power by a variety of disability specific sport groups and fear of "gigantism" at the Olympic Games'. He considered that there was still opposition within the International Olympic Committee and within the disability sport federations. The IPC President had been in the unique position of addressing a joint General Assembly of the IOC Executive Board and the Association of National Olympic Committees (ANOC) on the subject of disability. To this audience Steadward posed the important dilemma that continuing to include only demonstration events in Olympic Games for athletes with a disability was 'patronising and perpetuating the message of difference instead of advancing the message of full acceptance and legitimacy'. He went on to relate this attitude to discrimination: clearly against the Olympic Charter. It was not clear whether the IOC and ANOC reacted to this at the time.

Paralympic Games Preparation

A new experience awaited the International Paralympic Committee, in the form of the signing of the first major sponsorship deal in relation to the Atlanta Paralympic Games. On 14th October 1993

Bob Steadward was present when the Atlanta Paralympic Organising Committee signed the agreement with the Coca Cola Corporation. This first step made further sponsorship more likely.

The 2002 Winter Olympic Games had received ten bids. Of those, nine cities had indicated that they would also organise the Paralympic Games. But only six cities were then moved to submit a 'bid dossier' to the IPC to host the 2002 Winter Paralympic Games. These cities were:

- Ostersund, Sweden
- Quebec, Canada
- Poprad-Tatry, Slovakia
- Salt Lake City, USA
- Sion, Switzerland, and
- Tarvisio, Italy.

From this list it was necessary to elect the final four candidate cities. IPC members of the Executive Committee were encouraged by André Auberger to contact their national IOC member and canvass for the final four. Eventually the four selected candidate cities emerged as: Salt Lake City, Sion, Ostersund and Quebec. Some complications and ill feeling were created because François Carrard, Director General of the International Olympic Committee, wrote to Bob Steadward to inform him that the cities and the IOC considered that the IPC should not go ahead with site visits before the decision of the IOC was announced. Steadward was strong in his response to Carrard on 9th February. Carrard had said that the four bidding cities had affirmed their willingness to stage the Paralympics, but that they were all very busy at this time. Steadward made it clear that all four cities had already accepted that they would host a visit from an IPC delegation, and some travel arrangements had already been made. The main thrust of Steadward's concern was that a loose assurance to the IOC by a city that it was willing to stage the Paralympics did not equal a formal agreement that the city would host the Paralympics according to the International Paralympic Committee's contract and Handbook. When the results were announced on 16th June, Salt Lake City had won through the Olympic bidding process, but there was a problem as far as the Paralympics went. The other three bidding cities had signed the undertaking to organise the Paralympic Games as well as the Olympic Games, but Salt Lake City had not. The IPC President was, however, able to announce to the 1995 General Assembly that the Salt Lake City organisers had agreed to host the Winter Paralympic Games – but that they did not accept the terms of the IPC contract. As a result, the Organising Committee did not make a presentation to the General Assembly in Tokyo.

To ensure that all appropriate parallels could be drawn between Olympic and Paralympic Games organisation in future, Bob Steadward wrote to Howard Stupp, IOC Director of Legal Affairs on 31st July 1995, to request copies of recent contracts with host organising committees of the Olympic Games of Nagano, Sydney and Salt Lake City.

Following the signing of the contract between the IPC and the Sydney Paralympics Organising Committee (SPOC) in August 1995, another agreement was signed between SPOC and the Sydney Organising Committee for the Olympic Games (SOCOG), allowing a close relationship for shared benefit in preparation of both events. John Grant, a long-standing servant of the Paralympic Movement, had led the Sydney bid for the Paralympic Games, and he introduced Lois Appleby to the Tokyo General Assembly in November 1995. Appleby was Chief Executive of SPOC, and she stressed the need for high profile exposure in the build-up to attract the interest of sponsors. Grant and Appleby confirmed that all disability groups would be included in the Paralympic Games of 2000, providing they qualified under IPC regulations. The bid provided for 5000 participants offering 19 sports – the details of sporting programme and events were to be the prerogative of the IPC.

Relations with the Atlanta Paralympic Organising Committee were becoming more strained as a result of increasing frustration at the number of obstacles that were being encountered. APOC had not been successful in obtaining the funding that it had based the bid upon, and sought to alter its arrangements with the IPC. There had been a request to change the financial agreement between the two organisations. There were disagreements over interpretations of the contract in areas of rights fees and the sharing of revenue.

In Atlanta in April 1995, meetings took place between APOC and members of the IPC Management Committee. APOC said that it had not been able to reach the targets for sponsorship because the Paralympic name was not well enough recognised, and because the agreement between APOC, USOC and ACOG 'took them out of the free market'. The main wish of APOC was to renegotiate the contract with IPC relating to revenue share. The proposal was to pay a flat fee to IPC instead of using a formula of percentages. The discussions were quite enlightening in the apparent ease with which APOC leapt from one proposal to a doubled amount. The initial contract had suggested a formula of revenue to IPC based on: 5% on all cash received; 2.5% on the fair market value of goods in kind of any corporate sponsor; 20% on the net revenue of TV and radio broadcasting; 5% on surplus; and US$20 capitation 'tax' per participant. The first proposal of the Atlanta Paralympic Organising Committee was: US$250 000 plus a 10% on all surplus. This was not going to impress the IPC representatives, who came back with a testing reply: US$2 million, no surplus, but a capitation tax. The last round of these negotiations brought APOC to offer US$500 000; 10% on net surplus, and a capitation fee to IPC. When this process was discussed within the Executive Committee there was great concern that revenue was being lost to IPC, and that other significant problems seemed to be developing. One was the exact nature of the proposed establishment of a legacy fund that would benefit the people of the USA with a disability. This worthy cause was diverting revenue away from the IPC, and the Executive wished to be clear of the precise composition of the board of any such foundation. In all there was a concerted view that the line taken with APOC on the financial contract must be firm and forward-looking. It was agreed that the President and First Vice President should take up negotiations again, but with a minimum level of acceptance of a flat fee of US$2.5 million paid over five years, as well as a capitation tax.

A host broadcaster was still being pursued, and vital information was outstanding about rates for media services. Advertising was proving a concern, as was the restrictive agreement that APOC had with both the United States Olympic Committee and ACOG. The list of protected categories that had to be respected by countries seeking sponsorship had been extended by APOC. In effect this now put out of contention many of the larger companies identified as being appropriately inclined. All corporate sponsors of the Olympic Games were included. The lateness of the announcements about changes to sponsorship and advertising restrictions was definitely aggravating to representatives at the Tokyo General Assembly: financial support would wither away unless the sponsors were permitted some visible return. While all advertising and marketing rights had been transferred to APOC until after the Games, which some might have seen as restrictive, this put the International Paralympic Committee in line to receive direct payment from APOC.

Another significant issue was the decision of APOC, without any consultation or agreement, to shift the Opening Ceremony forward by one day. This was to impact upon the timing of athletes' preparation, as well as accommodation and the competition programme. In addition to these changes, the Atlanta Organising Committee had announced that it would be opening the Paralympic Village only three days before the Games were scheduled to open – the regulations in the agreement specified that the Village must be open between five and seven days beforehand. The compromise of APOC was to help in arranging for accommodation elsewhere for teams wanting to arrive earlier, but at the expense of national federations. Of course there were practical difficulties for athletes themselves to deal with: humidity that would average between 70% and 80%, and temperatures expected to reach between 35° C and 40° C.

Some very straight talking was the characteristic of the exchange between the Atlanta Paralympic Organising Committee and members of the IPC Executive Committee, meeting in Cairo for the 15th

Executive Committee meeting, from 3rd to 5th March 1996. On the financial side of preparations David Simmons, Chief Operating Officer, indicated that they still had a long way to go, although this was the best moment: all bank loans had been fully repaid. Bernard Atha reminded Simmons that APOC had produced a bid that promised a legacy for the future of the Paralympic Movement. Atha was concerned that there was no evidence that a financial legacy would be endowed. Andy Fleming, Chief Executive Officer and President of APOC, stressed that no specific amount was promised in the bid or contract, the obligations being percentage and revenue share. He expressed his disappointment that no compromise had been reached in producing an alternative formula for the finances, and pointed to the continuing disagreements about the interpretation of the contract. Simmons promoted the idea that the legacy could be considered in terms of the improved marketability of the Paralympic Games after 1996 due to the higher public profile that would be created by the Atlanta Games. Future Paralympic organising committees would be poised to insist on far higher fees for media rights. York Chow pragmatically reminded the meeting that the relationship between APOC and the IPC was a partnership, and the sponsorship possibilities of the future were only a small part of the benefits to be gained from the relationship. He was confident that the obligations of the Atlanta Paralympic Organising Committee could be fully met.

The tensions continued to be present when APOC moved on to the subject of television coverage and advertising on uniforms for the Atlanta Paralympic Games. Simmons told the IPC Executive Committee that CBS would be the network partner, proposing four hours of national broadcasting. CNN would also show highlights of the Atlanta Paralympic Games. But the production costs would necessitate countries to bid for the international feed. Some objections were raised to the rights fee: nations would have difficulty persuading their national broadcaster to bid. It was clear the there would not be the same attitude from the media to bidding for coverage of the Paralympic Games as for the Olympic Games. The IPC wanted a flat rate of cost, preventing a small number of wealthy nations pushing up the price for the poorer countries. Simmons explained that the bidding process would probably benefit more countries. There had never before been a rights fee for the Paralympic Games. He stated that the purpose of the bidding process was 'to provide educational experience, not an increase of benefits to APOC'. Andy Fleming said that IPC presented a paradox: advertising to reduce costs for TV broadcasting, while producing guidelines for advertisement on uniforms that 'jeopardises the broadcasting contracts'. The problem with advertisements on athletes' uniforms and equipment was explained by Simmons as sponsors needing 'a clean field of play' – no existing logos that might be considered to be competing. He asked for '100% compliance'. The professional field of marketing and advertising had given rise to some colourful language use, as was shown when Harald von Selzam, from APOC, talked of the need to prevent 'ambush marketing' from putting off potential sponsors. The established relationships that some nations had with sponsors needed to be considered by APOC, Carl Wang insisted. This was fundamental to the functioning of the national organisations, and affected the feasibility of their athletes' participation in the Paralympic Games. Von Selzam expressed frustration at the obvious lack of understanding by the countries of the rules in existence. He considered that some problems arose because each sport had its own rules. He suggested that these should be applicable to competitions other than Paralympic Games, but that there should be a discrete set of regulations governing Paralympic Games. This issue needed resolution, but there was no immediate answer at the Cairo meetings. When the representatives of the Atlanta Paralympic Organising Committee left the room, further discussion centred on the need to ensure that APOC complied with every aspect of its contractual obligations to IPC. While there was agreement with Bernard Atha's insistence, Hans Lindström wanted to voice his concern that any rift between APOC and the IPC could jeopardise the quality and impact of the sports event of the Paralympic Games – which should not be risked as that aspect of the Games seemed to be well established. The credibility of IPC and future Paralympic Games could be affected by the present problems not being firmly resolved. The Sydney 2000 organisers must see that they would not be able to manipulate things in the same way.

No presentation was made to the Cairo meeting by the organisers of the Salt Lake 2002 Paralympic Winter Games, because there was no valid contract in place. The Salt Lake group had rewritten the contract and the amendments were not acceptable to IPC, especially the financial aspects. The negotiations would have to continue steadily, but battle lines had been drawn. In contrast, the Nagano organisers were entirely positive in their update. The 1998 Winter Paralympic Games were firmly progressing, with no complications foreseen with regard to advertising, or the inclusion of athletes with intellectual disability.

When the Paralympic Games were starting in Atlanta there were still important differences between the Atlanta Paralympic Organising Committee and the International Paralympic Committee. Andy Fleming reported to the IPC Executive Committee on 12th August 1996, emphasising that there were some problems in Games operating that were currently being sorted out. But more fundamental was the absence of any reference in the Atlanta Media Information Guide to the athletes with intellectual disability at the Paralympic Games. Bernard Atha asked for this to be put right, and requested that the minutes should reflect the lack of response from Andy Fleming. Once the APOC officers had withdrawn the IPC Executive Committee talked frankly about their worries regarding the financial agreements with APOC. The arguments had continued, and now IPC delegates were anxious lest the organising committee wound up its affairs and put itself beyond reach immediately after the Games. The Executive Committee got as far as discussing the method of bringing an injunction against APOC if necessary. The Atlanta Paralympic Organising Committee had insisted on calculating figures based on balance results rather than a fixed sum. This was all most distressing.

Intellectual Disability

The Atlanta Paralympic Organising Committee had initially proposed a limited programme of events for athletes with an intellectual disability. The suggestion in April 1995 was for events with exhibition status only, direct finals for a maximum of 32 athletes. The costs were not to be borne by APOC, but would have to be picked up by the IPC. The IPC Management Committee rejected this proposal, and pressed the President and Vice President to renegotiate. The fruits of this were much more satisfactory. The Atlanta Paralympic Organising Committee eventually accepted that events would be provided for 56 athletes, semi-finals and finals to be available. The competition programme would consist of: swimming – 50 metre freestyle (men and women), 100 metre freestyle (men and women); athletics – 200 metre (men and women), long jump (men and women). Flexibility in the numbers would have to be possible due to the qualification issue. Another success was the agreement of APOC to absorb the cost of the additional events. There was further agreement from APOC that it would accept participation in the equestrian events from athletes with an intellectual disability, as was consistent with IPC rules.

No one could suggest that the subject of inclusion of athletes with intellectual disability had become any less controversial or emotive by the 1995 Tokyo General Assembly. This was demonstrated clearly by a motion sent in by the International Stoke Mandeville Wheelchair Sports Federation with the following wording: 'The ISMWSF requests the adoption of a policy by the IPC that restricts participation in the Paralympic Games to the qualifying athletes of four international federations: ISMWSF, IBSA, CP-ISRA and ISOD'. The details of the debate are not recorded, but the ruling is equally clear: 'The motion was not accepted as it violates the constitution'. It is inconceivable that the international federations would have been unaware of the inadmissibility of such a motion, causing us to consider the real intent behind bringing the subject to the Assembly. If the officers of the ISMWSF were oblivious to the IPC constitution they would be guilty of a casual understanding of their own purpose that is impossible to accept. This could only mean that there was a wilful attempt to provoke a rift within the IPC – between those who believed passionately that the Paralympic Movement was all about equality of opportunity, and those who wished to exclude certain groups for fear of public reaction or negative association. The ISMWSF motion emanated from a survey that it conducted among athletes, coaches, officials and organisers during 1994. The rationale is important to examine, as it permits an understanding of the nature of the objections. Although some details of the statistics were not available, it is significant that 72.5% of the 360 responses did not approve of the inclusion of athletes with intellectual disabilities. In a preamble to the motion, the ISMWSF put forward reasons for the suggested ruling:

- INAS-FMH athletes at elite level are not physically or sensorially disabled. The Paralympic Games were meant for and should be restricted to those disability categories
- INAS-FMH athletes being non-physically disabled, have the possibility for integration into regular sports and should be encouraged to pursue integration on that level
- INAS-FMH athletes are already participating in the International Special Olympics which have far greater funds and resources for organising quadrennial competitions than IPC. In addition, the media attention given these athletes far exceeds that paid to physically and sensorially disabled athletes. Their needs are more than sufficiently met. Thus there are no additional benefits in their participation in the Paralympic Games
- Identifying physically disabled athletes in the Paralympic movement with Special Olympics athletes by the media and the public is difficult enough even when their competitions are separate. To combine them tends to reinforce the identification which troubles a great many athletes as evident in the responses to the survey
- The addition of non-physically or sensorially disabled athletes to the Paralympic Games programme will severely displace physically disabled athletes.

Technical Matters

By November 1994 the Sports Council had approved the awarding of Paralympic Sport status to wheelchair rugby. The sport had convinced the experts that it met with the criteria for inclusion under this banner, and the Executive Committee unanimously agreed to the exciting and visually attractive sport of Wheelchair rugby being welcomed into the 'family'. The status would not automatically lead to the sport's inclusion in the Paralympic Games, but the Atlanta Paralympic Organising Committee had been asked to consider offering wheelchair rugby as a demonstration sport.

During 1994 there had been a successful range of high profile world championships in IPC sports. Hans Lindström proudly presented the details in his report to the 1995 General Assembly:

- athletics: Berlin, July – 1077 athletes, 57 nations over 9 days;
- equestrianism: Hartbury, UK, July – 10 days of competition, 15 countries;
- powerlifting: Uppsala, 1st to 5th September, 141 athletes, 30 nations;
- shooting: Linz, Austria, 21st to 31st July, 23 nations, 145 athletes;
- cycling: Hasslet, Belgium, 30th May to 5th June, 238 athletes, 20 nations;
- swimming: Malta, 3rd to 8th November, 600 athletes, 40 nations.

While the sport of wheelchair dancing was denied its place alongside wheelchair rugby for the moment, the 1995 Tokyo General Assembly received clarification of the three levels of affiliation of sports in relation to the International Paralympic Committee. André Raes explained that the levels were:

- Paralympic sport: 'sports fulfilling criteria for inclusion in the Paralympic Games. Financial support is given by IPC for all matters relating to the Paralympics';

- IPC sport: 'sports fulfilling criteria for inclusion in the IPC Championships programme. Financial support by IPC';
- IPC-affiliated sport: no financial support is given by IPC but the affiliation increases the development possibilities of the sport'.

A number of important technical decisions came before the General Assembly in 1995 and were referred to the overview of the Task Force. It was much more sensible to delay some structural changes until time had been spent on an appraisal of the whole picture. This was not popular with all factions within the IPC. For example, when a motion to approve a vote for each of the Paralympic Sports within the General Assembly was put off until the Task Force had reported, the reaction from the Sports was politely disgruntled. Howard Bailey, as a representative of the Sports Committees, read an agreed statement:

> We would like to express our regret in the apparent lack of trust in our integrity and ability by delaying a firm decision on Motion 1. However, for our part we will continue to strive for the enhanced development of our individual sports and to ensure the success of the sports programme for the forthcoming Paralympic Games. We recognise that our presence at the General Assembly has improved relationships between ourselves and the member nations and we, for our part, will continue to strive to further improve greater understanding and knowledge.

The allocation of athletes to the Paralympic Games underwent a change. Until 1994 there had been concern that the number of entrants for each sport was climbing to overwhelming levels. As discussions with the International Paralympic Committee proceeded about inclusion of events in the Olympic Games, the IPC could see the IOC working to establish manageable participation levels and the IPC needed to do the same. Restricting entries or the number of sports could do this. The Sports Council Executive Committee (SCEC) looked at earlier proposals of the Paralympic Programme Committee for change from entries limited by country to entries limited by sport. The SCEC discussed this with the Atlanta Paralympic Organising Committee, which subsequently proposed a structure. National quotas of earlier days were swept away. Qualification became the watchword. There would be a limited number of opportunities for athletes unable to compete in qualifying events, especially for 'new' countries. This created opportunities and burdens for regional committees to run qualifying events prior to the Paralympic Games. Another adjustment for the 1995 General Assembly's information was that events that had been cancelled for two Paralympic Games, due to a having too few entries, would be deleted from the Paralympic programme.

A permanent staff would be needed very urgently to service the growing workload of the Technical Department. This was similar in other heavily laden areas of the IPC's operation. But his employer – the Swedish Sports Organisation for the Disabled (SHIF) – supported Hans Lindström to an unprecedented extent. The running of the Technical Department was effectively a full-time job, with no specifically dedicated secretarial help provided. Soon this would have to be addressed.

Sport Science and Medicine

Towards the end of 1994 Bob Steadward had cause to write to Juan Antonio Samaranch on several subjects. One was to ask that Michael Riding should be given the opportunity of working more closely with the IOC Medical Commission. Samaranch was aware that the IPC was basing its procedures for drug testing and regulation on those of the International Olympic Committee. When Steadward addressed the IOC Executive Board and the Association of National Olympic Committees, he suggested to Samaranch that Riding might even be appointed to the IOC Medical Commission as a full member. Samaranch suggested that he would be able to act on this suggestion all the more effectively if Steadward wrote a more formal request. This was composed on 4th January 1995, asking Samaranch to speak to Prince Alexandre de Mérode, Chairman of the Medical Commission. In the run-up to the Atlanta Games there was a need for approval from the IOC for the laboratories that would carry out the dope testing, and at the Tokyo General Assembly in November 1995, Michael Riding had to report that he had still not received notification from the IOC of this approval. The preferred laboratory was the Smith Kline Beecham facility in Atlanta itself. With approval expected before February 1996 it was hoped that testing would be carried out on a total of 15% of participants at the Atlanta Paralympic Games, as was desirable. Riding had a tough job keeping up with the modifications to the International Olympic Committee's doping policies, and adapting them to the context of the Paralympic Games. But the legitimacy of this 'piggybacking' was very desirable, because the IOC had more extensive resources for scientific research and broader cooperation. Basing the IPC policy on that of the IOC served to add weight to the International Paralympic Committee's policies and procedures.

Sport science was always going to involve sharing of information and resources, and the IPC Sport Science Committee asked the Executive Committee to move towards membership of the International Council of Sport Science and Physical Education (ICSSPE), the umbrella organisation coordinating the dissemination and implementation of findings of research. The Sport Science Committee also recognised that ICSSPE could be the source of research funding, and suggested a cooperative approach between IPC and the International Federational of Adapted Physical Activity (IFAPA) to bid for ICSSPE support. The IPC was accepted as a member of ICSSPE at the latter's meetings in conjunction with the International Pre-Olympic Scientific Congress in Dallas in August 1996.

Areas for exploration within the Medical Committee in the future would include ethical guidelines for classifiers, advice on athlete retirement and the development of a database for sports for persons with a disability. Trevor Williams, based in Loughborough, UK, would pioneer this important initiative. Consideration of ethics would need an expansion into many areas of the work of the IPC. Protocols and codes would become a part of several aspects of the daily routine. Regular research was to be carried out at Paralympic Games, and the Medical Committee drew up guidelines for the types of research that should take place, as well as its conduct. The arrangements for Atlanta were too well advanced to consider any implementation of these guidelines for 1996, and the contract in place with APOC would preclude any imposition of IPC preferences.

The International Olympic Committee did approve the use of the laboratories in Atlanta as the centre for testing samples during the Olympic Games, so Michael Riding was able to proceed with plans for the same laboratory to serve the Paralympic Games. Riding was kept busy with modifications to the IPC doping regulations as a result of the recommendations of the International Court of Arbitration's recommendations, following the conclusion of the case of the US Wheelchair Basketball Team.

A Task Force to Steer the IPC Onwards

The future success of the International Paralympic Committee depended on regular review of its structure and function, along with a willingness to submit itself to modification. So far the IPC had demonstrated such willingness in broad terms – certainly it had remained relatively close to its democratic goals. A sort of pluralism had overtaken the organisational configuration, with too much duplication of effort and authority structures. The IPC Congress in Tokyo in 1995 was seminal to this review and redefinition process. Just as in the past, a congress provided the stimulus for change: dedicated participants in organisational and scientific aspects of the Paralympic Movement met on 6th and 7th November. As a theme for the meetings the organisers took: 'A Call for Dialogue: unity and partnership – a vision for the future'. All speakers were passionate about the subject matter on which they spoke, but many articulated grim apprehension about the way the International Paralympic Committee was functioning, and in particular about the rapid expansion of the phenomenon of elite sport for athletes with a disability. A Task Force was invited to prepare a report for the Atlanta meetings in August 1996. The Executive Committee, meeting on 11th November 1995, just after the General Assembly, agreed to direct US$15 000 towards the work of the Task Force.

The International Paralympic Committee was not afraid of change. It was now a question of trying to rebuild the boat in the middle of the ocean. Bob Steadward suggested to the Tokyo General Assembly in 1995 that a congress such as the one they had just experienced should become a regular element of its procedures – linked to the period of the General Assembly. This would mean that the review of the 'health of the nation' in a congress could lead to resolutions being passed in the General Assembly, coupled with the elections of new officers – who would then have to carry out the tasks for the next era. The fruitful debate that had led to the Task Force coming into being should continue to enable reassessment of the structures and functions of the IPC. The Task Force, comprising Brendan Burkett, York Chow, Phil Craven, Helen Manning and Donald Royer, was entrusted with the responsibility of investigating current practices to assess the effectiveness of the IPC in achieving its objectives. The Tokyo Congress in 1995 produced frank and revealingly passionate views from the people most directly involved in the workings of the IPC. Each member of the Executive Committee had been asked to submit a paper, as well as other papers being welcomed from other quarters of the IPC membership.

André Auberger put a paper before the delegates at the IPC Congress in Tokyo entitled 'Development and Solidarity'. This laid out his ideas for a Solidarity Programme that would support developing countries in ways that would even up some of the effects of their economic limitations. He proposed that a Development Committee would undertake the following.

- Foster sport activities in countries where sports for the disabled do not yet exist
- Ensure basic education and training of staff and technical, medical and administrative trainers in countries where sports for the disabled are only just starting, and in those countries that do not have the means to develop them
- Set up a programme of indispensable equipment in those countries
- Administrate the organisation of competitions so that their best athletes could be singled out. They could then participate in high-level training programmes.

Auberger put forward a possible structure for such a committee, and a financial and operating plan. He informed the meeting that there would be a scheme in place for the Atlanta Paralympic Games, with the support of the IOC President. The target was to facilitate the sending of three people from each developing country – possibly enabling competitors from 35 nations to compete.

As hard-hitting as ever, André Raes chose to present direct criticisms to the IPC members attending the IPC Congress at the time of the Tokyo 1995 General Assembly. He entitled his paper 'We All Recognise the Diseases, But We Don't Recognise the Remedies'. The main points made by Raes were that there was a real need for greater unity in the Paralympic Movement. The effectiveness of the IPC was being hampered by duplication of effort, multiplied cost and shared leadership. The 'diseases' he referred to were 'mistrust and power', and the 'remedies' were 'rationalisation and unification'. Raes pointed to the separate headquarters of the international federations, the duplicated meetings and fundraising that overlapped and reduced effectiveness. He suggested that there should be only one headquarters, the IPC headquarters from which all secretariats would operate. The international federations should be reduced to the status of 'small working groups'. Another of André Raes's initiatives was to present a further paper on the 'Vision for the Future'. He said that: 'The political power must be reinstated in the General Assembly, and the nations have to realise that the power belongs to them'. This was a more acceptable message for the delegates to receive. He did not mince his words when he said: 'The Executive

Boards of IPC (Executive Committee and Sports Council Executive Committee) must be depoliticised and brought back to efficiently working executive bodies'. The way to do this was to reduce the number of officers and to entrust each officer with a specific task. A positive suggestion was for the sports to agree to clear requirements for competition. They must accept integrated classification, minimum disability, minimum number of participants in an event, and a quota system and rankings.

In contrast to the demanding nature of the Secretary General's papers, the joint position paper from ISMWSF and ISOD called for a freeing of the international federations from the restrictive agreements relating to the staging of competitions. They wanted liberty to engage in reciprocal agreements to arrange multi-disability competitions without hindrance or obligation to a third party – the IPC.

The French members submitted a paper on the possible impact of the inclusion of athletes with intellectual disability. Bernard Verneau was the speaker, and his paper entitled 'Paralympics for everyone?' examined the effect on other athletes and the phenomenon of the Paralympic Games of adding to the existing population of athletes and events. The thesis was that the Games could not expand very much more before having to limit participation in a way that was inappropriate to the objectives of the Paralympic Movement. Dealing also with the inevitable increase in participation from the severely disabled (referred to by Verneau as the 'heavily handicapped'), the suggestion was to have a four-year cycle that allowed Summer and Winter Paralympic Games to be interspersed with specific 'Mentally Disabled World Games' in one year and 'Heavy Handicapped Games' in the other year.

At the Tokyo Congress, Phil Craven impressed the delegates with an impassioned paper that spelt out the difficulties ahead under the present structure, while celebrating the achievements of the past. As President of the International Wheelchair Basketball Federation, Craven had proven his willingness to immerse himself in the tough issues of his own sport, and the political side of international organisations. His assiduous analysis was characteristic of his openness and fighting spirit. These talents would be recognised a few years later, when Craven was to be elected to the Presidency of the International Paralympic Committee. Craven's paper was entitled: 'The IPC – where lies the future?' He assessed the origins and purpose of the International Paralympic Committee:

- to build on the work of the ICC, and to mirror the IOC in the organisation of the Paralympic Games;
- to bring together widely disparate existing disability sports federations;
- to encourage the coming together of certain sports under a pan-Paralympic banner, particularly with regard to common classification systems;
- to reduce the financial burden on countries paying membership fees to several different disability sport federations by paying to only one.

In his comments, Craven pointed out that some progress had been made in the first and third goals above, while the second issue had failed to disperse the apprehension of the international federations about their own security and integrity – even survival. Craven suggested that the IPC had not done enough to reassure these organisations. However, other contributions to the Tokyo Congress would confirm that the fears of the international federations had been entirely appropriate, as calls were heard for the subsuming of the international federations to become minor committees of the International Paralympic Committee. The subject of membership fees led Craven to comment that many members had very limited funds and needed to get value for money from membership fees, and that many countries still had a medical/disability/rehabilitation approach rather than a sport approach to the Paralympic Movement. This was identifiable in the people they nominated for elections. These countries, in Craven's opinion, also tended to want as much 'service' as possible for as little outlay as possible – not appreciating that investment was necessary in the IPC to enable the best returns.

Craven had the ability to ask good questions. Referring to the elected representatives in the IPC he asked whether, after six years, the IPC was too large and unwieldy. How many of its members had an agreed, achievable and time-limited workload? He felt that the two-tiered structure of Paralympic Sports and IPC Sports was ineffectual, although he acknowledged that it had been a result of the attempts to bring together the sports under the pan-Paralympic banner. Craven saw the system as divisive. He called for sports to have 'headroom and breathing space in order to further their development'. But independence was not suitable for all Paralympic sports. He also suggested that direct financial support from IPC to all the sports would reduce the necessity for the sports to impose membership fees themselves. Continuing his excellent observations, Phil Craven looked to the future in term of the core principles of the IPC. He projected that they should be:

- to ensure the continuing development of the Paralympic Games – one of the few jewels in the crown of world sport;
- to protect against unwelcome bidders the very special ideals and philosophies that have developed within the Paralympic Movement over the last fifty years;
- to have a sport-specific work ethic rather than a disability-specific ethic and work to finally banish the 'rehabilitation syndrome' from high performance Paralympic competition at world and zonal level.

To the principles, Craven added his projected functions of the IPC:

- to negotiate with potential and actual organisers of the Summer and Winter Paralympic Games;
- to maintain close liaison with the IOC;
- to support Paralympic sports which initially may not seem attractive to Paralympic Games organisers, but which with proper marketing and explanation would attract spectators and would show more impaired athletes that they are just as important to the Paralympic Movement
- to remove legal restrictions on the development of individual Paralympic sports;
- to undertake corporate marketing;
- to undertake corporate fundraising and sponsorship acquirement;
- to undertake corporate public relations.

Further suggestions for the future included possibilities for funding and an action plan 'that is owned by everyone involved with international Paralympic sport'. Craven's idea of an action plan would contain clear, measurable and realisable objectives that were transferred into specific responsibilities of individuals which had a time frame for completion.

Carl Wang submitted some ideas from the European Regional Committee – EUROCOM. Wang identified clear lines of development within the IPC.

- There was an increasing numbers of national members.
- There was uncertainty over the development of a more sports-specific organisation, due to the retention of control by international federations over their own disability group. Wang emphasised that unity was still missing as a result.
- The role of national 'units', such a major feature of the new organisation, was still too weak. Wang attributed this to the IPC not having a specific policy for the regions.
- Integration was developing too slowly, even though signs were clear that there was a more positive acceptance of disabled people in society. There was evidence that integration was best maintained on the basis of sport rather than by emphasising handicap.
- There was still confusion regarding the IPC's position in the relationship between elite sport, mass participation (recreational) sport and sport for development. Wang asked whether the IPC could cope with 'this double challenge'. He used the term 'gigantism', as had been applied to the Olympic Games.

Carl Wang proceeded to discuss the challenge of integration and then to emphasise that the IPC had to grasp the challenges that lay ahead in promoting the participation of more women with a disability, as well as stimulating the involvement of the athletes with a severe disability. He voiced concern at the tendency to split up sports into separate organisations. In competitions other than the Paralympic Games, Wang expressed the view that the IPC needed to take greater control of the events, distributing the allocation of regional and world championships more evenly around the nations. He promoted further reductions in the number of classes, looking to the IPC Sports Councils to come up with ways of making this possible.

Wang ended his astute presentation by stressing the most important factors that began the ball rolling in Arnhem in 1987: the strengthening of national influence; athletes having a greater influence in a democratic process; and the building up of regional units – now needing more power and a clear mandate.

When Juan Palau Francas, President of the Federación Española de Deportes de Minusválidos Físicos (Spanish Federation of Sport for Persons with a Disability), submitted his paper, it was clear from the beginning that the tone was going to be highly critical. His first main concern was the insistence that the International Paralympic Committee should organise more than the Paralympic Summer and Winter Games. He felt that it was too ambitious, especially if the world and regional championships were to be run as truly multi-disability events. He put his views plainly: 'This model has no future, it is a true administrative chaos, and goes against the model of World Sport, against the interests of the International Federations and of the affiliated countries, which are, in short, those who work day by day for the development of sport'. Francas used the examples of the Berlin Athletics World Championships and the Swimming World Championships in Malta, to illustrate his concerns. He said they: 'only serve to confirm that we are not on the right track'. In looking forward, Francas described the proposals of his national federation:

- that IPC only organise Paralympic Games;
- that there should be, as members of the IPC Executive Committee, influential people: 'of the highest financial position, Presidents of International Foundations and Monarchical representatives';
- that the international federations should organise world championships, not the IPC;
- that the IPC should not seek to be an international federation, 'but rather an international organisation at the highest level';
- that IPC should seek resources for the Paralympics;
- that it should coordinate, support and respect international federations;
- that it should 'sustain international representation of the Paralympic Sports';
- that it should encourage the creation of Paralympic Committees in every country;
- that it should reaffirm its desire to establish adapted, normalised and integrated sports within the context of world sports, under the guidance of the IOC:
  o Having a professional Secretariat in Lausanne
  o Working closely with the IOC so that the city organising the Olympic Games will also be obliged to organise the Paralympics
  o With Olympic and Paralympic flags
  o With the same design of medals
  o With the same rights and obligations as the Olympic Athletes.

Francas considered that the International Paralympic Committee 'should act as an IOC for those with disabilities and work to achieve this, leaving each international federation to organise its competitions according to their respective handicaps'. His suggestions for the future included revision of the membership fee structure to allow for a sort of proportional scale according to number of participants, wealth of the country and so on. Even with the exhortations for the IPC to hand over the control of world and regional championships to the international federations, Francas still asked that the IPC do more to promote sport for all and work in developing countries. This critical presentation was still focused on rebuilding and redirecting the work of the International Paralympic Committee.

The scale of the demands on the IPC was the central focus of the paper presented by Hans Lindström, the Technical Officer. He put before the Congress an overview of what actually happened,; so that the members could consider a structure 'which best serves their interest and needs'. His paper was a morass of facts and figures – convincing delegates of the overwhelming growth of the Paralympic Movement. Nine international organisations in the world organised sports 'for athletes with locomotive disabilities, visual impairment, mental handicap and deafness'. IPC provided two different programmes: the Paralympic Games and the championships of 13 multi-disability sports. The five international organisations of sport for people with a disability (IOSD), which were the international members of IPC, provided their own championship or games programme. The number of meetings of each separate organisation had become unmanageable, as had the funding of the different administrations. His summary was: 15 General Assemblies in each 4-year period; 6 Executive Committees, with about 48 meetings in each 4-year period; one Paralympic Sports Council, with 4 meetings in each four-year period; 6 Sports Technical Committees with about 35–45 meetings in each four-year period; 6 medical committees; about 35–45 Sports Assemblies every fourth year, with another 10–15 every second year; approximately 73 Sports Committees/Sections/Coordinators for 31 sports, 57 of them covering 15 of the sports! After all this, Hans Lindström subtly put the question of whether national member organisations considered that the formation of the IPC had led to the fulfilment of the aims and objectives in terms of sports structure.

The IPC Magazine was in its infancy at this time, although newsletters had been regularly produced throughout the days of the International Coordinating Committee and the first days of the IPC. The issue of the Magazine that followed the Tokyo Congress and General Assembly had a sensitive article from Bob Steadward, expressing his satisfaction with the openness demonstrated by members in Tokyo. There was certainly a reservation in the tone of Steadward's writing, less convincing enthusiasm than he had been renowned for. André Raes, on the other hand, was more blunt. His article told of the dreams of many delegates, and of himself: 'there is no place in IPC for dreams, the future is uncertain and gives no guarantees. Struggling and fighting to survive is the IPC way of life.' In the same magazine issue Raes conveyed his annoyance that the delegates at the Congress and the General Assembly had shown such lack of political sophistication – ironic when one considers his calls to de-politicise the Executive Committee. He suggested that the main theme of the Congress had really been 'authority'. Bitterness was shown for the unwillingness of the international federations to give up the heritage of authority they had gained under old regimes. Raes resented the wish for the international federations to dominate with: 'a heritage from the past inspired by great leaders indeed, but sport was not the principal goal'. When Raes turned to the specific problems of the past meetings he focused on the tendency of member nations to arrive without the circulated papers having been read at all, without having studied the proposals and motions in advance. Raes accused the members of being naïve: 'many voted without really knowing the content and consequences of their decisions . . . One member told me that the nations have to be taught and literally brainwashed to understand and see the consequences of the various motions in the General Assembly.' This was not the most promising position from which to launch a restructuring of the International Paralympic Committee.

The Tokyo Congress of 1995 produced essential questions that drove the inquiries of the Task Force. Barbara Campbell and Gudrun Doll-Tepper produced a precise summary of the Tokyo discussions as follows.

- Can the IPC really fulfil its proclaimed mandate of coordinating and governing sports for persons with a disability for the whole world?
- Would it be more realistic for the IPC to focus on the Paralympic Games?
- Is the current IPC structure appropriate for its functions?

- What are the roles of the IOSDs/regional bodies?
- What are the roles of the sports sections within the IPC?
- Who should coordinate development in different regions?
- How can the IPC balance and address the needs of equity in sports, events, disability categories, degrees and severity of disability and sexes?
- What should the IPC's external policies be – for example, its relationship with IOSDs, regional federations, IOC and other sports or international bodies?

The Task Force was given the mandate of bringing some solutions to the membership so that an invigorated organisation could take the Paralympic Movement on to the next stage of development. The specific directives were:

- to review and compile the results and issues raised in the IPC Congress and direction arising from the General Assembly, Tokyo 1995, and to provide guidance for focused topics for the next IPC Congress;
- to review the roles and functions of the IPC and its officers and constituents (that is, departments and committees);
- to recommend future roles and functions of the IPC and the delineation of responsibilities, guided by the recommended IPC objectives, shared values and principles and structural recommendations proposed to the IPC Congress and General Assembly;
- to make recommendations on options to restructure IPC with a view to improve its effectiveness and efficiency.

Atlanta Olympic Games, 19th July to 4th August

Izzy, the mascot of the Atlanta Olympic Games, was much in evidence as athletes numbering more than 10 000 settled into their accommodation. These elite sportspersons would compete in 26 sports over the 16 days. This was the first time that all 197 member National Olympic Committees were represented. Sadly, the Olympic Games would be rocked by tragedy with the bombing in Centennial Olympic Park on 27th July.

Muhammad Ali lit the Olympic Flame at the Opening Ceremony. There were two main venues for the events: Olympic Park and the Olympic Ring. Among the feats accomplished in the Atlanta Olympic Games were Donovan Bailey's (Canada) 100 m run in 9.84 seconds and Michael Johnson (USA) taking the demanding double of 200 m and 400 m. In the women's events Junxia Wang (China) won a convincing 5000 m race, signalling the arrival of a new nation of distance runners; Stefka Kostodinove (Bulgaria) won the high jump with a new World and Olympic Record of 2 metres and 5 centimetres. The flamboyant Florence 'FloJo' Griffith Joyner (USA) won both the 100 m and 200 m sprints. Carl Lewis achieved his ninth Olympic Gold Medal. The exhibition events at the Atlanta Olympic Games were well received by the many spectators, especially as they were scheduled close to other prime track events. In the men's 1500 m wheelchair race the results were: 1st Claude Issorat (France), 2nd Scott Holonbeck (USA), 3rd Franz Nietlisbach (Switzerland). In the women's 800 m wheelchair race the expected close race between Chantal Petitclerc and Louise Sauvage did not materialise, with Petitclerc only managing 5th. The results were: 1st Louise Sauvage (Australia), 2nd Jean Driscoll (USA), 3rd Cheri Becerra (USA).

The motto of the Atlanta Games was well chosen as the Triumph of the Human Spirit, symbolising the significant obstacles that need to be overcome to achieve the elite level of sporting prowess represented by the Olympic and Paralympic Games. When the Paralympic Games opened on 16th August, those gathered for the Opening Ceremony could not have considered it possible that the Paralympic Movement

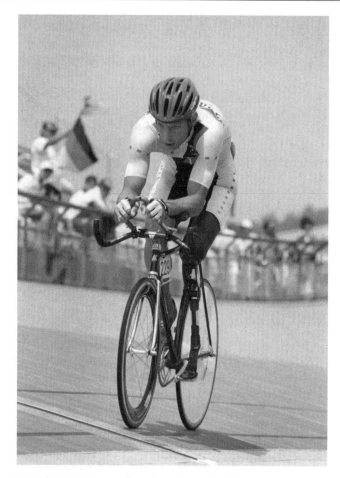

Figure 6.1   Atlanta 1996 (photograph courtesy of Lieven Coudenys).

had developed so phenomenally. In the period from 16th to 25th August 1996, Atlanta would encounter 3195 Paralympic athletes representing 103 countries in 20 sports. Of these athletes, 2415 were men and 780 women. A total of 1717 team officials were accredited. There were a staggering 10 330 volunteers. Classification was done on 890 athletes, with 186 of them being reclassified. The statistics suggest that 2088 members of the media attended the Paralympic Games, and they saw a total of 1574 medals awarded. Demonstration sports were racquetball, sailing and wheelchair rugby. Athletes with intellectual disabilities took part in swimming and athletics.

Most outstanding on the track was Louise Sauvage (Australia), winning 400 m, 800 m, 1500 m and 5000 m. Béatrice Hess (France) beat World and Paralympic records in winning the 200 m individual medley. Swimmer and elementary school teacher Trischa Zorn (USA) won two gold, three silver and three bronze medals, in addition to her ten gold and two silver medals from Barcelona and 12 gold medals from Seoul. Zorn was born with aniridia, the absence of irises, and is legally blind.

This was the first Paralympic Games to benefit from worldwide sponsorship, even though there had been monumental difficulties in establishing an acceptable agreement between IPC and the Atlanta Paralympic Organising Committee. The Paralympic Congress held between 12th and 16th August explored issues connected with the 'political and economic empowerment of persons with a disability'.

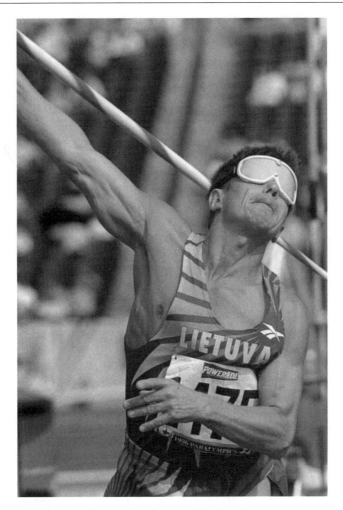

Figure 6.2   Atlanta 1996 (photograph courtesy of Lieven Coudenys).

Returning to some early intentions of Pierre de Coubertin, founder of the Modern Olympic Games, the Paralympic Games in Atlanta hosted a Cultural Pyramid: artworks entered for competition and display throughout the period of the sporting celebrations.

It was with some surprise that IPC officials were informed that the wheelchair basketball athletes from Iraq had not turned up at all in Atlanta. Their actions had the effect of preventing other competitors from being able to participate – another team would have filled their places willingly. André Raes was asked to prepare a letter to the national organisation in Iraq, stating that their failure to attend or to communicate had caused serious disruption to the media scheduling of coverage, as well as excluding others from participation in the Paralympic Games. A satisfactory explanation was essential in order for Iraq to avoid sanctions.

While the sporting competitions at the Atlanta Paralympic Games were tremendously successful, there were some facets of operation that did not go totally without a hitch. The transportation system came in for much criticism. In one instance the driver had no idea of his route and took an equestrian team into another state by mistake. At the very start the athletes felt as though they were not being

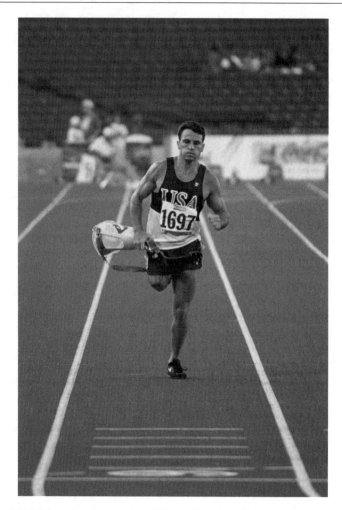

Figure 6.3 Atlanta 1996 (photograph courtesy of Lieven Coudenys).

treated with the respect that should be accorded to the best in the world: the British athletes were presented with a bucket full of unmarked keys when they arrived at their accommodation – and were told to sort themselves out! Anger replaced mere frustration when they saw that even the televisions provided for the Olympic athletes in the Olympic Village had been ripped out prior to the arrival of the Paralympic athletes. In response to the criticisms levelled at the Atlanta Paralympic Organising Committee by Bob Steadward after the Games, Andy Fleming admitted that his organisation had not been able to deliver the quality expected. But in mitigation he cited the legacy of inheriting 'thoroughly trashed' athletes' rooms and delegation offices from the Olympic Games organisers. He claimed that they had spent hundreds of thousands of dollars trying to put things right – from replacing consignments of bed linen that had disappeared, to replacing keys that couldn't be used. The conditions at some of the sporting venues were similar, according to Fleming. Swimmers described their surprise at seeing holes in walls of the building – where television crews had removed cabling they would not be using as they were not covering the Paralympic Games.

In the cycling there had been a lapse in the police security system and accidents resulted on the road. A number of protests had to be dealt with in the equestrian events, due to the disqualification of several

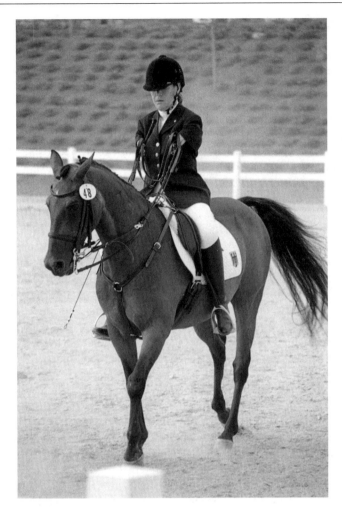

Figure 6.4   Atlanta 1996 (photograph courtesy of Lieven Coudenys).

horses. The swimming pool was the location of an unusually high number of disqualifications due to a 'stringent rule, enforced for the first time'.

After all the controversy and effort to gain inclusion of athletes with intellectual disability in the Atlanta Paralympic Games, there was still more trouble to come. The Atlanta Paralympic Organising Committee, APOC, intended to all but ignore the presence of the 56 athletes given leave to attend. Bulletins like the *Spectator News*, published and distributed during the Games themselves, managed to run issues throughout the Paralympic Games without once mentioning athletes with intellectual disability. Even in the most obvious circumstances, such as in explanations of the systems of classification, only four categories were outlined: visually impaired, amputees, cerebral palsy and wheelchair athletes (17th August 1996). The Opening Ceremony was the greatest insult to athletes with intellectual disability. While all other disability groups were welcomed and praised in turn, these athletes were emphatically denied the honour of being embraced within the Paralympic commu-nity through being mentioned. As Bernard Atha said: 'It was a gratuitous and childish insult'.

Even the daily 'Event Sheet' failed to show the classification of athletes with an intellectual disability, until a public outcry by Bernard Atha brought the subject to the attention of the Atlanta newspapers. *The Atlanta Journal* reported the insult in an article on 19th August. The Atlanta Paralympic Organising Committee refused to respond to official communications from Atha, President of INAS-FMH. Once the newspapers took up the cudgels APOC immediately apologised for its 'unintended oversight'!

When the Athletes' Committee reported to the Executive Committee following the Atlanta Paralympics, there was a perception that the competitions and sports technical matters were well organised and professionally run, but the accommodation was considered to have been 'unacceptable'. This was quite a tame assessment, as when Steadward wrote directly to Samaranch in September 1996 to thank him for supporting the Games with his presence, Steadward put the situation plainly: 'Although performances by our athletes were the "best ever", the operation and administration of the Games was less than satisfactory for the athletes, and this included *everything*, from transportation to Village conditions, to food, and on into protocol matters as well'. Steadward took the opportunity of urging a closer working arrangement between the two host organising committees. But there had been a strong athletes' protest during the Games, about the poor standards of accommodation and services. They had intended to unfurl a banner very publicly during the Closing Ceremony so as to draw large-scale media attention. The persuasive intervention of IPC representatives led to an agreement that the banner would be on full display throughout the next Executive Committee meeting. This would serve as a reminder that the athletes had not been content with the provision given by the organising committee. The athletes had their way, and the banner was prominent during the meetings of 18th to 21st March 1997 in Lisle, even during the report of the Atlanta Paralympic Organising Committee.

At the IPC Executive Committee meeting, Bob Steadward asked that a little group should sit together and record the specific issues so that they could provide feedback to the Atlanta organisers, as well as advising the Sydney Paralympic Organising Committee in its planning.

A total of 318 doping tests were carried out, without a single positive result. Michael Riding, Medical Officer, told the Executive Committee at its meeting on the morning of 25th August 1996 of his displeasure with the attitude of the 'Chairman of the International Wheelchair Basketball Federation, for trying to interfere with doping tests in the women's final' (IPC EC VIII/16/11 Item 7). Some testing was done on athletes for boosting, but no one was withdrawn from competition – just what was learnt from these tests is not so obvious. The Sport Science and Medical Committee drew up regulations relating to boosting among athletes, with clear emphasis on the health risks of stimulating autonomic dysreflexia.

The Task Force Reports Back at Atlanta

The five-strong group that made up the IPC Task Force were to provide the sort of appraisal of the structure and function of the organisation of an order parallel to the work done in Arnhem and Düsseldorf. The differences were that this time the investigation was entirely structured, covering an acceptable time frame. Enough information could be gathered to inform the members appropriately of the most suitable proposals to put forward to the General Assembly. Of course, this also enabled the motions submitted in Atlanta in 1996 to have a very good prospect of being accepted.

The Task Force report took a familiar analytical structure from the business world as a model, assessing strengths and weaknesses. As the Task Force appraisal moved on to the more negative characteristics of the IPC's existence, the weaknesses were identified as including: a 'clear lack of unity among different stakeholders with regard to the mandate of the IPC' – this tended to pull the membership apart. The simple size and complexity of the IPC's present mandate caused problems, and controversy was also sometimes a product of its actions. The Task Force quoted the scope of the IPC's objectives, and suggested that: 'the reality may be that no one organisation can take on such a large area of responsibility – certainly a young, under financed organisation will experience great difficulty in satisfying such a task'. With agreement about the IPC's responsibility for Paralympic Games, there was still disagreement over the responsibility of IPC to organise regional and world championships and development programmes. The Task Force added that: 'this has created considerable mistrust among officers of different organisations and thus has affected the image and credibility of the IPC'.

Low levels of funding and a lack of public exposure had tended to reduce the power of IPC to encourage further financial support, as well as making the position of the IPC weaker when negotiating contracts and insisting on quality levels for Paralympic Games. Threats to the International Paralympic Committee in the future were assessed as part of this process of review. Quite obviously, the greatest threat to the IPC was to ignore the concerns raised at the Tokyo Congress. This would have been foolish, especially as the concerns came from within the membership itself. The Task Force stressed that the existing divisiveness would spread, and 'would become very destructive to the IPC, our athletes and the Paralympic Games'. Another threat was to the maintenance of quality in the Paralympic Games. This was proven by the difficulties encountered in dealing with the Atlanta Paralympic Organising Committee, and the fact that 'the Salt Lake Olympic Organising Committee has very little intention of hosting a Winter Paralympics in 2002 – certainly no intention of hosting a Paralympic Games of the quality we have come to expect'. Subscription issues featured among the threats to the IPC: some countries were being put under considerable strain as a result of increases. The question had to be whether members were receiving value for money: 'without resolution of this conflict within IPC, we might further lose the loyalty and trust of our members'.

The Task Force spelt out the opportunities that stood ahead for the International Paralympic Committee. The first of these was the opportunity to redefine its mandate – particularly suggesting a narrower focus, in order to better utilise its resources. It was more likely, in the opinion of the Task Force, that members would back such a narrower and more achievable goal. The relationship with the international organisations of sport for disabled needed to move towards a more obvious partnership. The suggestion was for clearly defined roles and joint strategies to be developed. Partnership should also be developed with the mainstream international federations and the IOC, looking for clarity and consistency. The Media Committee would be a vital organ in the new operation, ensuring appropriately high-level exposure for the IPC and its activities, especially television. A consistent marketing strategy was seen to be the foundation of a secure funding base, and members should also receive guidance on how to market their resources professionally.

Proposals made by the Task Force for the International Paralympic Committee were predictable to a reasonable degree. Their main thrust went along the lines of discontent most clearly expressed at the 1995 Congress: professional staff in a permanent secretariat; concentration by IPC solely on the Paralympic Games rather than world and regional championships; the Paralympic bid to be part of Olympic bidding procedure; and restructuring of the Executive Committee to allow a smaller, task-driven body.

The Task Force envisaged the IOSDs concentrating on the disability-based sports, promoting grass roots development as well as organising competitive programmes. With IPC's support, the IOSDs would cooperate to manage the multi-disability championships at national, world and regional levels, allowing the IPC to bring the greatest attention to the Paralympic Games. While the international disability sports organisations had been asking for something similar, they were unlikely to welcome such a marginal role in the Paralympic Games organisation. They had worked their way on to the stage of the second largest sporting event, and would be reluctant to hand over control. This was a proposal to reverse the power base of the early years: under the International Coordinating Committee the IOSDs had totally managed the Paralympic Games. The Arnhem Seminar that had effectively created the International Paralympic Committee was looking to establish a more democratic, sport-based organi-sation with a focal base on the nations. This was obviously not to the liking of the international federations. Now, according to the Task Force proposals, they were finally going to be part-players.

The Sports Sections of the IPC would be encouraged to be independent if they had the resources, or they could work more closely with the IOSDs. The implication was that they were being released from the restraints that some considered were limiting their development. But for some sports this would mean that survival would be dependent on rapidly acquiring new skills, especially marketing and management structures. The IPC Sports Council would bring them together, and some funding would emanate from IPC as well. Regional organisations would have more prominence under the Task Force's proposals, and the relationship of national federations and Paralympic committees would alter so as to reflect the purposes of the IOSDs and the IPC's proposed mandate. In practice the hope of the Task Force was probably unrealistic – a significant number of smaller countries would simply have lost any ability to function under this system.

The group circulated a draft of its findings and recommendations in March 1996, requesting feedback from member nations, international federations and members of various committees by 30th April. The response of the membership was good, although the numbers sending in their comments still repre-sented a relatively small proportion: 23 nations, six sports, all five IOSDs, five members of the Executive Committee and nine individuals. York Chow seemed satisfied with this level of response, including comments that were: 'positive, critical and also with some alternative suggestions'. He received opinions from some members who did not want anything changed, as well as one who disagreed with every section of the Task Force's report. The Task Force then met in Manchester and prepared a final report for the Extraordinary General Assembly in Atlanta.

Colin Rains wrote to York Chow on 28th March 1996 to put on paper the views he had been expressing in meetings. The proposals of the draft Task Force Report would cut the international organisations out of the central decision making for the IPC. Rains appeared saddened that: 'the international federations within any new proposed structure appeared to have lost their identity'. Rains called this a 'retrograde step', because the IOSDs 'have been and still are likely to remain the backbone of any new IPC arrangements and structures'. Rains proposed an addition to the suggested twelve members of the Executive Committee, to include the representatives of the IOSDs.

The European Region of IPC met to discuss the Task Force's report on the occasion of the IPC Ice Sledge Hockey Championships in Nynashamn, Sweden, in April 1996. Twenty countries deba-ted the merits of the draft report, and strong opinions were expressed. This was an excellent forum for exchanging viewpoints, and the particular concerns of member nations were summarised as follows.

- They did not wish the IPC to be concerned only with the Paralympic Games.
- Understandably, they wanted the regional structures to be strengthened, with responsibility for regional championships automatically being given to them.
- Regions should not have to support classifiers and technical experts coming in to help run regional events – they should have their own.
- They did not support the idea of independent sports organisations at this stage. If sports were to separate into autonomous groups, it needed to be done gradually and after much more investigation about the consequences. An important point was that the nations had originally wanted to create the International Paralympic Committee because they wanted fewer organisations to deal with, fewer membership fees and less administration. Unity within IPC could also be further threatened by fragmentation.

- The European region had no argument with the proposal to remove the IOSDs from the Executive Committee, but it did want stronger sports representation and defined functions for Executive Committee members. IOSDs should focus on development and recruitment.

These views were communicated to the Chairman of the Task Force in various letters after the European Conference. Hans Lindström urged the logical involvement of both the sports technical and the policy-making people within IPC to respect each other's knowledge and sphere of influence. He advocated voting rights for the Paralympic Sports Councils at General Assemblies because the delegates attending the General Assemblies so far had tended to be the political leadership of the nations, and not people with the technical knowledge from the sports sections – these representatives tended to be the ones to attend the Sports Assemblies. Lindström, later to stand down as IPC Technical Officer to take on the presidency of the European region, wrote his views in the IPC Magazine of June 1996. He was not suggesting that the sports technical representatives would hold opposing views from their other national delegates, but that they would bring a different angle to the General Assembly. Respect would also be shown to this group, acknowledging that there was more to the entity of decision making than policy matters. He was sceptical about the suggestion of making the sports into independent federations, repeating the European region's agreement that: 'it does not fit into the realities of the nations who participate in the sports'. National organisations cover most of the sports for people with a disability in their country in one way or another. The national organisation could accept that international federations such as the International Yacht Racing Union cater for athletes with a disability alongside other athletes, but Lindström could not accept that 'their sports subcommittee representatives with sports specific mandates' would move to establish international organisations – it was 'just a bit too far off key'. He acknowledged that the independence of sports could be investigated over a lengthier period, but decisions should only result from agreement of a majority of nations practising each sport concerned.

The response of the International Blind Sports Association to the draft report of the Task Force was predictably frosty. Enrique Sanz considered that the documents were 'disappointingly imprecise' in both the thinking and the expression. He did not mince his words, calling the whole process 'crude and unintelligent'. IBSA believed the proposals of the IPC to be a 'retreat'. He somewhat spitefully aimed criticism at Phil Craven and York Chow, and suggested that the intention appeared to be to offer prominence to activities such as wheelchair basketball, and to give power to FESPIC and possibly IPC Europe. The criticisms continued unabated: confusion between what was implied about IOSDs early in the draft and apparently different intentions later on; and calling the draft document an invitation for members to buy 'a pig in a poke'. A reasonably made point was that IOSDs, excluded from meaningful representation within IPC, would seek solace in each other's company – effectively reconvening a type of ICC from the past. Sanz concluded with a strong statement: 'It seems to be the work of people who never met, have quite different agendas, and who have not been forced to resolve their differences and confusions – except that is by stuffing them out of sight (almost) by fogging problems in generality'.

Elizabeth Dendy's response to the Task Force draft report was more restrained than that of Enrique Sanz. As President of CP-ISRA, Dendy also showed concern for the fragmentation of IPC through the distancing of the international federations from the central discussions and decision making. The same might be true of the sports and regional organisations. IPC would have only the Paralympic Games as its remit. This would, in her view, then require another umbrella organisation to bring everything together – she subtly pointed out the inconsistency in this logic. Another interesting comment of Dendy's was her concern at the language used in the Task Force report. The terminology employed was that of business analysis, not entirely suited to direct transfer to the current subject: 'our movement comprises people doing sport and people, mainly volunteers, working with them. Too close an analogy with business terms can affect the ethos and priorities.' The 'SWOT' analysis described the athletes as 'the product' of the IPC – perhaps not the most endearing language.

The members of the Task Force acknowledged that their investigations suffered from being unscientific in nature, although all constituent groups involved in IPC were consulted extensively. Credibility and strength were derived within IPC from the breadth of its membership: national members and international federations having been involved in its establishment. The commitment and resilience of the participants were also identified as major strengths identified in the IPC, including the nucleus of dedicated staff and committee members serving the diverse membership. Throughout the working period of the Task Force, the IPC Secretariat, in the form of Leen Coudenys and Barbara Vertriest as well as André Raes, provided great support.

The Extraordinary General Assembly Votes

To be able to start heading in the direction identified by the members as being most appropriate for the IPC, an Extraordinary General Assembly had been called for 16th and 17th August 1996, in Atlanta. The important occasion was hosted by Georgia Tech University, with its President, Dr Patton, welcoming delegates to the Marriott Marquis Hotel. Among the dignitaries present were Juan Antonio Samaranch, Walther Tröger, Andy Fleming and Leroy Walker, President of the United States Olympic Committee. The official opening of the Extraordinary General Assembly gave an opportunity for the presentation of the Gold Medal of the Paralympic Order to the IOC President, Juan Antonio Samaranch.

The total voting representation at the General Assembly was 363, representing 76 nations, 5 international organisations and the chairpersons of most Paralympic Sports. As was usual at these meetings, new memberships were ratified: Yugoslavia, Sierra Leone, Nauru, Burundi, Armenia, Tajikistan and Honduras were all accepted into membership of the International Paralympic Committee. York Chow, Chairman of the Task Force, gave assurances that they had worked very closely to the mandate given by the Tokyo Congress. Further opportunity was given to raise clarification on the official report of the Task Force.

All members had been sent the motions recommended by the Task Force in advance; they had been given the opportunity to respond directly with their comments and suggestions at earlier stages. It is not clear how many nations arrived in Atlanta with a full understanding of the implications of the votes they were about to cast. The actual process of presenting motions and the subsequent voting reveal much about the contemporary attitudes and tensions.

The first motion (5.1) was amended before being put to the vote: 'The IPC is the sole organisation to award, supervise and coordinate the Summer and Winter Paralympic Games' – the amendment did not alter the intended meaning, but replaced the original words 'assist in the coordination of' with the single verb 'coordinate'. By implication, the IPC was to stand alone in its responsibility, rather than to abrogate it to organising committees. Probably the most significant motion was proposed next. This related to the major change in IPC's outlook towards regional and world championships. The motion stood as: 'The IPC shall not have responsibility for the sanctioning or organisation of any world or regional games or championships'. From before the meeting itself it had become clear that this was a pivotal recommendation of the Task Force. Part of the wish to assign a manageable mission to the IPC included the reduction in scope of competitions other than Paralympic Games that the IPC would take responsibility for. The other line of argument also supported the handing of these events to the regional committees, IOSDs and sports organisations, giving them the type of specific role being recommended by the Task Force's consultations. The Swedish representatives suggested an amendment that would retain the multi-disability, multi-federational or IPC sports world championships, but excluding others. The international organisations would be free to run their own separate events in their own disability groups if they wished. But the discussion became even more animated at this point, with some accusations that the motion would impose direct dictation to the IOSDs by the IPC. The meeting agreed to vote on the original motion, without amendment. The result was defeat for the motion: the IPC was to retain responsibility for the sanctioning of regional and world championships. The Task Force had lost its first battle; some within the Executive Committee sighed heavily.

Immediately there was a sense that the earnest hard work of the Task Force might prove to bear little fruit. Enrique Sanz, President of IBSA, had already communicated his opinion of the earlier naivety of the Task Force documentation. Now he was disappointed and not a little angry at the response of the delegates to this groundbreaking motion. He spoke of his regret, and the sense that the blind were poorly represented within the national structures of IPC. The changes would have given greater coherence to the purpose of their organisation, and would have led to better communication and representation. Almost immediately Sanz announced that the IBSA would begin 'analysing their withdrawal from IPC'. As a technical point, Sanz moved that the result of this vote had effectively blocked the progress of all further motions, as the motions were presented in a logical and consequential order. He suggested that no further voting take place. Bob Steadward ruled this out of order, as the Extraordinary General Assembly had been called specifically to receive all the recommendations.

The meeting moved on to decide modifications to the structure of the General Assembly and to voting rights. The original motion had not allowed for representation by each of the Paralympic sports in the General Assembly, and a successful amendment from the INAS-FMH, seconded by Sweden, added these representatives. The Chairman of the Athletes' Committee did not succeed in his proposal to add the occupant of his post to the General Assembly as well – there would be great difficulty in holding back the tide if one Standing Committee was represented, as all others would call for similar rights. Each member of the General Assembly would have a single vote. The composition of the Sports Council received a favourable hearing, and the meeting adopted the motion after denying several amendments. Next came the important alterations to the balance of the Executive Committee. The Task Force had emphasised the need for identifiable and measurable roles for members of the Executive Committee, proposing a streamlined group compared with the existing body. The Task Force's motion was that: 'The Executive Committee shall consist of a President, 1st Vice-President, Vice-President (Strategy and Planning), Vice-President (Games Liaison), Secretary General, Treasurer, Chairman of the Sports Council, Chairman of the Sports Science and Medical Committee, a Summer Sports Representative and a Winter Sports Representative'. Bernard Atha, President of INAS-FMH and an astute and constructive contributor to this sort of process, wanted the delegates to consider amending the motion to include all the present members of the Executive except the three Members at Large. This would effectively add another 12 people to the ten members of the Executive Committee being proposed by the Task Force. Of course this would not in any way improve the unwieldy nature of the Committee, but it did bring the five international federations and the regional representatives straight back into the picture, when they would have been completely left outside the Executive Committee by the original motion. This was a major defeat for the nucleus of people trying to take the IPC towards a vitality so far elusive in the present larger structure. In effect it returned the 'old guard' of the international federations to the position that they were being carefully eased out of. It was perhaps surprising that the voting was so emphatically in favour of the amendment: 182 in favour, 41 against, with five abstentions. Perhaps the factor that influenced the vote was the built-in formation of a Management Committee that would collate reports from more diverse groups and prepare material for the Executive Committee. Although there had been a Management Committee in existence since 1991 it had not operated so as to draw together material effectively in the way being proposed. So far, those who had spent so much time drawing up the proposals for the Extraordinary General Assembly had no great sense of elation. Just how the members of the Executive Committee were to be elected became the next complicated decision. In the end there was agreement that the 22 members would be elected according to the formula:

- elected by the General Assembly: eight members (President, three Vice Presidents, Secretary General, Treasurer, Chairman Sports Council, Chairman Sport Science and Medical Committee);
- elected by the Sports Council: two members (Winter and Summer Representative);
- elected by the Athletes: one member (Chairman Athletes' Committee);
- elected by their own constituency: five members (IOSDs representatives) and six members (regional representatives).

Paralympic Solidarity received a priority rating from the Extraordinary General Assembly, which instructed resources to be allocated to its establishment and maintenance. Bob Steadward stressed that this important direction of the IPC's mandate would begin with close cooperation with the IOSDs and the regions. Other priorities that the Task Force had identified were also favourably acknowledged by the membership, passing with a unanimous vote that 'the IPC reaffirms its commitment to include in the Summer and Winter Paralympic Programmes, sports and events for athletes with a more severe disability, and female athletes'.

Representation of athletes was identified by Martin Mansell, the Chairman of the Athletes' Committee, as having been disappointing. He considered that the motions had effectively reduced opportunities for athletes to be represented as efficiently in the General Assembly and in the sports structures. Duncan Wyeth, who had been acting as Master of Ceremonies, considered that there was a contradiction between the decisions taken during the 1995 Tokyo General Assembly and the present Extraordinary General Assembly. He asked for the motions that had caused this contradiction to be reconsidered. Bob Steadward acknowledged the concern, but asked whether Wyeth would be satisfied if the Executive Committee looked in detail at the subject and brought it to the 1997 General Assembly, if they thought it warranted change. With Wyeth's agreement the matter was postponed.

As the work of the Task Force was being concluded with the last motions of the Extraordinary General Assembly, York Chow called on the leadership of the International Paralympic Committee to cooperate better and to unite in their work towards shared goals. Bob Steadward thanked the Task Force members wholeheartedly for their endurance and perception. He did not seem to show any emotion at the Task Force's having only achieved a limited part of the reshaping of the IPC's structure. As ever, Steadward managed to make each participant feel that they had contributed positively to a worthwhile enterprise. The IBSA position concerned him, but he expressed hope that it would show 'understanding of the need to work in partnership'.

CONCLUSIONS

The Atlanta Paralympic Games were still more phenomenal than Barcelona as a spectacle. The competitions were superb, although spectator levels were very disappointing. Bernard Atha commented: 'I think the universal feeling was that the Games themselves were splendid, the competition was excellent and the people of Atlanta as warm and supportive as one could possibly hope. The Games in that respect were an enormous success. On the other hand, the athletes felt that they had been very badly treated'. With loose ends still to tidy up it was not possible for Bob Steadward and his key officers to feel relaxed as the Games came to an end. There were still many hours of wrangling before the Atlanta Paralympic Organising Committee handed over the cheque for US$725 000 at the beginning of 1997. Andy Fleming, President of the Atlanta Paralympic Organising Committee, wished to emphasise that his colleagues had provided the opportunity to prove the financial viability of the Paralympic Games, showing the possibilities for the future. Although it was a point of significant displeasure within the Paralympic Movement, Fleming's organisation was able to transfer a kingly sum of US$3 850 000 into a newly formed US Disabled Athletes Fund, Inc. Steadward suggested that this payment was 'at the absolute expense of the IPC and the 1996 Atlanta Paralympic Athletes'. It had been likened to exploitation. But Fleming was correct in the sense that the organisation of the Paralympic Games should become more attractive to future bidders in the light of the proven marketing possibilities, and the reduction of risk.

The Task Force had returned to the wider membership with its findings, after lengthy and frank investigations. The proposals for change to the IPC's structure were aimed at the future vibrancy of an organisation that had seemingly been hampered by an inherited hierarchy. The rejection of the idea of a slimline Executive Committee was a blow, but there was a reasonable wish to retain the representation of the five IOSDs and the six regions. The Management Committee, however, came to fulfil the purpose of the slimmed down Executive Committee – albeit operating in addition to the Executive. While the Management Committee was then able to attend to the day-to-day operation, it did serve to make a top-heavy organisation. But the decision to create a Management Committee in 1997 overlapped with the decision to create a permanent headquarters with a permanent staff – thus adding to the possibilities of duplication.

The international disability sports organisations (IOSDs) had held on to their influence, shrugging off the attempt of the IPC to assign new but less spectacular roles: grass-roots development and the coordination of competitions other than Paralympic Games. In the end the major opportunity for change was not grasped. The members of the Task Force had reason to be disappointed at the results, but there had been a certain over-eagerness on their part to fix everything at once. There was a great deal at stake; the hard work of every different participant in the Paralympic Movement risked being undone by potentially rash and ambitious proposals. But the balance between radical and irresponsible proposals was difficult to determine. The International Paralympic Committee demonstrated emphatically that it was a democratic organisation, with the membership giving authority to make some alterations, but stopping short of the full-blown 'new look'. Whether this would hamper progress would remain to be seen. There were still very considerable problems on the horizon for the International Paralympic Committee, and the officers needed to be able to function within any constraints that might be laid on them. Without doubt the Task Force had aired vital concerns than would have to be addressed before long.

The next phase in the IPC's operation would have to address the urgent need for rigorous and enforceable agreements with Paralympic Organising Committees, the establishment of a permanent headquarters, and a closer tie between the IPC and the IOC in bidding procedures.

CHAPTER 7

Repair What Needs Repair?
1996 to 2000

OVERVIEW

The unsettling effects of the 1996 Extraordinary General Assembly were to prevent the International Paralympic Committee from getting into its stride immediately after the Atlanta 1996 Paralympic Games were finished. Without the restructuring proposed by the Task Force, there were still in-built problems relating to the ability of the IPC to function while managing such a big mandate, and with a relatively sizeable Executive Committee. However, the feeling among some members of the Executive Committee was one of relief that the nations had slowed down the proposed tempo of change. It was plainly unrealistic to make such drastic changes to a complex organisation in a single sweep. One participant has offered the opinion that the Task Force had been unable to really 'take the temperature' of the membership, instead bringing proposals that might have reflected a utopian inclination. The direct clash with the IBSA needed resolution; the other international federations would also watch this closely.

By the time the nations met again at the 1997 General Assembly in Sydney, the International Paralympic Committee had pressed on with some reforms, as well as developing some new strategies for the future. It was important to show the membership that the central officers were deserving of the trust accorded them. When Bob Steadward opened the first meeting of the General Assembly, on 6th November 1997, he informed the delegates that his main purpose was to 'encourage and renew our devotion to the advancement of our beloved organisation'. Although his welcome was friendly and sincere, his words reflected the tough path that he had travelled over the past year. Steadward asked that the constituents should not: 'dwell wastefully on negativism, or regretfully on past disappointments, but it is time to constructively repair whatever needs repair and continue to build a positive and sound structure upon our foundation'. As if his words had not been clear enough, Steadward urged everyone to work on 'the age of improvement'. He entreated them to focus their goals 'on building, promoting and performing something worthy of being remembered ... and our building must be done together, with one design, and one team principle. The image we project to the world must be one of unity'. Extending his metaphors, the IPC President asked the International Organisations of Sport for persons with a Disability (IOSDs) to act according to the principle of unification: 'Inasmuch as we are respectful of one another's views, it will not be one player who wins the game, it will be the team'.

Athlete First: A History of the Paralympic Movement   Steve Bailey
© 2008 John Wiley & Sons, Ltd

FROM ATLANTA TO NAGANO

IBSA Presents its Concerns

While the key members of the IBSA Executive Committee were still in Atlanta, they gathered for a meeting to draw up their formal response to the disastrous outcome at the IPC Extraordinary General Assembly. The President of IBSA, Enrique Sanz, put together a letter that set out the concerns and needs of the organisation for blind and partially sighted athletes. Principal issues included the lessening of voting representation through the adoption of the motion that gave each nation only one vote. Sanz's letter emphasised that IBSA would have been content with the motion delegating organisation of world and regional championships to IOSDs and regional representatives. His organisation was asking to be able to nominate one representative to each Sports Assembly Executive Committee, where blind athletes participate in that sport. Sanz wanted the IPC to agree that IBSA would have sole authority over the establishment and maintenance of rules in sports practised by blind and visually impaired athletes. He repeated that Bob Steadward's closing remarks at the Atlanta Extraordinary General Assembly were about unity and respect: 'It is our purpose now to establish in what ways and to what degree that respect exists in the specific case of the IPC's attitude and policies towards IBSA and blind associations and athletes who are part of the larger Paralympic Family'.

In an interview for the *IBSA Magazine* (no. 11), Enrique Sanz made it clear that it was up to the IPC to demonstrate a willingness to acknowledge the needs to blind and partially sighted athletes through their organisation:

> Every alley undoubtedly has, sooner or later, some way out. But IBSA, at this time, cannot take any further steps towards reaching an agreement, without receiving an explicit commitment from the IPC to the effect that it will respect IBSA's right to organise its own World and Regional Championships; to have a representative on the Sports Committee of those events practised by the blind and visually impaired; to elaborate and develop – without external interference – the sports rules that must prevail in these sports and establish the consequent classification systems.

The magazine concluded that the IPC membership's unwillingness to accept the changes promulgated by the Task Force meant that: 'the Paralympic Movement is now heading towards a period of instability, division and inefficiency and, as a result, the conclusion that IBSA feels obliged to undertake an analysis of its possible withdrawal from the IPC'.

The IPC Executive Committee called an additional meeting in Atlanta, on 25th August, just before the Closing Ceremony of the Paralympic Games. Although André Raes was tied up with medal ceremonies and Martin Mansell was in the Athletes' Assembly, they still collected 13 members.

When the Executive Committee discussed the position of IBSA, Bob Steadward expressed his anxiety that the IOC's wish to have a single form of representation was being eroded. The letter from Sanz was looked at in detail, and Jens Bromann, together with Bernard Atha, considered that all IBSA's worries were adequately covered by the IPC's rules already. Hans Lindström came to a different conclusion: that separate agreements would be needed between the IPC and each of the international federations, taking into account their differing requirements. Lindström proposed a meeting between Steadward and Sanz to examine future cooperation.

IBSA immediately presented its apprehension to the World Blind Union, meeting in Toronto at the end of August 1996, and received resounding support for its action. It called on the IOC to cease financial aid to the IPC until the problems had been resolved.

Communication and the Future Structure of IPC

Some displeasure was soon officially expressed at the manner of communication of some IPC members. André Raes had apparently circulated a paper in the wider community containing his personal views on the proposals of the Task Force. This was considered inappropriate given his position as Secretary General. Jens Bromann commented that he felt constrained to have to refer all media enquiries to the Media Officer. He thought it important that he should be able to speak freely and personally once the Paralympic Games were concluded. The concord of the International Paralympic Committee was being comprehensively tested.

A number of national representatives had expressed grave regret to Bob Steadward about the result of the Extraordinary General Assembly. He told the assembled IPC officers that some member nations had informed him that they might propose the reduction in size of the Executive Committee at the General Assembly in Sydney in 1997. York Chow stressed that there were flaws in the process both of the Task Force's research, and in the voting of the Extraordinary General Assembly. The widest possible consultation had been undertaken, but only 24 nations had responded with written feedback to the report – albeit with strongly expressed views. This didn't equate well with more than 80 nations voting in the Extraordinary General Assembly. But among the nations were many new members, inexperienced in IPC organisational matters, and possibly susceptible to suggestion and persuasion. It was possible that these relative novices in the world of Paralympic politics had affected the outcome of decisions in the General Assembly.

The Executive Committee discussed the outcomes and the way forward. Bernard Atha was of the opinion that a Management Committee should take on the daily running of the IPC, and the Executive Committee need not be slimmed down further. He had written to York Chow to suggest this as a way of improving the IPC's effectiveness, as part of the consultation process to the Task Force's proposals in 1996. A Management Committee would meet more frequently and report to the Executive Committee. While there was a wish for a slimmed-down operation, the IPC still managed to create this additional body. There was a second irony: that the new Management Committee came into being in 1997, just when decisions were being taken to establish a permanent headquarters precisely for the daily operation of the IPC. This was to lead to some duplication of effort and some confusion about mandates between the elected officers and the employed staff of IPC.

Hans Lindström pointed to the clear decision of the Extraordinary General Assembly that the Sports Sections should not be independent – there being relatively few nations with appropriate sports structures within their organisations. Lindström was concerned that some countries would lose more than they would gain by pushing for independence of sports.

Bob Steadward reminded the Executive Committee, at its first brief meeting after the Sydney General Assembly, of the members' agreement to be loyal to a decision once it had been passed in their body. Steadward wanted to emphasise the need for a united voice.

André Raes Stands Down

Personality conflicts between the Secretary General and other members of the Management Committee led to André Raes standing down as Secretary General prior to the Executive Committee meeting in Nagano in May 1997. Problems had been brewing, and Raes's firm approach made it difficult to repair the situation. But the difficulties had come to a head during the early part of 1997, and the President called on the wisdom of Michael Riding, Jens Bromann and Colin Rains to hit upon a suitable outcome. In the end Raes did not get to present his Secretary General's report at the Nagano Executive Committee meeting, and his involvement with IPC ceased. At the 1997 Sydney General Assembly in November,

Bob Steadward expressed his thanks to Raes for his contribution over many years to sport for people with a disability in general and to the IPC in particular. A tenacious but challenging character, André Raes had tended to cut straight to the heart of any matter, not suffering fools gladly. At times his abrupt manner had upset individuals to the extent that remedial work was sometimes necessary, but in organisational matters André Raes had driven the International Paralympic Committee forward. A military rigidity and concern for following rules helped the IPC out of the 'ICC years'. Hans Lindström was appointed Acting Secretary General, with Leen Coudenys taking responsibility for operational matters. Miguel Sagarra succeeded André Raes as Secretary General following the new elections. As a point of information, the Executive Board of the International Olympic Committee was informed that André Raes was no longer Secretary General of the International Paralympic Committee, when they met in Lausanne on 30th and 31st August 1997. The brief comment was accompanied by the minuted statement that: 'relations within the IPC and with the IOC will certainly be made easier by this'.

New Headquarters for IPC Cause Trouble for the Executive Committee

In Sydney, the IPC President reported to the General Assembly on the subject of the proposals for a new IPC Headquarters. He informed the members that the Management Committee had examined the six bids in detail, and decided to put forward one city for ratification by the General Assembly. The requirements were for the Paralympic Movement to have 'a place . . . to call home, a promise of long term residence, the assurance of prominent visibility, and the potential for employing multilingual staff'. Steadward included in his preamble the idea of inaugurating a Paralympic Hall of Fame and Museum 'in order to recognise and preserve the outstanding accomplishments of athletes with a disability and other individuals who have made extraordinary contributions to advancing the cause of the Paralympic Movement'. But the discussions about the new Headquarters ran into trouble rather sooner than the Executive Committee expected. While the President described the examination of the bid materials as having been conducted in a 'very unbiased, open-minded and business-like manner', some members of the General Assembly believed that the decision should rest with them after hearing a summary of recommendations.

There had been a clear distinction between two groups of bids: Oslo, Ferney-Voltaire and Colorado Springs were judged not to meet the criteria to the extent that Bonn, Paris and Madrid did. Within the evaluation group, made up of members of the Management Committee (excluding André Auberger, who disqualified himself as having an interest through the Paris bid), there was a clear understanding of the potential effects of presenting the case of each city to the General Assembly, or even to the Executive Committee. The Management Committee had agreed in April 1997 that the finalists would be asked to make a presentation to the General Assembly in Sydney. But this was not the way things emerged. The evaluation group was later in agreement that Paris and Bonn were placed close to each other in terms of potential, with Paris perhaps offering a more attractive financial position, but with Bonn offering a better long-term investment. They agreed that 'it would be best if the Management Committee would present recommendation on only one bid'. While still giving the outward appearance of considering all six bids, Paris and Bonn were asked to clarify certain specific issues. Should the Management Committee not be able to decide on just one city after that process and a conference call, the two cities would be asked to make a presentation to the Management Committee.

Steadward informed the General Assembly that Paris and Bonn had been considered in the final rounds of discussions. He made it clear that it was the recommendation of the Executive Committee that the General Assembly accept Bonn as the city to host the IPC Headquarters. When put to the vote in the General Assembly it could hardly have been closer: 43 in favour of Bonn, 38 against and 13 abstentions. A short time after the proposal was laid to rest as having accepted Bonn as the host city, there was a discrepancy identified by the Russian delegate, recognising that the total number of votes appeared to have been 94, when there should only have been 92 delegates eligible to vote. Steadward accepted that there was an irregularity, but was firm in suggesting that even if the two 'drifting' votes were deducted from the total votes in favour of the motion there would still be a majority – the integrity of the motion would stand. Immediately after this declaration, Phil Craven, representing the International Wheelchair Basketball Federation, together with the Swiss representative, challenged the ruling of the chair. This forced a vote on the ruling made by the IPC President – a very delicate matter, with the possibility of leading to a vote of no confidence. At the moment of this vote there were 95 eligible delegates: 53 voted in favour of the motion and 38 voted against. There were four abstentions this time. The complaint was really to do with an apparent sideways shift in the decision-making process, removing the General Assembly's potency by effectively asking it to 'rubber stamp' an earlier decision of the Executive Committee.

The matter was allowed to rest until the next day, when Chris Cohen, Athletics Representative, proposed a motion 'to express complete confidence in the President of IPC'. This motion was carried, with two abstentions. The long process of repairing the damage done the day before then started: a good deal of information was provided for the General Assembly about the three leading candidate cities, with advantages and disadvantages laid out for the members to consider. The Executive Committee had met the evening before to decide on the best way of calming things, and had agreed on this strategy. The General Assembly was then asked again to consider the recommendation of the Executive Committee that Bonn was the most suitable city to host the Headquarters of the IPC. Tactfully, Miguel Sagarra announced the withdrawal of Madrid from contention. André Auberger reaffirmed the French Government's commitment to offer its services as host to IPC, and the details of how Paris and Bonn were evaluated were given to the meeting. After an unexpected amount of time, Colin Rains moved that the General Assembly 'in due consideration of the information presented, reconfirms the decision to support Bonn as the city for the new Headquarters'. The clarity of the voting was a relief to everyone: 59 votes in favour, 31 against, with five abstentions.

This particular issue, the apparent disregard of the usually democratic procedures of the IPC, was revealing in several ways. It demonstrated that Bob Steadward was willing to sidestep some of the conventions that normally marked the IPC's practices and exert more personal influence than had been publicly obvious before this point. It also highlighted the protagonist's role that Phil Craven was willing to play, in his challenging the ruling of the Chairman – that is, the President. The attention of the membership was certainly drawn to this action. Although the Executive Committee rallied around, some damage had been done to alter the relationships within the closest circles.

Membership, Solidarity and Elections

Membership was steadily climbing, and the 1997 General Assembly received six new members: Belarus, Benin, Cambodia, Guinea Bissau, Uganda and Palestine. Only Belarus and Palestine had sent delegates to the meeting, so they immediately received voting rights.

André Auberger took pleasure in describing the solidarity projects that had permitted 78 athletes to take part in the Atlanta 1996 Paralympic Games, and to help 40 countries send representatives to the Sydney General Assembly. There was some feeling at the 1997 meeting that the funds directed towards Paralympic Solidarity should be used to aid athletes in competition rather than for delegates to attend meetings such as the present General Assembly. This was a lively topic of discussion, and one unlikely to bring the opposing sides into agreement. To this information Auberger added that there had been a favorable memorandum of cooperation signed with UNESCO and the Conseil International de Sport Militaire (CISM) that would bring the organisations together in matters of development. This sort of outreach was a healthy sign; recognition from organisations such as agencies of the United Nations that the IPC was a valued partner. While the gesture existed with the memorandum signed, no tangible action resulted.

The election of members of the Executive Committee at the Sydney 1997 General Assembly was an important part of the changing face of the IPC. Among those standing down from lengthy continuous involvement from the beginnings of the IPC, even via the ICC, was Hans Lindström. He had indicated his candidacy for the position of Vice President Policy, Planning, and Development, as well as standing for Secretary General. He withdrew from both elections, as did François Terranova for the same Vice Presidency. Colin Rains withdrew from the contest for Vice President Paralympic Games Liaison; Sverre Bergenholdt stood down from the Secretary General candidacy, and Karl Quade withdrew from the position of Technical Officer. Three positions were elected without a need for a vote as there were solitary candidates: Bob Steadward as President and André Auberger as Treasurer, and Carol Mushett took over from Hans Lindström as Technical Officer. Those positions that required votes to be cast also allowed the candidates to address the Assembly for two minutes in support of their candidacy. In the ballots, the following were returned:

- York Chow   Vice President Policy, Planning, and Development
- François Terranova   Vice President Games Liaison
- Duncan Wyeth   Vice President Marketing and Communication
- Miguel Sagarra   Secretary General
- Michael Riding   Medical Officer

International Olympic Committee

Following the Atlanta 1996 Paralympic Games, Gilbert Felli (IOC Sports Director) and Pere Miró Sellares (IOC Technical Director) had written to congratulate the IPC on the success of the Atlanta 1996 Games. While complimenting the 'top management' of the IPC, they also observed that the positive development and growing importance of sport for people with a disability was helped by 'the close cooperation and contact with the International Olympic Committee over these past years'. They looked forward to even better cooperation in future.

When Bob Steadward had written to Juan Antonio Samaranch after the Atlanta 1996 Paralympic Games, Steadward asked Samaranch not to agree to separate meetings with each of the international federations in this field, with a view to ensuring the identity of the IPC as the sole voice of sport for people with a disability. He made it clear that there must be no interference in the internal operation of the IPC, and that he would try to ensure that there were 'effective and open communications with all international federations so that they can grow and develop in a way in which they can both be proud and satisfied'.

The next meeting between representatives of the IOC and the IPC took place in December 1996. This was a well-attended meeting, with the key people showing respect for the other organisation. From the International Paralympic Committee, the representatives were Bob Steadward, Jens Bromann, André Raes, André Auberger, Hans Lindström, Michael Riding and Leen Coudenys. Representing the International Olympic Committee, the representatives were Juan Antonio Samaranch, Walther Tröger, Gilbert Felli and Pere Miró Sellares. The agenda was wide-ranging and the exchange of views was straightforward and frank. Finances were covered first: the IOC accepted that the operating costs of the IPC had climbed with the expansion of the Paralympic Movement, and the IOC agreed to increase its contribution by 20%. This projected the total made available by the IOC from 1997 to 2000 to be US$1.2 million (that is, US$300 000 a year) – an increase of US$50 000 per year. The IOC

President was thanked for his willingness to help send participants from 40 countries to the Atlanta 1996 Paralympics with an infusion of US$100 000 towards the Solidarity project. The IOC President indicated that the IOC would contribute US$60 000 for two athletes and one official per country to attend the Nagano 1998 Winter Paralympic Games. While not wanting to commit to definite levels of financial support for the Sydney Paralympic Games at this early stage, Samaranch did agree to Steadward's request for IOC funding for member nations to attend the IPC General Assembly in 1997.

The most significant offer of direct help from the IOC came in mediating between the IPC and the Salt Lake Organising Committee (SLOC). There was agreement about the technical side of the Paralympic Games, but stalemate over the financial matters. SLOC was insisting that the delegations would have to pay all the real costs of food, accommodation, internal transport and ski lifts. This might amount to more than US$2000 per person, as opposed to the preferred significantly lower amount. Another thorn in their side was the inability to agree over the revenue share to the IPC: Previously suggested a sum of US$150 000 plus 5% of sponsorship and ticket income, with a share of overall profits. The Salt Lake committee was not considering offering this. At the Lillehammer Paralympic Winter Games, the income to IPC had been US$250 000, and at Atlanta over US$725 000. Nagano was expected to yield US$500 000 and Sydney US$2 million. Samaranch said that he would act upon this situation on receipt of a formal written request from the IPC. It would lose no time in sending a letter.

In another very positive move, the IOC President suggested that it should be possible that 'in future, the IOC would oblige host cities to organise the Paralympics'. This pronouncement, made at the meeting in December 1996, was an invitation for the IPC to draw up the basic technical requirements for bidding cities to consider. In the words of the minutes of the meeting: 'this modus operandi would have the advantage of settling the somewhat unclear situation as regards marketing and . . . at the same time the financial relations as regards repayments and basic deposits, and the costs for athletes and delegations should be discussed and established'. The 2004 arrangements would have to be played out, as the process was already underway. But Samaranch suggested that host cities could be pressed for their ideas on how they would host the Paralympic Games after 7th March 1997, when the International Olympic Committee's Executive Board was to meet. The next step would be a questionnaire to host cities, and the establishment of a joint IOC/IPC delegation for site visits. These were very positive offerings to the Paralympic Movement.

In the end Samaranch did manage to broker an agreement between Thomas Welch, President of SLOC, and Bob Steadward, writing to both of them on 18th February 1997 to confirm the terms of this agreement: acknowledging that SLOC would host the Paralympic Winter Games, taking responsibility for the entire organisation. The main financial stumbling block was removed by the statement of agreement that: 'In consideration for the use of all of IPC's TV, sponsorship and other marketing rights relating to the 2002 Winter Paralympic Games, SLOC will pay to IPC a total amount of US$400 000'. There was a further $100 000 sanctioning fee to be paid to IPC in addition. Samaranch set the date for the signing of this agreement as 26th May 1997, in his presence at the IOC Headquarters in Lausanne. Steadward had travelled in March 1997 to Salt Lake City to try to release the deadlock, and the IOC President had provided strong intervention that had made the difference. What Steadward described as a gloomy time had turned into 'positive vision'. He was able to write to Samaranch on 2nd May 1997, saying that Tom Welch, Chief Executive Officer of the Salt Lake Organising Committee, agreed to the conditions IPC had wished, particularly due to the intervention of Samaranch.

On the same date as his letter to Samaranch and Welch about the Salt Lake 2002 Paralympic Winter Games, Samaranch issued a press release announcing the agreement signed in Lausanne between Bob Steadward and Enrique Sanz, President of the International Blind Sports Association. This agreement, signed on 17th February 1997, was described as applying particularly to 'participation of blind athletes in the Paralympic Games and the development of future world championships for blind athletes under the responsibility of the IBSA, whose first World Championships will be held in Madrid in 1998'.

Progress in Establishing a Headquarters in Bonn

With the rather rocky reception for the process of selecting Bonn as the host for the new IPC Headquarters, it was important to ensure that the office was fully functional as soon as was feasible. Miguel Sagarra gave a progress report to the Executive Committee in Nagano on 4th March 1998. The IPC had to be registered under German law, and this was being promulgated. There was a draft contract being discussed with the City of Bonn, and all seemed to be moving along well. The Executive agreed to delegate authority to the Management Committee for the employment of the first three people essential to the Headquarters: a receptionist/secretary, an administrator and a Chief Operations Officer.

Inclusion and Integration

The inclusion of events in the Nagano Winter Olympic Games had been a troublesome subject covered in preparatory meetings, with the Nagano organising committee not wishing to organise exhibition events due to other operational problems they were already having to deal with, and also because they considered that they had 'invested a great deal in the Paralympics', due to start soon afterwards. They clearly did not understand the purpose of each of these events. In December 1996, Samaranch was not optimistic that he could persuade the organisers to change their minds.

The IPC had applied in 1996 for the inclusion of two wheelchair races in the Sydney Paralympic Games of 2000, as full medal events rather than exhibitions. The IOC President explained two considerable problems facing them in this quest: that there could reasonably be a claim of discrimination against those athletes with other disabilities who were not being catered for in the Olympic Games, and that the numbers involved caused other troubles. The fact that only eight competitors raced in the wheelchair events meant that the normal open competition the Olympic Movement strived for was not possible. In order to find parity they would have to expand the number of athletes involved in earlier stages, which was contrary to the present trend within the Olympic programme to reduce the scale of the Games. Sydney had been forced to reduce the total numbers of athletes from 10 700 to 10 200. These discussions continued, but there was a measure of calmness about them.

Paralympic Games Preparation

A number of IPC representatives, including the President, attended the IAAF World Athletics Championships in Athens. This gave them the opportunity of renewing their acquaintance with the bidding committee for the 2004 Paralympic Games, especially now that the decision for awarding the Games to Athens had been taken. Negotiations could begin in earnest.

At the Executive Committee meeting of 9th November 1997, Paul Griffiths, Media Director, reported that although the Sydney Paralympic Organising Committee was sure that a host broadcaster would be in place for the 2000 Games, the Nagano organisers had still not secured a host. This was worrying for the nations and for the IPC more broadly. The marketing opportunities were consequently limited by this lack. NAPOC had agreed to provide for two videotape crews at each event, but this was still not enough reassurance of good coverage – without the distribution being commercially attractive.

In October 1997, 'Lizzie' the frill necked lizard was adopted as the mascot for the Sydney 2000 Paralympic Games. Native Australian creatures had been selected as the mascots of the Olympic Games as well: Millie the echidna, Syd the platypus and Olly the kookaburra. Community Relations Manager for the Paralympic Games and captain of the women's wheelchair basketball team, Donna

Ritchie, said of Lizzie: 'She strives for the same things our Paralympians strive for – power, performance and pride'.

Technical Matters

Demonstration sports at the Paralympic Games were discussed in Lille, France, when the Executive Committee met in January 1997. Hans Lindström explained the difficulties of having demonstration sports in the Paralympic Handbook: that the Paralympic Games become a testing ground for sports that might not be completely ready for this sort of exposure, and that the arrangements create two separate classes of participants. If only full medal status events were included in the Paralympic programme there would not be any problems. There was a weakness in permitting Paralympic organising committees to nominate demonstration sports. Lindström also pointed out that the IOC had deleted demonstration sports from its programme. The integrity of the Paralympic Games would be served best by removing the process of new sports entering the Games via demonstration. The Executive Committee unanimously agreed to remove the section from the Handbook referring to demonstration sports. New events and disciplines would be considered by application four years before their entry in the Paralympic Games, with a decision being given three years before the Games. The decision to do away with demonstration sports at future Paralympic Games called for stringent procedures for assessing the inclusion of sports and events in the Paralympic programme. For the 2008 Paralympic Summer Games and beyond, the principles would be that individual sports would have to be widely practised in at least 24 countries and three regions, while team sports would have to be practised in 18 countries and three regions. The definition of a team sport needed clarification as well. The Sydney meeting of the IPC Executive Committee agreed that a team sport must include 'multiple players interacting', and that an individual sport can have team events, but team sports cannot be played by an individual.

Once the IBSA agreement had come into place, there was a need to provide representation on the Sports Council Executive Committee (SCEC). The proposal was that one seat on the SCEC would be provided for 'an IBSA liaison person'. If an election to this position was needed, only those countries with blind competitors in that sport would be permitted to vote. The Sports Chairmen opposed this motion, but it was passed through. There was some feeling that this representation was 'forced' and therefore was inappropriate, but the requirement arose directly from the IPC–IBSA special agreement, and had to be honoured.

At the brief meeting of the Executive Committee after the Sydney General Assembly in November 1997, Hans Lindström presented a new staff ratio for Paralympic Games that would improve provision for athletes with severe disability. The Sports Council had adopted the idea that the ratio of staff to athletes of 35%, which had been employed in Atlanta, should be increased to 50% for the Sydney 2000 Paralympic Games. The Sydney Paralympic Organising Committee was happy with the idea, and the Executive Committee unanimously approved the alteration to the IPC Handbook. This was very positive.

Minimum Disability

Greater precision was being achieved in the search for the most appropriate way of identifying minimum disability, a current focal point of the IPC Executive Committee. The Sports Council Executive Committee had proposed that each Paralympic sport should tender its operational definition on minimum disability. This could then be used as a guide for all competitions in these sports. At the March 1998 Nagano Executive Committee meeting, Carol Mushett was commissioned to go ahead with the Sports Council Executive Committee's recommendation. There were legal implications to take into account, especially considering the climate of litigation, and so it was thought sensible for the Executive Committee to ratify the definitions.

Sport Science and Medicine

The adopted regulations concerning competitor fitness came into effect after the Atlanta Executive Committee meeting of 12th to 14th August 1996. The definition of boosting that was being employed for the purpose of these rules was 'the deliberate precipitation of autonomic dysreflexia leading to elevation of blood pressure in athletes whose spinal cord lesion is at T6 and above. Boosting may be achieved by using cutaneous, visceral or proprioceptive stimuli below the level of the cord lesion'. In order to ensure that competitors were not participating in this dangerous practice, examination was to take the form of testing of 'systolic and diastolic blood pressure, pulse, levels of sweating, presence of skin blotching, cutis anserine [goose flesh], dyspnoea, anxiety and tremors'. Anyone showing signs of boosting would be reassessed after ten minutes had elapsed from the first testing. Should the symptoms confirm boosting with no satisfactory explanation being provided, the athlete might be withdrawn from the event in question. Although autonomic dysreflexia is a natural phenomenon in tetraplegia there was an obvious need to respond to the intentional self-inducement of this response.

A medical code had been drawn up, and this was in draft form for consultation. Michael Riding informed the Executive Committee that the review process would allow for the code to be ratified at the Nagano Executive Committee meeting, and could be operational for the Nagano 1998 Winter Paralympic Games. However, the code was still being discussed within the international federations, and formal adoption was moved to May 1998. Meetings were taking place in 1998 between Michael Riding, Michael Ferrara and Xavier Gonzalez to make proposals for the establishment of a classification databank.

The controversial subject of marijuana testing was raised by Michael Riding at the Nagano Executive Committee meeting of 4th March 1998. He described the debate that had taken place within the Management Committee. The IPC rules were clear that testing may take place on the request of international federations, and sanctions may be imposed. But it was also acknowledged that the legal ground was too unstable to make the position secure with the Court of Arbitration of Sport, should there be an appeal. The difficulty was that of ascertaining whether marijuana was performance enhancing. The result of all this uncertainty was that the Management Committee decided that no testing for marijuana would take place during the Nagano 1998 Paralympic Winter Games. Michael Riding and Paul Griffiths, as Media Director, would need to draw up a suitable statement for use by the media, conveying the clear discouragement of the use of marijuana.

The classification database had moved on by the Executive Committee meeting of May 1998. Collaboration with the Sydney Paralympic Organising Committee was proving effective. It hoped to achieve its target of classifying 88% of athletes before the Sydney 2000 Paralympic Games. Out-of-competition drugs testing was going to begin, with assistance from the IOC – funding from the IOC Medical Commission had been requested. Michael Riding reported that no positive results were recorded at the Nagano 1998 Paralympic Winter Games, out of 60 tests. As the Court of Arbitration for Sport was now to be involved with all appeals against positive drugs test, it was considered that representatives should be present at the Paralympic Summer Games.

Sports News, not Disability News: Nagano, 1998

The 6th Winter Paralympic Games opened in Nagano, Japan, on 3rd March 1998. With the modesty of the Japanese organising committee first showing a quiet intention to manage a good Paralympic

Games, this event soon became a stunning sporting revelation. As the months had led into the start of the Games themselves, the Japanese media picked up on the phenomenon of the Paralympic Movement and began to report the event in a highly charged manner. The same had been true of the Tokyo Paralympic Summer Games in 1964: enthusiasm for the great good done through this sporting competition. Tickets had been sold out in advance, and Japanese people were very well informed before the Paralympic Games opened.

The conscious aim of the Japanese Government over the previous two years had been to address the needs of a society with increasing numbers of elderly people. The consequences of this trend were to lead to significant investment in facilities that would benefit both the elderly and people with disabilities. The Nagano sites were developed with access in mind – perhaps even more so than some other Paralympic Games venues. The Deputy Secretary General of the Nagano Paralympic Organising Committee (NAPOC), Fumio Miyake, indicated how their preparatory work was very tough at first: 'When we began our preparations, public interest both in the disabled themselves and in barrier-free facilities was low. We had great difficulties procuring transportation vehicles and obtaining cooperation from various facilities. There were not enough step-free buses available, for instance'. But attitudes shifted within the country, and resources were pooled so as to bring together all existing amenities for Nagano, while also building fresh with long-term provision for people with a disability in mind.

Following through with the theme of 'Friendship and Warmth', some 3195 volunteers provided an essential service for the successful operation of the Paralympic Games. This first Winter Paralympic Games to take place outside Europe was a resounding success for competitors and for the Paralympic Movement. Some statistics from the official report illustrate the scale of the undertaking:

- 32 nations
- 571 athletes
- 575 officials
- 5 sports (biathlon and cross country were disciplines of Nordic skiing)
- 34 events
- 151 376 spectators in total
- 1468 media representatives
- 9274 games operational staff
- 35 000 police officers
- 754 runners in torch relay
- 7.7 million hits on official website during the Games.[1]

The Nagano Paralympic Organising Committee was dynamic in capturing the imagination of the population of Japan leading up to the Games, and public relations events were very successfully managed. The mascot of the 'Parabbit' began to show up in all sorts of places. This mascot, representing the three *Tae-Geuks* of the IPC as the body and ears of a rabbit, had been selected from an entry of more than 10 000 to a competition to find a suitable mascot for the Nagano 1998 Paralympic Games. As had been the case with the Tokyo Paralympic Summer Games in 1964, the Japanese Royal Family honoured the Paralympic Movement with a great deal of attention. His Imperial Highness the Crown Prince agreed to act as the Honorary Patron of the Games, attending in Nagano on 5th, 6th, 7th, 13th, 14th and 15th March 1998. The Emperor and Empress even spent two days in Nagano, watching several events. Quite remarkable in their support, the Empress

---

[1] Official Report, 1998 Winter Paralympic Games, Nagano. Organising Committee of the Nagano Paralympics.

even joined in a 'Mexican wave' at the ice sledge racing, as spectators stood up in sequence around the stadium.

An Experts Congress was organised by NAPOC, to run in the afternoons of 7th and 8th March. The selected theme was 'Trends and Issues in Winter Paralympic Sport'. Some 217 participants represented 20 different countries at the Congress, also attracting media attention from 16 organisations nationally and beyond. The keynote address was given by Hal O'Leary (USA), with invited lectures from Inge Morisbak (Norway), Wolfgang Ott (Austria), Mirre Kipfer (Switzerland), Birgitta Blomquist (Germany) and Jerry Johnston (Canada).

The ice sledge hockey provided spectacularly energetic support from spectators, and the energy was tangible on the ice as well. Norway beat Canada in the final, 2–0, although the Canadians felt that their heroic struggle against the confident Swedish team for the semi-final was probably the most satisfying moment. In the ice sledge racing, the host country had surprising success, taking nine of the 16 available gold medals.

The helpfulness of the volunteers and officials was remarked upon by many participants at the Nagano Games: 'There were times they were overly friendly, overly nice and, being in a wheelchair, they were overly helpful', commented Stacy Kohut (Canada) in an interview with the *Calgary Sun*. 'Some of us were joking the last couple of days over there – "I can't wait to get back to North America where people slam doors in your face"'. The spectators took one particular local competitor to their hearts: Masahiro Shitaka became the first Japanese man ever to win gold in an Alpine event at the Winter Paralympics. The first gold medal for the host nation came in the women's sit-ski race, in which Kuniko Ohbinata finished ahead of the defending champion, Sara Will from the USA.

The Closing Ceremony, on 14th March 1998, saw a pulsating programme of music and movement, culminating in the release of more than seven and a half million folded, colourful paper cranes, traditional Japanese symbols of peace and the realisation of one's prayers. The origami cranes also represented the wealth of cooperation, as more than 350 000 people had responded to the organising committee's request to the public to make these decorative objects.

Where there were technical and administrative hitches during the Nagano 1998 Winter Paralympic Games, they were effectively dealt with due to the positive attitude of both the local organisers and the delegates appointed by IPC. In the Alpine Skiing there was supposed to be a limit of three competitors per event from each country. For reasons still unclear, the US team entered five athletes in the downhill LW5 class, all of whose entries were accepted. This was not spotted until the last moment, and all five were disqualified, then three of the athletes were reinstated. This untidy process was necessary because of the lateness of the decision – possibly attributable to the computer-generated draw, and the lack of specific guidance for appropriate action to be found in the IPC Handbook. Of course the root cause was the lack of attention to the sports rules by the US team officials when submitting their entries.

Classification also caused some consternation in Nagano. It was suggested that some of the classification had been conducted by the IPC Alpine Skiing Committee, rather than by the nominated classification team. There were also later changes in classes: there were to be two classes for sit-skiers (LW10 and LW11). But another class (LW12) was introduced just before the Games began, and further sub-division took place within this category (LW12/1 and LW12/2). The safety of athletes was a major concern during the Alpine events. Some competitors had major crashes and falls, and there were real delays in the competition programme as a result of the number of people requiring assistance. Barriers and safety controls had to be checked after all these incidents, further slowing the competitions. The incidents were sometimes caused by the steepness of the gradient and the snow conditions, but they were also considered to have been a result of the eligibility criteria not being stringent enough. Nagano was spectacular and the people of Japan were warmly embracing. Many of those who could remember told of the similarity of feeling when reflecting on the Tokyo Paralympic Games in 1964.

FROM NAGANO TO SYDNEY

Administration

The IPC Sports Council held a Strategic Planning Session on 5th and 6th June 1998 to examine a programme for the future. The organisation had undergone some major changes in the recent past, and there was a need to re-evaluate the effectiveness of services to member countries and to athletes. York Chow, as Vice President Policy, Planning and Development, led the discussions. A list of 'critical factors for success' emerged from the productive meetings. The statement of intent is a sign of modernity; acknowledgement of essential tightening up of practices and accountability. The critical factors were identified as:

- improvement in sport operations and development of sport infrastructures;
- development of a diverse funding base to increase financial resources;
- enhancement of marketing support;
- recruitment of bids and organising committees for championships;
- improvement of internal and external communications;
- coordination of championship programme calendar between IPC Sports, IOSDs and independent sports;
- ensuring voting rights of the Sports in the IPC General Assembly;
- a systematic evaluation of new sport/discipline applications for Paralympic status within Paralympic organisers' limitations on number of athletes and sports.

In order to help the prioritisation of sports technical services, a mission statement was constructed:

> The IPC Sport Technical Department will promote elite competition and coordinate Paralympic Sport through an athlete-centred, sport specific model which recognises the diverse delivery systems serving athletes with disabilities and member nations. The focus of the Sport Technical Department includes:
>
> 1. Fostering the growth of Paralympic Sport by increasing the number of athletes and nations while improving the caliber of athletic performance;
> 2. Enhancing the quality of Sport Technical operations and administration; and
> 3. Ensuring diversity in Paralympic Sport.

While the discussions were wholeheartedly constructive, the participants went through a soul-searching process of identifying realistic weaknesses in their structure, as well as celebrating the strengths. The most important weaknesses limiting the performance of the Sports Technical Department centred on issues of communication, financial resources, depth of human resources and expertise. But they extended into concerns about perceived political influence, understanding of responsibilities and lack of consensus regarding ideology. More broadly, the Sports Council demonstrated that it was concerned about 'potential fractionalisation of the Paralympic Movement, program stagnation, and the realisation that accelerated growth has exceeded current resources'.

Most positively, strategic goals were proposed in a draft report presented to the IPC Executive Committee in December 1998 in Bonn. Again, the tide had turned for the International Paralympic Committee, now in need of clear statements of realisable targets. These goals are worth stating:

- HUMAN RESOURCES: To improve the quality and efficiency of our Sport Technical service to athletes, nations and games organisers by enhancing our human resource base
- FINANCIAL RESOURCES: To increase financial resources for Paralympic Sports and improve fiscal responsibility

- ADMINISTRATION: To provide high quality, professional sport management and functional administrative support mechanisms in all sections of the IPC Sports Technical Department
- POLITICAL: To improve the level of influence of the Sports within IPC through advocacy, education, and voting rights.

The last part of the Strategic Planning Session was to develop initiatives at the short-, medium- and long-term levels, to enable the Sports Technical Department to achieve these goals. Some immediate responses from international sports organisations for athletes with a disability were critical of the marginal role that these initiatives permitted them to play. It was an understandable reaction to a loss of hands-on involvement in central decision making, and even in implementation of strategy. Once again the international federations rekindled their discussions about the construction of a more formal liaison mechanism among themselves – when in doubt they returned to the familiar model of the International Coordinating Committee of the past.

At the Extraordinary General Assembly of EUROPC, the European Paralympic Committee, held in Malmö, Sweden, early in September 1998, it passed a motion to register itself as a non-governmental, non-profit organisation. This process was completed on 2nd July 1999, when EUROPC was founded and registered according to German law in Düsseldorf, Germany. At the next IPC Executive Committee meeting, EUROPC was adopted as the IPC Standing Committee for the IPC European Regional Committee.

Voting Rights

The matter of voting rights became highly complex with the transfer of the International Paralympic Committee's Headquarters to Germany. The voting procedures had been changed in 1997 to permit all sports, including the IPC sports, to have a vote in the General Assembly. A result of the move was the need to register the IPC under German law. As the organisation prepared the ground for a General Assembly in November 1999, it seemed that the IPC had one constitution in place as a result of the 1997 General Assembly (reflected in the Handbook), and another constitution that was now registered in Germany. There were several points of conflict between the two. The complicating element of the latter constitution was that, under German law, only members have voting rights in a registered organisation. The alterations made to the constitution in 1997 did give the sports voting rights, but did not alter the status of the sports – they were not members of the International Paralympic Committee. The potential existed for a disastrous series of meetings if the Legal Committee could not come up with a solution. Decisions made in the General Assembly could be challenged and could be deemed unlawful, leading to lawsuits if relevant. Thomas Reinecke, who had been appointed IPC's Chief Operations Officer in October 1998, worked hard to provide a number of possibilities: one was to put an emergency motion to the 1999 General Assembly to create a new category of membership, and to accept the duly registered Paralympic Sports and non-Paralympic IPC Championship Sports into membership of that category immediately. The sports would not be entitled to vote on this motion, should it be proposed as the solution. For the purpose of the business to be conducted at the General Assembly in Salt Lake City, Bob Steadward intended to operate on the basis that the right of the sports to vote was given by a ruling of the chair. Anyone objecting would have to challenge this. Those delegates who accepted the rule of the chair should ward off the possibility of subsequent decisions being legally challenged at a later date. When the General Assembly heard the explanation given by Bob Steadward, no objections were raised to the temporary position.

When the Legal Committee got together in Crans Montana in January 2000, at the time of the Skiing World Championships, Thomas Reinecke and Mr Pauly, the IPC lawyer, had found a way of solving the guaranteeing of voting rights for the sports without needing to register them as legal entities. An amendment was required to the constitution registered in Germany. Although complex in its wording, it would have the effect of ensuring that the sports had the privileges guaranteed at the 1997 General Assembly, while keeping the differences clear between the sports, the nations and the IOSDs. There were still important aspects of the legal position of the IPC to be resolved: particularly the fact that the organisation was legally operating according to the constitution registered in Germany, in German, and not according to the constitution that the General Assembly had officially adopted. The plan was to amend the German constitution through the involvement of those 'founding members' who had been signatories of the registration in Bonn, so as to bring it as closely in line as possible to the General Assembly's adopted constitution.

The new IPC Headquarters is Opened in Bonn, September 1999

The opening of new IPC Headquarters in Bonn took place on 3rd September 1999. The official ceremony took place in the former plenary of the German Parliament, followed by lunch there. Many dignitaries visited the building that had been donated by the German Government, at 212–214 Adenauerallee, for the inauguration. The event also coincided with the tenth anniversary of the founding of the International Paralympic Committee, so the scale of celebration was double. The German Paralympic Committee created a lavish gala event for the Friday evening, bringing more than a thousand guests together. Bonn's Mayor, Bärbel Dieckmann, hosted a dinner. Shortly afterwards, the German Chancellor, Gerhard Schroeder, held a reception to welcome the IPC to Germany and its new seat in Bonn. The IOC donated an exquisite statue to be displayed in the new IPC Headquarters. Staff were recruited steadily to the Headquarters to tackle essential tasks. With the plush new building at the disposal of the International Paralympic Committee, it is important to note that the administration of the organisation had been sustained for more than a year largely out of home-based offices. The rental contract for the Brugge offices ended in December 1997 and the IPC moved out. Leen Coudenys was mandated by the Management Committee to bring to a close all contracts in Belgium and gradually to work towards the transfer of assets and registration to Germany. All contracts that had been signed with organising committees of championships and Paralympic Games had to be sound in their transfer to a new headquarters for the IPC. The final liquidation process was only formally concluded with the publication in the *Official Journal* of the Belgian State on 11th March 1999.

Executive Meeting in Bonn

The Executive Committee took the opportunity of its attendance at the opening ceremony of the IPC Headquarters in Bonn to hold a business meeting. Among a number of routine matters, there was fairly energetic debate over the recommendations to restructure the Management and Executive Committees. A move towards a professional staff in IPC should mean that many day-to-day tasks would be taken from the shoulders of these committees. It was possible that an elected Secretary General would become unnecessary now that a Chief Operating Officer was in post. There was certainly a view that the Executive Committee might only meet once a year. Several delegates continued to feel that the two committees needed to be streamlined, as recommended by the Task Force, but the Presidents of IBSA, INAS-FMH and ISOD were emphatic about their opposition to a reduction in the size of the Executive Committee or a reduction in the number of meetings. A good deal of time had been wasted in contemplation of the alignment of these two committees, according to these three international federations' leaders. They suggested that it was only inside the Executive Committee that the role of the IOSDs had been brought into question – the General Assembly had not questioned the IOSDs' permanence on the Executive Committee. They suggested that if this were brought in these terms to the General Assembly, they would see it as a measure of disunity. The ensuing debate was very productive of a range of ideas. Bob Steadward proposed that IPC should have an Executive Board and a Board of Directors. The Board of Directors would resemble the present Executive Committee, but would only meet once each year, giving leadership and direction. The Executive Board would be composed of officers elected by the General Assembly – starting with nine identified positions, but possibly more. Further discussion of this scheme showed that there was general agreement for the concept, and that it should be worked on to arrive at a proposal to be presented at the Salt Lake Executive Committee meeting and then the General Assembly. The Executive Committee voted to proceed with the plans by a margin of 13 votes in favour to five votes against, with two abstentions. As the Chairman of the recent Task Force, York Chow was eminently well qualified to produce a discussion paper, eventually titled: *The IPC for the New Millennium*.

One weakness of the Task Force proposals had been the apparent urgency to embark on radical restructuring. The organisation's key individuals appeared to recognise that this was to be avoided in the current climate. Greater success was likely, and success that was to be long lived, if there was wide consultation and steady decision making over time.

General Assembly at Salt Lake City, 1999

When the Executive Committee met just before the Salt Lake General Assembly, in November 1999, Hans Lindström proposed that there should be a new 'Arnhem Seminar' to offer extensive opportunities to bring debate into open forums. This was a vital characteristic of the International Paralympic Committee – overt democracy, sometimes perniciously inefficient, but fundamental to the objectives of the organisation. Time needed to be taken to allow for preparation of a strategic planning seminar, possibly looking to bring IPC members together in 2001 for Lindström's 'new Arnhem'. At the Salt Lake General Assembly, York Chow made several recommendations, all agreed by the Executive Committee, to the gathered IPC members. These were:

- to retain the existing Executive Committee and Management Committee structure for this and the next tenure (2001–2005);
- to identify and prioritise the important strategies, policies and tasks for IPC for the next six years, and establish relevant commissions to address, develop and implement these policies;
- that the Management Committee and staff should develop a more detailed and revised Manual and Schedule of Delegate Authority to streamline all operational functions of IPC, with clear delineation of the roles of all members of the Executive Committee and IPC staff;
- that the above recommendations would remain under constant review;
- that the IPC should actively promote an overall review of the functions of the IPC. To that purpose a formal IPC seminar/workshop was recommended for the spring of the year 2001.

New members welcomed into the Paralympic fraternity at the 1999 General Assembly, held in Salt Lake City on 19th and 20th November 1999, included Azerbaijan, Barbados, Cabo Verde, Namibia, Samoa, Sao Tome and Principe, Tonga, Turkmenistan, Vietnam and Vanuatu. Another 18 applications were pending, but without documentation having been received. These would need to be scrutinised, but the Executive Committee could award provisional membership until the next General Assembly.

Some membership matters brought greater complexity to the administration than others. The position of membership in Colombia vexed the Secretary General for some time. Although the matter was resolved suitably, a great deal of time was taken to determine which of two different bodies was the legitimate claimant of IPC membership in that country. Another perspective of membership was the flurry of nations trying to secure their recognition so as to enable their athletes to participate in the forthcoming Sydney 2000 Paralympic Games. It was always heartening to receive membership payments and applications, but some of the paperwork was simply not submitted correctly, and sometimes vital portions were absent. There were numerous countries that had applied for membership some years before, but that still had not submitted comprehensive constitutions or obligatory details that would advance their admission. The Secretary General wrote reminders to these countries, but with only limited success.

The IPC Code of Ethics was submitted to the General Assembly, but the delegates were put under unfair pressure because they had only just received the papers – the final details had only been settled in the Executive Committee meeting the day before. York Chow explained that the intention had been to lean heavily on the general principles of honesty, human rights, non-discrimination, fairness and justice. He suggested that a Commission for Ethics be set up to tune the document and the principles further. The General Assembly voted to accept the code in principle, while a commission would use the texts as a framework for a definitive document.

World Summit on Physical Education, November 1999

The International Council of Sport Science and Physical Education (ICSSPE) organised the first ever World Summit on Physical Education from 3rd to 5th November 1999 in Berlin. The intention was to bring to the attention of governments, through their Education and Sports Ministers, the need for positive action in relation to the provision of physical education as a life-long process. The Summit attracted over 250 delegates from 78 countries. The *Results and Recommendations of the World Summit on Physical Education* were presented as an official working document to the 3rd International Conference of Ministers and Senior Officials responsible for the Physical Education and Sport (MINEPS III) that took place in Punta del Este, Uruguay, from 30th November to 3rd December 1999. The United Nations Educational, Scientific and Cultural Organisation (UNESCO) was geared up to use the recommendations contained in the Declaration of Punta del Este as a guideline for its programmes of development and activity in physical education and sport, including individuals with a disability.

International Olympic Committee

Bob Steadward was in Seoul, Korea, in June 1999 to take part in the IOC's 109th Session and to be present at the 2006 bidding city presentations and final discussions. Steadward was also appointed to the IOC 2000 Commission on Ethics and Reform. His assignment was to Working Group II, examining the role of the IOC.

There was an increasing connection between the IPC and the IOC as the Sydney Games approached. Gilbert Felli wrote to Bob Steadward in May 2000 to ask him to nominate IPC delegates to sit on the IOC Coordination Commission and the IOC Evaluation Commission. Steadward had already been appointed as a Board Member of the International Foundation for the Olympic Truce. The impetus for this sort of involvement came firstly from the IPC President, suggesting to Samaranch at various times that the IPC should have a more direct role in helping take the Olympic Movement forward. Of course, this would also serve the future of the International Paralympic Committee very well. It was important that Steadward should not lose sight of the IPC's main business, while the security of closer alignment with the IOC was seductive.

The major work between the IPC and the IOC was concerned with drawing up an agreement or memorandum of understanding, formalising the affiliation between the two bodies. This document would give the International Paralympic Committee the opportunity of defining what it saw as the most beneficial connection between itself and the IOC in future. A meeting with Gilbert Felli had led to plans for a two-part contract dealing with the relationship between the two organisations. The first part would include matters of protocol, accreditation, funding, representation on commissions, administrative relationships with staff and information technology. The second part was concerned with Olympic and Paralympic bidding processes and procedures, Olympic and Paralympic contracts with the host Organising Committee, the international TOP sponsorship and marketing programme, host broadcaster and television rights, and Olympic and Paralympic Games operation manuals and other publications. Bob Steadward asked Samaranch whether it might be possible to employ someone to help with related administrative and operational matters relating to the implementation of this agreement. He suggested Xavier Gonzalez, who was due to finish his contract as General Manager of Sport and Venues with the Sydney Paralympic Organising Committee before the end of 2000. Within the agreement, the marketing issue looked like being the stickiest. This would require careful attention.

Following Recommendation 15 of the IOC 2000 Commission, a strong future connection was proposed. The recommendation related to the IOC–IPC relationship, and detailed some important principles:

- The Paralympics must be organised in the same city as the Olympic Games. The obligation for the host city to organise the Paralympic Games must be included in the Host City Contract
- The Paralympic Games will always follow the Olympic Games
- The IPC will have a representative in both the IOC Evaluation Commission and the Coordination Commission
- The Paralympic Movement, through a member of the IPC and Paralympic athletes, could be represented in the IOC. Similarly, the Olympic Movement could be represented in the IPC.

This highly significant proposal was a coming of age of the relationship between the International Paralympic Committee and the International Olympic Committee. At times in the previous ten years, the IOC had considered it undesirable to locate the Paralympic Games particularly close to the Olympic Games, either geographically or philosophically. The IOC Executive Board had wavered over time, but had always commented on the public image that was so crucial in the IOC's dealings with the disabled sport community. Juan Antonio Samaranch had been steady in his support for the International Paralympic Committee, although he had sometimes shown some concern for the possibility of overlapping marketing strategies.

In October 2000, Samaranch wrote to Bob Steadward to confirm officially his election as an IOC member. This decision had been taken at the IOC's 111th Session in Sydney. Earlier discussions between the two leaders had looked at whether Steadward should be elected via the new regulations permitting members to come from the international federations, or as an individual member. Steadward was bound to prefer election as an individual member, although there would be complications ahead as Steadward's time as IPC President was coming to an end. He was duly put forward as an individual member. Samaranch had informed Steadward that the IOC Nominations Commission had proposed him as a candidate in July 2000.

Finances

The marketing programme for the Sydney 2000 Paralympic Games appeared to be falling short of its target, when the IPC received its regular report to the Executive Committee in Sydney in April 1999.

A suggestion was made that an International Paralympic Foundation could be a way of generating significant resources, while retaining an ongoing structure for the future. The idea was discussed in a closed meeting, when York Chow, Bob McCullough and Thomas Reinecke were commissioned to work together with the Sydney Paralympic Organising Committee to look at more concrete possibilities. With further research and discussion with SPOC, it was decided that the idea could be pursued at a national level, and the Australian Paralympic Foundation was established. It was still thought desirable to proceed towards an International Paralympic Foundation, but for now the fundraising for the Sydney Paralympics would be paramount.

André Auberger was definitely proud of the achievements of the IPC in relation to its financial position. He should also have been proud of his own management, when he described the strong base to the General Assembly in 1999: when he first accepted the position of Treasurer in 1989 the IPC had no funds. Now, after ten years, the projected revenue in the accounts for 1998 was US$1 792 000, although the final result was US$1 302 612.55. The aura of success was marred by the acknowledgement that the marketing report showed a distinctly Spartan return. For the outlay of more than US$103 000 to Optimé International, there had been no income from the marketing programme since its inception in 1998. This certainly was 'cause for concern', as one member of the Executive Committee put it. The gentle tone of Nabil Salem's report on marketing was not well received by the delegates at the General Assembly. Salem, whose position as Vice President Marketing and Communication had only just been ratified earlier in the meeting, was slated because the contract with Optimé International had recently been renewed until February 2000, despite a dismal performance by the appointed marketing experts. Salem's appointment had arisen from the resignation of Duncan Wyatt.

These criticisms, principally voiced by the representative of the Netherlands, Switzerland and Denmark, also took the discussion towards the need for the IPC Executive to present a more transparent planning projection to each future General Assembly. This should map out the strategies for advancing IPC's major policies in the next period. In view of the serious discontent of the General Assembly, and the real failing of the marketing programme, the Executive Committee had agreed to propose an emergency motion at this point in the meeting. The motion included the termination of the contract with Optimé International at the end of the current agreement; and the establishment of an Ad Hoc Marketing Task Force made up of Phil Craven, Andy Scott, Tony Sainsbury, Chris Donaldson and Serge Valentin, with Thomas Reinecke coordinating from IPC Headquarters. The Marketing Task Force had as its remit to produce a report covering: the image of the IPC; marketing deliverables of IPC, including media/TV exposure and so on; strategic options for marketing for IPC; and marketing and advertising policy for IPC and its member constituencies.

Financial planning also required a longer-term view, and the General Assembly of 1999 heard the IPC President announce that a four-year budget would be presented for approval at the next General Assembly. This would necessarily need to have some flexibility built into it, as the predictions would have to be based on a portion of expectation and hope, as well as sound experience.

The 1999 to 2000 Paralympic Solidarity programme was extended due to additional IOC funding and the improved IPC financial position. Before this it had been available only to support athletes attending the Paralympic Games, and some attendance of delegates at the General Assembly, but now the support was extended to regional championships as well. Eligibility was determined by a calculation of the gross national product of the applying country.

Paralympic Games preparation

As soon as the IOC announced that Torino, Italy, would be the host of the 2006 Winter Olympic and Paralympic Games, Bob Steadward immediately made contact with the organising committee. There would be an acceleration of effort to ensure that the Paralympic Winter Games could receive the very best cooperation from the Organising Committee.

The original plan for television coverage in Sydney was for Channel 7 to provide the Australian broadcasting of content from the Sydney 2000 Paralympic Games. But it later became clear that there was to be a paucity of television coverage, with only late night summaries of under an hour a day in Australia. The Sydney Paralympic Organising Committee (SPOC) was not happy with this and committed to fund the host broadcasting at a higher level of delivery. The Australian Broadcasting Corporation (ABC) successfully negotiated to secure the position of domestic rightsholder. SPOC appointed London-based Media Content plc as the exclusive worldwide (excluding Australia) TV rights sales agent for the Sydney 2000 Paralympic Games.

Juan Antonio Samaranch was informed by Bob Steadward on 5th April 2000 that it was the intention of the IPC to do away with entry fees for athletes at all future Paralympic Games. But there were problems in negotiations with the Athens 2004 Organising Committee because they had spotted that the contract with Sydney included entry fees, whereas there was no mention of them in the proposed contract between IPC and the Athens 2004 Organising Committee. Another cause of disquiet was that the Athens 2004 organisers were planning to pay for all travel expenses of the Olympic athletes, but not to offer the same facility to Paralympic athletes. Steadward told Samaranch that he was going to hold out for a payment of at least US$1.5 million from the Athens 2004 Organising Committee for the television and marketing rights for the Paralympic Games. He claimed that these rights were really worth about $4.5 million, given the higher status and improving visibility of the Paralympic Movement worldwide, but he would settle for the lesser amount.

Another concern for the IPC was the prominence of Special Olympics Inc. in Greece, rather than the International Paralympic Committee or INAS-FMH. The political influence of Special Olympics might be a contentious issue should the IPC representation not be increased in the preparations for the Paralympic Games in Athens in 2004. There was a supplementary complication in the form of membership of IPC by a Greek organisation. Before a Paralympic Organising Committee could be formed to start work on the 2004 Paralympic Games, it was essential to have a bona fide IPC member organisation for Greece. At the Cairo meeting of the Executive Committee in May 2000, the decision was taken to accept the application of a hurriedly constituted Hellenic Paralympic Committee to IPC membership. Because the new organisation was struggling to create the paperwork, the IPC Executive agreed that the Hellenic Paralympic Committee should have three months in which to submit a legally impervious constitution for scrutiny.

Intellectual Disability

Michael Riding described the successful work aimed at classifying 88% of competitors prior to the Sydney 2000 Paralympic Games. When he presented his report to the Executive Committee meeting in Salt Lake City in November 1999, he expressed some concern at the progress of athletes under the direction of INAS-FMH. There had been some delays with registration of athletes, but IPC had an agreement in place with SPOC that no one would be permitted to compete in INAS-FMH events in Sydney without being registered INAS-FMH athletes. Some of the sports had also requested a classification appeal process to be put in place for INAS-FMH athletes – just as there was for each other group of athletes at the Paralympic Games. Riding would work on these wrinkles together with the Medical Officer of INAS-FMH.

By the time the IPC General Assembly took place in November 1999, the International Association for Sport for Persons with Mental Handicap (INAS-FMH) had undergone a restructuring: a permanent commission was now in charge of the day-to-day running of the organisation. It had also changed its name to the International Sports Federation for Persons with Intellectual Disability (INAS-FID).

Technical Matters

Efforts to increase the involvement of the international federations in the organisational bodies of the Paralympic Games were evident in a motion put to the 1999 General Assembly in Salt Lake City. The Greek delegate proposed that if a country is entrusted to hold the Paralympic Games, then the Paralympic Organising Committee must include five members proposed by the National Paralympic Committee, that is, one representative from each IPC disability group. This motion was defeated after a busy discussion. The grounds on which it lost the vote included the fact that the disability groups would have an input of a technical and operational type in the organising committee anyway. An important consideration was that there was already a requirement for certain specific position-holders to be included on a Paralympic Organising Committee: the President or Secretary General of the National Paralympic Committee and any IPC Executive Committee members of the host country would have to be included. There was not complete freedom in the make-up of the organising committees, especially as there was a move for greater overlap between the Olympic Games Organising Committee and that of the Paralympic Games. Increasing the numbers might make it difficult for some countries to consider bidding for the Paralympic Games, and there could even be legal restrictions within a country on who could be included in a board such as this. When all this had been covered, it still appeared as though the IOSDs were working to guarantee their prominence, or at least their inclusion in the high-level decisions pertaining to the Paralympic Games. Later on in the same meetings, Sweden moved to alter the structure of the Executive Committee, effectively by removing the representatives of the International Federations and the regional representatives. The motion was defeated, particularly as there had already been agreement that there would be a detailed scrutiny of the IPC's roles and responsibilities before altering its structure.

Women in Sport, 2000

The 2nd IOC World Conference on Women and Sport was held in Paris on 6th and 7th March 2000. IPC delegates to this conference were Carol Mushett (IPC Technical Officer, USA), Katarina Brandoburova (athlete and Secretary General of the Slovak Paralympic Committee), Andrea Scherney (athlete and Sport Manager, Austrian Paralympic Committee), Béatrice Hess (athlete, France) and Dr Susanne Reiff (IPC Media and Communication Manager). The focus was on the 21st century, and the place that women should have in all aspects of participation and administration. The IOC President, Juan Antonio Samaranch, opened the Conference with some powerful comments:

> The challenge will remain until women hold positions of responsibility at all levels of national, regional and international sports leadership. The challenge will remain until girls have the same opportunity to practise sport as boys. In all cases, the IOC is determined to make a concrete contribution so that this century will mark the start of a new era for women and sport with a better representation in sport administration and a parity in the Olympic Games programme.

'Women in sport' was identified as requiring a more active level of support from the IPC. Carol Mushett examined the details of women's participation in the Paralympic Movement, with some startling results. The Atlanta 1996 Paralympic Games saw women making up only 24% of competitors, whereas the Olympic Games had 34% female athletes. Remarkable also was the statistic that showed that 47% of nations did not have any female competitors at the Atlanta 1996 Paralympic Games (only 13% of nations in the Olympic Games failed to enter women). The IPC Executive Committee could only boast one woman on its 22-strong body. Only one of the 24 Paralympic Sport Chairs was a woman. The IPC Executive Committee wholeheartedly endorsed the Brighton Declaration on Women in Sport, emerging from the first IOC conference in 1995.

As a result of the more recent discussions, the IPC Sports Council strongly approved a definitive statement that aligned the IPC with those other organisations striving to increase opportunities for women to participate in sport. The Sports Council noted that there had been a decline in levels of participation by women, a consequence in part of what it saw as a reduction in opportunities for women in Paralympic sport. There had been a decline in the percentage of nations entering women in the Paralympic Games. The Sports Council recommended the establishment of a working group on Women and Sport, and to 'advance sport technical initiatives which promote equity and ensure opportunities for women in Paralympic Sport'. They urged the Executive Committee to consider the establishment of a standing committee of this sort, taking responsibility for developing a strategy for improving opportunities for the full involvement of women in Paralympic sport.

A policy was established to use the solidarity allocations of funding to promote participation for female athletes. In early 2000 Bob Steadward asked André Auberger to earmark one third of the solidarity funding for such support. But it was immediately evident that in some countries that would qualify for this sort of funding, there were not enough female athletes who would qualify for the Paralympic Games. A lengthier process of development would be needed to bring the competitor numbers and levels up. It was left in principle that gender considerations would be a factor when deciding solidarity funding in future. Gender would also be a marker in future decisions about wild card entries to the Sydney Paralympic Games.

Carol Mushett urged all constituents of the International Paralympic Committee that: 'for access to become true opportunity, IPC needs a systematic, organisation-wide strategy to mobilise institutional change. Awareness must be translated into commitment and philosophical support into strategic action.'

Development

There had been a reduction in the number of worthwhile applications for development funding during the period 1999–2000, according to York Chow, speaking at the Management Committee meeting in Bonn in February 2000. In particular it was pointed out that IPC needed to be responsible to the International Olympic Committee for the appropriate use of the funds it had given. Chow felt that some applications had not been in keeping with the original intent of the development theme: ISOD's week long classification seminar; INAS-FID's training of basketball officials. The representatives at the meeting considered that future funds should not be evenly shared out among budget holders, but should be allocated according to the priorities of the IPC Executive Committee. These would include projects to meet the 88% classification target, and to improve participation of female athletes and athletes with a severe disability, for example.

National and Regional Representation Issues

The 1999 IPC General Assembly had identified a need to reinforce the duties and responsibilities of the National Paralympic Committees, and a document was drawn up and approved by the Management

Committee in February 2000. The outline mission of the National Paralympic Committees was clarified as: 'to undertake the coordination of all IPC member disability sport groups in order to develop and protect the Paralympic Movement in their respective country in accordance with the following ethical principles, business responsibilities and sport guidelines'. There then followed a number of specific tasks that were either constitutionally mandatory, or principles of the IPC philosophy. It was certainly a clear statement for the National Paralympic Committees to use in taking their work forward, as well as giving a very timely opportunity to introduce important aspects of the code of ethics at the end of the document. Some National Paralympic Committees might need a significant amount of support from the IPC Headquarters in carrying out the identified mission to the full, but this would facilitate a positive interaction as a by-product.

Regional development had gone on apace in the past two years, with numerous initiatives being supported from IPC Headquarters. The alignment of countries' regional membership was being reviewed to see the best configuration to ensure the best service. There were several nations that had been admitted as members of one region which might be better served by membership of another region. The particular countries being discussed included Kazakhstan, Turkmenistan, Uzbekistan, Kyrgystan and Tajikistan. The idea of repartition was explored at a joint meeting of the IPC Middle East, South Pacific and East Asia regional committees, together with FESPIC Executive Committee members in Seoul, Korea, in December 1999.

Proposals were put to the 1999 General Assembly for the creation of an Asian Paralympic Council, and then also a Pacific Paralympic Committee was added. It was agreed that more consultation should take place among the constituents who would benefit from these changes, as many were not represented at the Salt Lake General Assembly. It was agreed that the proposals would be tabled in order to allow more specific plans to be made and submitted later.

Sport Science and Medicine

In his regular report to the IPC General Assembly, Michael Riding described the awkward situation that the International Olympic Committee had found itself in at the Nagano Winter Olympic Games, when a competitor tested positive for cannabis. The absence of a policy on the use of so-called 'social' drugs had led to the decision that the IPC would not declare any positive tests for cannabis in Nagano. Riding was clear, however, that the responsibility of the IPC was not solely to ensure that competitors presented themselves in the sporting arena free from substances that might give them an unfair advantage. There was a fundamental ethical position that the IPC should maintain in the protection of the health of competitors. Riding told the gathering of the proposed World Anti-Doping Agency that was being established, independently of the IOC. The IPC Medical Officer connected the issue to out-of-competition testing that was vital to the credible maintenance of a thorough anti-doping policy. However, Riding made it clear that the IPC could not finance this process, and was looking for sources of funding. The National Paralympic Committees were asked to set up and maintain out-of-competition testing on their own Paralympic athletes. Testing procedures could cost up to US$1500 per test. There was some merit in researching the use of hair testing rather than blood or urine testing.

The IOC World Conference on Doping had been a highly significant occasion for Bob Steadward and Michael Riding. There had been the opportunity for them to be reassured that the IPC had procedures in operation, but they gleaned clarification of important issues. Doping was defined as contravening sport and medical ethics. The athletes' health needed to be prominently protected through anti-doping controls. The 600 delegates were largely agreed on the desirability of standardised procedures and standardised penalties for doping offences. There was a strong view that any new agency should not be an offshoot of the IOC, but should be independent. It remained to be seen whether this independence could be achieved.

Vista '99

The Second International Conference on Sport for Athletes with a Disability took place between 28th August and 1st September at the German Sport University in Cologne. The event was made possible by the patronage of the International Council of Sport Science and Physical Education and the IPC, with significant financial support from the Government of the Federal Republic of Germany, the Government of the Federal State of North Rhine Westphalia, the Deutsche Forschungsgemeinschaft (German Research Council) and the IPC. Toyota Deutschland GmbH also sponsored the conference. As a central theme, this large-scale conference took the title: 'New Horizons in Sport for Athletes with a Disability'. Delegates included 170 athletes, coaches, administrators and sport scientists from 38 countries. Gudrun Doll-Tepper, President of ICSSPE, acted as Conference Chair, with Michael Kröner as Secretary General and Werner Sonnenschein as overall coordinator for the conference. The conference underlined the need to remain athlete-focused in all aspects of Paralympic administration and management. The delegates arrived on the Saturday ready for a welcome buffet dinner. On Sunday 29th August the presentations and discussions began in earnest at 8.30 am. The conference was divided into sections, with a number of papers in each section and sub-section:

- sport performance:
  - exercise physiology
  - advances in training techniques
  - technical developments (equipment)
  - sports medicine;
- classification;
- integration, development and recruitment;
- organisation and administration;
- ethics;
- media, marketing and sponsorship.

During the afternoon of Monday 30th August, technical demonstrations were put on, followed by poster presentations and films. On the Tuesday, after a morning of papers, there was a round table discussion with the Presidents of the International Organisations of Sport for the Disabled. The final day mopped up the remaining presentations and then delegates went into 'special topics' sessions before everyone gathered again for a summary and conclusion. Fundamental topics emerged in discussions during the conference that would become important issues for the International Paralympic Committee and the IOSDs:

- 'the athlete's voice in an athlete-centred organisation';
- gender equity;
- ethical issues (including doping and boosting);
- objectivity in classification;
- optimisation of sports performance;
- progress in integration and inclusion;
- challenges for developing countries;
- marketing and funding realities.

Testing Times

The IPC Medical Officer, Michael Riding, reported to the Executive Committee in Sydney just prior to the start of the 2000 Paralympic Summer Games. He made several fundamental comments about the need of IPC to accept a shift in its structure to recognise the scale and importance of the work that IPC does at the start of the new millennium. Riding was also very critical of the Sydney Paralympic Organising Committee (SPOC), for its refusal to handle the accreditation of the Anti-Doping Commission. Other aspects of discontent expressed by Riding included the contrast with the Sydney Olympic Games Organising Committee's willingness to pay for the whole of the IOC Medical Commission's expenses, numbering more than thirty members, while SPOC was not willing to cover the IPC Medical Commission – six members only. This was not entirely an accurate representation of the situation: SPOC had agreed to fund a total of 50 representatives from IPC, and IPC was left to decide who was paid for. Inevitably Riding was not happy when told that the pressure of numbers meant that only six members of the IPC Medical Commission were being allocated funded places. This was more of an issue for IPC than SPOC.

Testing of erythropoietin (EPO) was expensive, and the IOC was providing payment for this level of testing at the Olympic Games. As a result of the costs involved, the IPC Commission was expecting not to do any EPO tests. Erythropoietin is a hormone that stimulates the body to produce more red blood cells, thus aiding in the transportation of oxygen. It is naturally produced in the kidneys, but sometimes is given to combat anaemia and other related problems. EPO was at the heart of the doping scandal that shook the 1998 Tour de France, and the problems had become more widespread.

Strategic Matters and Preparations

The International Paralympic Committee would not become a subsidiary, but a partner of the International Olympic Committee, under the terms of a Memorandum of Understanding between the two organisations. The first part of the agreement was signed during the Sydney 2000 Paralympic Games, covering the basic principles and relationship between the two bodies. The second part of the Memorandum of Understanding (2001) related specifically to the Paralympic Games. The agreement arose from the work done in the IOC 2000 Commission, of which Bob Steadward had been a member. Contained in the Memorandum were statements of shared philosophy, evincing that the two bodies support the 'right of all human beings to pursue their physical and intellectual development', and that 'the IOC and the IPC believe in international solidarity in accordance with their respective mandates and principles'. The Memorandum specified that the IOC would invite IPC representation on a number of IOC commissions, and that the IPC President would be invited to become a member of the IOC – a goal already achieved in the case of Bob Steadward.

As the International Paralympic Committee prepared itself for the Sydney Paralympics to begin, officers were also looking at the plans for their Strategic Planning Congress. There had been initial offers from five countries to host the congress: United Kingdom, Cambodia, Spain, Malaysia and the Netherlands. York Chow had been working with the proposal of this taking place in Cambodia, a war-torn country, but one needing support. Chow told the IPC Management Committee in August 2000 of the security and health measures that delegates would be advised about. Unfortunately, problems began to brew up in Cambodia, not least of which were natural disasters that put the wisdom of planning to hold the IPC Strategic Planning Congress there in doubt. The Executive Committee of IPC discussed the plans for the Congress at its September meeting in Sydney. First announcements had been sent out by this time, and a structure was in place for the running of the Congress. The Executive Committee made some adjustments, and discussion was directed at the implications of the Congress. There was a possibility that the members would call for an Extraordinary General Assembly to be held in conjunction with the Congress. There was some disquiet about this because the 1999 General Assembly had agreed that this Congress would only be concerned with long-term policy, rather than leaping immediately into decisions about the implementation of ideas newly formulated at the Congress. They were mindful of the problems that followed the last Task Force's presentation to the General Assembly.

Even though a major re-evaluation was just ahead of it, the IPC could not wait before implementing some changes that would take time to execute. Because of this, a number of commissions were established. Initially these included Ethics, Athletes with Severe Disability, Women in Sport, Development, Marketing and Media, and Solidarity.

A more formal delineation of awards made by the International Paralympic Committee was desired, as well as there being a wish to expand the range of recognition offered. The IPC Executive Committee had agreed to a review of the system of awards when it had met in Cairo in May 2000. The Paralympic Awards Committee was composed of François Terranova (Chairman), Bob McCullough, Ali Harzallah and Carol Mushett. The recommendations of this group were that there should be four types of award, in the following order of importance:

- the Paralympic Order
- the IPC Sport Award
- the IPC Medal of Merit
- the IPC Diploma of Recognition.

Further development of the awards scheme was considered. François Terranova also put forward the idea of an Association of Paralympic Order Members, to promote friendship and to strengthen the link between recipients. Those already dedicated to service of the Paralympic Movement would be inspired and encouraged to take their contribution further, especially as there would be a notion of progressing over time to the next level.

Other preparatory details included decisions that East Timor could compete under the IPC flag, just as it had competed in the Olympic Games under the flag of the IOC. The Olympic Torch relay had begun in Greece, as usual, but there was some concern on the part of the International Olympic Committee that too close a symbolic association between the two events could be drawn if the Paralympic torch was lit from the sacred Olympic Flame. The Paralympic Torch Relay began on 5th October 2000, with a lighting ceremony in Canberra, Australia's Capital Territory. Members of the Ngunnawal community in Canberra lit the torch from a flame ignited using traditional Aboriginal techniques. More than 900 people carried the torch on its way via all capital cities of Australian States by air, then on a 750 kilometre land relay around the Sydney area.

Ticket sales for the Sydney Paralympic Games were double those for Atlanta in 1996, a total of 1.1 million tickets in all. Trying out a new strategy for the Paralympic Games, the Sydney Paralympic Organising Committee sold reserved seats for the semi-finals and finals of competitions, but sold day passes for all other events. This had the effect of permitting spectators to see more and to be flexible in what they attended. Particularly noteworthy was the spectator profile at the Sydney 2000 Paralympic Games. There were, of course, the expected people supporting their athletes or their countries at the Paralympic Games. But the vast majority of these massive crowds were local Australians who were drawn to the phenomenon of elite sports. The Australian public had developed a unique passion for sport in their life; it is only necessary to cast a glance at the mass participation at all sporting venues around the country. The benefit for the Paralympic athletes on the occasion of the Sydney Paralympics was that they received precisely the same acclaim as their counterparts in the Olympic Games a few weeks before. These highly trained and dedicated athletes now had the opportunity to compete in the charged atmosphere of full venues, with the roar of vociferous crowds to spur them on. Several hundred thousand schoolchildren enjoyed organised outings to the Paralympic Games, along with other community and social groups. John Grant, President of the Sydney Paralympic Organising Committee, said: 'the next generation now understands the Games, the sports, and the disabilities. Adults can still be uncomfortable with people's disabilities, but children are wonderful! Kids are going up to athletes and not saying: "what's wrong with you?" they ask "what sport do you play?"'

A very promising agreement between the IPC and WeMedia was announced on 27th October 2000, giving the media company worldwide television and Internet webcasting rights to the Paralympics for six years. The IPC had the prospect of developing this relationship into a true goldmine. John Da Cruz had been working on marketing for the Sydney Olympic and Paralympic Organising Committees, and there was a possibility the IPC could employ him after the Paralympic Games, should this seem desirable to both parties. Da Cruz was promoting the Sponsors Visitors Programme at the Paralympics. He had also been responsible for working out the details of the arrangements with the New York company WeMedia. The proposals were to include valuable payments in installments from WeMedia to IPC amounting to what the IPC newsletter *The Paralympian* called 'a multi-million dollar deal' (no. 4, 2000). The agreement granted the New York company worldwide television and internet broadcasting rights for the Paralympic Games up to and including Torino 2006. As we will see later, this very desirable arrangement faltered at the first hurdle.

Sydney 2000 Paralympic Games: The Best Yet

The Sydney 2000 Paralympic Games provided the first opportunity for the full professional staff of IPC to be involved. The Headquarters staff would be located on the 8th floor of the Wentworth Hotel during the Games, along with the members of the Executive Committee.

As the world's media researched stories for their coverage of the Paralympic Games, the subject of boosting became a curiosity. When reporters discussed the subject with the athletes themselves, they found that the disturbing theories were realities among a small band of competitors. Newspapers and magazines told of the willingness of elite athletes to harm themselves in the name of competitive sport – the journalists did not always relate this to the conscious decision of other athletes to take banned substances for the same purpose. Rick Reilly, writing in *Sports Illustrated* (11th December 2000), described the worrying extremes to which wheelchair athletes would go. His introductory comments were damaging enough: 'You thought there was a boatload of cheaters at the Sydney Olympics? You should've seen what happened when the Games were *over*. That's when the worst cheaters of all arrived – the Paralympians.' Reilly went on to summarise the writing about boosting during the Paralympic Games:

> there were reports in respected newspapers in Sydney, London and Toronto of what some wheelchair track athletes were willing to do to win, including sit on tacks, stick themselves with pins, sit on ball bearings, tie piano wire around their scrotums or tie off their catheters until their bladders were nearly ready to burst. These advanced training methods gave these paralysed athletes no pain but caused their sympathetic nervous systems to drive their blood pressure straight up, kick in the fight-or-flight response and improve performance by as much as 15%.

US wheelchair athlete Bert Burns was quoted by Reilly as saying that competitors could tell who was boosting: 'I can tell at the start line which runners are clamping their catheters. They get goose bumps all over. Their muscles spasm so their legs are hopping up and down by themselves, and they're sweating. Quadriplegics don't sweat much'.

The initial standpoint of the media appeared to be that the Paralympics must be a virtuous and charitable happening that transcended human nature, unlike its seamier, earthy elder brother, the

Olympic Games. There was little logic in this view; rather it emphasised a lack of understanding about the maturity of the Paralympic Games and the nature of elite sport in any population. Mike Brace, Chairman of the British Paralympic Association, spoke about this in a radio interview: 'I don't know why they would be surprised in that it is elite sport and it's all of its glory and all of its downsides. The will to win for some people is such that they will do anything in order to achieve that'.

Four powerlifting competitors were sent home as a result of the pre-competition doping controls. Ali Mahmoudi-kordkheili (Iran) and Aurel Berbec (Romania) were found to have anabolic steroid metabolites in their system, and Marina Diakonova (Russia) and Radko Radev (Bulgaria) were sent home for using diuretic masking agents. Three more powerlifting competitors tested positive for having elevated levels of testosterone in their bodies. They were caught as a result of a new type of test that was able to detect the difference between naturally produced testosterone and the substance taken as a drug. The procedure employed carbon isotope ratio mass spectrometry for its levels of accuracy. Eleven competitors in total received bans as a result of testing positive for banned substances, nine of them in the out-of-competition testing. The only positive test in the post-competition testing that was not related to powerlifting was by Brian Frasure (USA), who tested positive for nandrolone. Frasure had won a silver medal in the athletics 200 m (T44) event, and was disqualified, with his medal withdrawn. Although he had already won a silver medal in the athletics 100 m final, Frasure did not test positive at that time. Frasure had been a high-visibility athlete, holding the 100 m sprint world record since 1998. Frasure was one of three athletes to be nominated for the 2000 Laureus World Sportsperson of the Year with a Disability Award, won by Louise Sauvage. He, along with the powerlifting competitors, was banned from IPC competitions for four years, including the Athens 2004 Paralympic Games.

In August 2000, the Paralympic Programme Committee submitted its recommendations for the qualification of sports for inclusion in the programme to the Sports Council Management Committee. The sports that were unable to meet the qualification criteria were: sailing, men's basketball for athletes with intellectual disability (both sports had provided insufficient documentation), and men's standing volleyball, which could only attest to being played in 12 countries. When this matter came to the Executive Committee in October 2000, the motion was put forward to remove standing volleyball from the Paralympic programme. The vote was not unanimous, but it was passed. It was 'regretted that such a decision had to be taken at this time when standing Volleyball athletes are participating in the Paralympic Games'. However, the evaluation process had been meticulously followed. The Executive wanted to make plain that the removal decision related only to the 2004 Paralympic Games, and that those involved in the sport could work to ensure that it was sufficiently developed to guarantee involvement beyond Athens.

The IPC Executive Committee approved the introduction of three new events for the Athens 2004 Paralympic Games: boccia class BC4 (for severely disabled), women's basketball (for athletes with intellectual disability), and women's sitting volleyball. Diane Craft, writing in *Palaestra*,[2] was less than sympathetic to the decision of the IPC to remove standing volleyball from the next Paralympic Programme:

> IPC issues reflect Paralympic growing pains. Controversy arose following the IPC announcement that men's standing Volleyball has been dropped from the 2004 Summer Paralympic Games. Carol Mushett, IPC Sport Technical Director explained, "The requirements for inclusion of team sports in the Paralympic program needs at least 18 nations in three regions to qualify a sport. It has been found after looking at official records that standing Volleyball doesn't fulfill the criteria to be included at the next Paralympic Games." Oliver Gutfleisch, member of the German Standing Volleyball Team, expressed dismay over the decision. According to a SPOC press release, he argued, "There are so many countries such as Cambodia and other Eastern Asia regions that suffer from land mines, and this

---

[2] Winter 2001, Vol. 17, No. 1.

type of sport is very strong there. Some countries in Africa play standing Volleyball, but they can't get the sponsorship for the team to join the IPC because their country is so poor. If this decision goes through, then it could mean the end of standing Volleyball in many countries." In a subsequent press conference, IPC President Dr. Robert Steadward said the decision to drop the sport was final. He directed athletes back to their own countries to gain support for playing the sport on a national level. Steadward suggested that standing Volleyball look to Tennis as a model, referring to the way Wheelchair Tennis is administered under the International Tennis Federation.

Diane Craft went on to berate the leadership of IPC for erasing sporting opportunities from the most needy, while claiming that the 'real estate value' of the Paralympics was rising. Steadward spoke in a press conference of the greater professionalisation, sophistication and financial attraction of the Paralympic Games. Craft sliced into Steadward's words, writing that the time may not be far off when: 'athletes with very limited function or with disabilities who do not fit the stereotypical beautiful people image may find it increasingly difficult to compete successfully in the collapsed categories. The Paralympic Games may be going Hollywood and some athletes are going to be left behind.'

The Sydney 2000 Paralympic Games Begin: 'The Things that Unite Mankind Far Outweigh the Things that Divide'

The Paralympic Village opened on 11th October, allowing a good orientation and acclimatisation for competitors. This was also the start date of the three-day Scientific Congress: 'Pushing the Limits: optimising potential through science and technology'. The launch of the most exciting 11 days of the Paralympic Games so far was via the Opening Ceremony on 18th October. Louise Sauvage raised the Paralympic Flame to bring back to life to the cauldron that had harboured the Olympic Flame only days before. The light and fire seemed to reside alongside the music that rang around the Homebush stadium throughout the night. The three-hour gala set the scene for a magnificent sporting spectacle. Graeme Connors' words, 'Being here is what it is all about', rang in the ears of the welcoming crowd. Australian superstar Kylie Minogue warmed the enthusiastic crowds with her sparkling performance, along with thousands of children who daubed paint on slabs in different colours according to a carefully planned routine. Professor Stephen Hawking sent a recorded message to all participants in the celebration of the

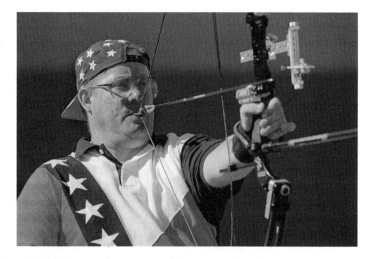

Figure 7.1   Sydney 2000 (photograph courtesy of Lieven Coudenys).

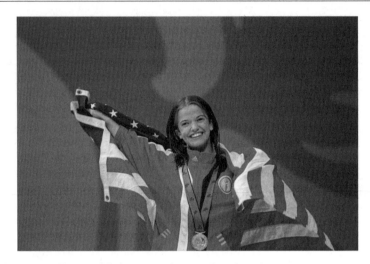

Figure 7.2   Sydney 2000 (photograph courtesy of Lieven Coudenys).

Paralympic Movement. He struck a note immediately shared by everyone at the Opening Ceremony when he talked of the 'fire in our hearts and our minds and our spirits'.

Athletes representing 122 countries (plus East Timor participating independently of Indonesia) took the number of delegations up from the 103 that attended the Atlanta 1996 Paralympic Games. The total number of competitors was 3824, with 2315 team officials and 804 technical officials. An army of 15 000 volunteers, long seen as the mainstay of the Paralympic Games, gave remarkable service throughout the Games, as well as in the many months of preparation. The number of nations participating at the Paralympic Games in Sydney was greater than the number of countries that entered competitors in the Olympic Games in 1972 in Munich.

Still quite difficult for unconnected spectators to understand was that the Paralympic Summer Games offered 561 gold medal events from 18 sports, while the Olympic Games only provided a total of 300 gold medal events from 28 sports. Of course the classification system was the answer, and the Sydney 2000 Paralympic Organising Committee produced excellent explanatory information to help visitors fully understand the spectacle they were witnessing. An advantage was that 14 of the 18 sports at the Sydney 2000 Paralympic Games were also common to the Olympic programme of sports, albeit with some specific modifications.

John Grant was able to boast honestly of having been in attendance at every Paralympic Games since the 1960 Rome Games. Grant had had extensive experience of dealing with the politics of international sport as a past President of the International Stoke Mandeville Wheelchair Sports Federation. The Sydney Paralympic Organising Committee benefited from the shared resources of the Olympic Games, but its own resolve and dedication were limitless. Lois Appleby, Chief Executive of SPOC, provided endless updates and responded to frequent requests for changes to already established arrangements with little show of frustration.

Stuart Devlin had designed the medals for the Paralympic Games, which depicted the Sydney Opera House and the Sydney Harbour Bridge. The reverse of the medal had the logos of the IPC and the Sydney 2000 Paralympic Games in relief. Controversially, the medals did not have any Braille lettering, as past medals have. This led to complaints from the IBSA representatives to the International Paralympic Committee. At all medal ceremonies, the medals would be carried on hand-made trays called coolomons – traditional Aboriginal artefacts, made at the Gavala Aboriginal Art and Cultural Education Centre in Sydney. While the gold and silver medals were being made from the expected

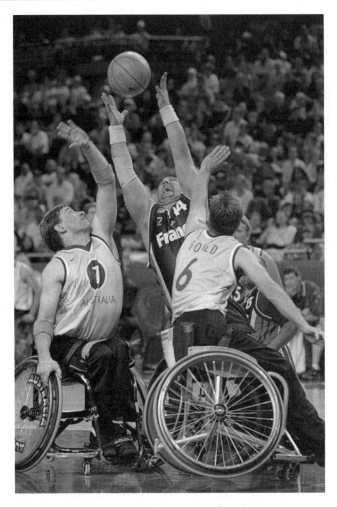

Figure 7.3   Sydney 2000 (photograph courtesy of Lieven Coudenys).

precious metals, the Australian Mint was busily melting down old 1 cent and 2 cent coins to make the bronze medals for the Paralympic Games!

Although the actual number of nations entering the Paralympic Games had been 128, seven countries had not arrived by the eve of the Opening Ceremony. Burkina Faso was late arriving, but Cameroon, Guatemala, Guinea, Niger, Sierre Leone, Sudan and Uganda had withdrawn.

Not all press reporting was favourable to the feats of athletes with a disability in Sydney. The *Sunday Independent*, a newspaper in Ireland, seriously insulted the competitors who had been participating in the Paralympic Games, calling the Games 'perverse' and 'grotesque'. In the column published on 22nd October, the newspaper suggested that the Paralympic Games bore no resemblance to serious sporting competition. Elite competition was not about a person who can: 'wobble his way around a track in a wheelchair, or can swim from one end of a pool to the other by braille'. The Editor of the *Sunday Independent* issued an apology for the distress caused by the article.

The recently completed Olympic Games had seen the superstar acclaim of Ian Thorpe (Australia) in the swimming events, and of Cathy Freeman (Australia) and Marion Jones (USA) on the track.

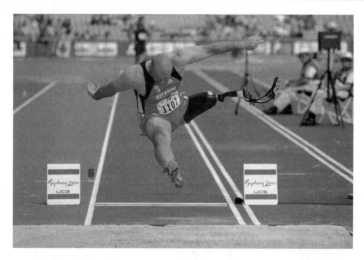

Figure 7.4   Sydney 2000 (photograph courtesy of Lieven Coudenys).

Lithuania gave a big fright to the USA's Basketball Dream Team, pushing them right to the wire before the Americans eventually took the honours. Once the Sydney 2000 Paralympic Games started in earnest, there were obviously going to be wholly parallel superstars identified as well. Canadian swimmer Jessica Sloan won six gold medals, establishing six world records at the same time. Another swimmer, Jason Wening (USA), proceeded to his third gold medal in successive Paralympic Games in the 400 m freestyle. He had not been beaten in this event since 1991. Experienced Paralympic athlete Tanni Grey-Thompson (UK) brought her phenomenal career to a peak with her victories in 100 m, 200 m, 400 m, and 800 m races. Louise Sauvage (Australia), reigning Laureus World Sportsperson of the Year with a Disability, beat the disappointment of a controversial collision in her 800 m track race, when Chantal Petitclerc went ahead of her to take the gold. Sauvage marked her place in the world of elite sport by winning the 1500 m race in style – with Petitclerc back in 5th place.

Wheelchair rugby proved to be the equivalent of the spectacle of ice sledge hockey of the Winter Paralympic Games. As a demonstration sport in Atlanta, Wheelchair rugby had sown its seeds as a potential crowd-pleaser. Now on the programme as a full-medal event, the gladiatorial determination of the players made this the most hard-fought of tournaments, with tickets as scarce as hens' teeth. In the final game, the USA defeated host nation Australia, 32 to 31.

Equestrian events had a particularly successful exposure in Sydney. The 72 competitors demonstrated outstanding poise and control, while competing at an elite level in demanding conditions. The equestrian competitions were the only ones to provide opportunities that catered strongly for women (75% of competitors) and athletes with a severe disability (45% of competitors). Franz Venhaus, The Sydney Paralympic Organising Committee's Equestrian Competition Manager, put together a highly professional facility, with excellent supporting staff and volunteers. The horses came from Riding for the Disabled Australia, with many of the owners attending the event as grooms.

Jim Thompson, Edinburgh-based Chairman of the International Boccia Commission, wrote of the Sydney Paralympic Games: 'The worldwide exposure that all sports received was unprecedented but for Boccia it was nothing short of miraculous. Spectator capacity was full every day; crowds were queuing to get into the venue, was this really Boccia?' There were five gold medals available in the competitions in Sydney, and they were all hard-fought. Thompson described the game of boccia as requiring: 'skill, accuracy, control and concentration'. Highs and lows of emotion were present throughout the competition as the spectators got behind favoured athletes to urge them on to victory.

Amalgamation of ISMWSF and ISOD at Sydney

The International Stoke Mandeville Wheelchair Sports Federation (ISMWSF) and the International Sports Organisation for the Disabled (ISOD) agreed at a joint General Assembly during the Sydney 2000 Paralympic Games that they would formally amalgamate – the completion took place in 2004. This brought together the representation of wheelchair, amputee, dwarf and 'les Autres' athletes in a single international federation. This was a very suitable union, especially as both organisations had been created as a result of the inspiration and direct action of Ludwig Guttmann more than 50 years before. An Interim Steering Commission would lead the joint body for six months, so that a suitable series of recommendations could be put before another General Assembly in mid-2001.

Sydney Closing Ceremony – a Big Party

Appropriately described by the Australian Broadcasting Corporation as 'informal, irreverent and one big party', the Closing Ceremony of the 11th Paralympic Summer Games was a true celebration of the hearty and wholesome enjoyment of the past 11 days. Over 100 000 revellers crammed into the Sydney Olympic Stadium for the colourful and noisy farewell. Bob Steadward, IPC President, declared the Sydney Paralympic Games to be 'the best ever'. Steadward spoke from the heart when he took the podium to bring events in the stadium to a close: 'It came as a sheer delight but no surprise that you excelled yourselves in hosting our Paralympic athletes to an absolutely outstanding event. Thank you, Australia, for enhancing the profile of our athletes, more than at any time in our history.' Compliments and encouragement were flowing that evening, as the Australian Governor-General, Sir William Deane, addressed the members of the Paralympic Family: 'You, the Year 2000 Paralympians, have particularly inspired us by your skill and commitment. These Games have brought the people of the world a little closer together and demonstrated that the things that unite mankind far outweigh the things that divide'. The inevitability of the progress of time saw the Paralympic flag handed over by Australian Minister for the Olympics and Paralympics, Michael Knight, to the deputy mayor of Athens, Nikos Yiatrakos.

Major Disgrace at Basketball for Athletes with Intellectual Disability

The Sydney 2000 Paralympic Games would not be able to avoid one further major upset: the allegation that members of the victorious Spanish basketball team for athletes with intellectual disability did not meet the eligibility criteria. After the Paralympic Games had ended, Carlos Ribagorda, a journalist with the financial journal *Capital*, made claims that were substantiated after some investigation. He alleged that a number of the Spanish players, including himself, did not qualify as having an intellectual disability, and therefore they had swindled the Paralympic Movement by competing fraudulently. The rules for minimum disability had to be applied differently for members of INAS-FID compared with other disabilities. The criteria for intellectual disability are that registered athletes must have a tested IQ of 70 or below, and have limitations in two or more adaptive skills such as communication, self-care, home living or functional academics. They must also have acquired their condition before the age of 18. Ribagorda claimed that he, and other Spanish athletes in Sydney, had never been assessed. As claims of more extensive duplicity reverberated around the sports world, the International Paralympic Committee established an investigative commission. The results of these inquiries would seriously mark the standing of sport for athletes with intellectual disability. The implications would tarnish the reputation of all athletes with intellectual disability, and would render them all ineligible for involvement in IPC competitions for a time to come.

CONCLUSION

The Sydney 2000 Paralympic Games had raised the Paralympic Movement to astounding levels of competition, administration and public awareness. Alongside the breathtaking spectacle and the energised athletic festivities, the Sydney 2000 Paralympics also saw controversies and upsets. These were entirely in keeping with the coming of age of a highly complex phenomenon; the meaning of Paralympic competition was now synonymous with the high stakes of all elite sport. With the immense growth and development of the IPC would come some new challenges that went hand in hand with the higher profile. As with other successful high-profile groups the IPC could be vulnerable to the political rivalry and tensions that can embroil organisations that are deserving of the level of attention it had acquired. In the same way, some of the athletes would deviously act in harmony with those Olympic athletes who chose to put their own health at risk in order to reach the ultimate goal: Paralympic Gold.

The next period in the history of the Paralympic Movement would have to address the 'fallout' from the Sydney 2000 Paralympic Games and the continuing work of establishing the long-term stability of the International Paralympic Committee.

CHAPTER 8

Sport is About Emotion: 2000 to 2004

OVERVIEW

Bringing an account of the Paralympic Movement up to the end of the Athens 2004 Paralympic Games is the purpose of this final chapter. In doing so we shall also try to project what lies ahead in sport for people with a disability, and for the International Paralympic Committee – now more than ever inextricably directing the Paralympic Movement.

Just as many of these themes have remained the same from year to year, the specific issues that command the greatest attention have shifted only slightly. The fiscal vigour of the International Paralympic Committee was greatly improved as the formal relationship with the International Olympic Committee was cemented in place. After disappointing results in the first marketing steps leading up to Sydney 2000, a greater confidence was evident as relative guarantees appeared to be reliable. There was to be a period of hardship, with pledges of support for the future rather than cash now, but with a very much more rosy future ahead.

The controversy of INAS-FID basketball players' disqualification in Sydney would lead to careful investigation of the claims and of the eligibility criteria employed by the international federation. There was a need for a reliable system of verification of intellectual disability before its impact on specific sports performance could be effectively evaluated. This subject was going to remain a thorny one.

Preparations for future Paralympic Games continued apace. The frequent meetings of the IPC Paralympic Games Liaison Committee and the organising committees would keep a finger on the pulse, and would give opportunities for attention to be drawn to areas that needed greater consideration on all sides. The procedures for bidding and selection of Olympic and Paralympic Games host cities were to become unified during this phase. The IPC had been invited to provide representation on the International Olympic Committee's commissions responsible for evaluating the various bids for Olympic and Paralympic Games.

In 2001, Kuala Lumpur would play host to the most important conference the International Paralympic Committee had organised in the period in question: anticipating the future of the Paralympic Movement through a decisive appraisal of the structures of the IPC. Part of the process would have to include critical review of how the organisation had arrived at the present point, as well as discussing where stakeholders believed the Paralympic Movement should be heading – then to find the mechanism for achieving these goals.

A new generation of officers of the International Paralympic Committee stepped up to the plate in 2001 – a 'changing of the guard' ready for the demands of new mandates and challenges. Their first actions

Athlete First: A History of the Paralympic Movement   Steve Bailey
© 2008 John Wiley & Sons, Ltd

were to promote an extensive search for the most appropriate structures of governance and management for the International Paralympic Committee in the years to come. There was acceptance of a need to address some issues immediately, but to take time and care to put long-term systems in place.

TOWARDS THE KUALA LUMPUR CONFERENCE

Not Just a 'Spanish Ulcer'

In the world of intellectual disability, the 'fallout' from the revelations of journalist Carlos Ribagorda was massive. He exposed his own scam, and the complicity of others, that a number of the Spanish basketball players had competed in Sydney without having an intellectual disability. The immediate response of the International Paralympic Committee was to announce its grave concern, and to begin to coordinate a meticulous investigation via a special commission. The Spanish Paralympic Committee was asked by the IPC to begin investigations into the allegations on 27th November 2000, and Bob Steadward met with its senior officials early in December to review progress. Following this visit to Madrid, the IPC President issued a press statement saying: 'It is our responsibility to all Paralympic athletes to provide fair competition. The IPC has taken a firm stand with regard to the doping offences that occurred during the Sydney 2000 Paralympic Games. It will take a similarly strong stance, if these allegations are proven to be correct.' The Spanish Government indicated its wish to be thorough in shedding light on the affair. Not long afterwards, the International Paralympic Committee announced that, due to the seriousness of the assertions, it would be setting up its own commission. The members of the IPC Investigation Commission were announced as:

- André Nöel Chaker, former Secretary General of ICSSPE and lawyer, specializing in sports legislation;
- Colin Rains, President of CP-ISRA;
- Thomas Reinecke, IPC Chief Operating Officer;
- Donald Royer, IPC Legal Committee;
- Lutz Worms, sports physician.

When this group lodged its first report on 27th January 2001, it was decided that immediate suspension from the International Paralympic Committee of the International Sports Organisation for Athletes with an Intellectual Disability (INAS-FID) was essential. INAS-FID President, Fernando Martin Vicente, was also suspended from the IPC Executive Committee. There had long been concern about the integrity of the systems of eligibility verification for athletes with intellectual disabilities, expressed even by those responsible for classification and registration of these athletes; but the essence of sporting endeavour had to include the philosophy of fair competition, and the IPC needed to stamp its mark of resolve in dealing with fraudulent behaviour – whether through doping or cheating by other means.

As more details were released of the content of the investigations, it became clear that 10 of the 12 members of the Spanish basketball team had not met the minimum disability standards set out for athletes with intellectual disability.

On 7th February, Bob Steadward released an open letter about the suspension of INAS-FID. He stressed that the action was preliminary: 'pending the conclusions and final report of the IPC Investigation Commission'. This report was due to be put before the IPC Executive Committee on 9th March 2001. When the report was published there was an even greater shock: it was discovered that over two-thirds of the registration forms for intellectually disabled athletes competing at the Sydney 2000 Paralympic Games were invalid for one reason or another. This did not mean to imply that two-thirds of the athletes had been wrongly assessed or had knowingly committed fraud, but that the eligibility verification form had been significantly mismanaged and administered both on a national and international level. The Investigation Commission was careful to point out that the mechanism for approving registrations was at fault, leading to the possibility that bogus athletes could have been admitted as eligible. Donald Royer commented: 'This is a dramatic and global problem, which cannot be reduced to only one national team or to one specific sport'. The IPC President had to demonstrate a strong and tough line: 'The participation of ineligible athletes at the Paralympic Games must never happen again. The IPC Executive Committee asks the INAS-FID membership to review their eligibility criteria and processes.' Although it was thought possible, at first, to provide a system of provisional certification for athletes with intellectual disability, enabling them to compete in planned events, their inclusion in Paralympic Games would still have to be confirmed later. The negative publicity generated was enormous, and led to an inevitable oversimplification of the issues involved.

Athens 2004 Paralympic Games Contract

There were issues worrying the IPC members as they headed towards a firm agreement with the Athens Organising Committee, ATHOC. In particular, the IPC wanted to watch closely to ensure that the Greek authorities addressed the provision of suitable access for people with a disability. The contract for the Athens 2004 Paralympic Games was signed on 5th April 2001. In a characteristically upbeat and optimistic statement, Bob Steadward looked forward to the challenges ahead:

> This contract is an important step towards the success of the next Paralympic Summer Games. We have experienced some delays, so the signing of this contract is a happy occasion for all our athletes. With only three years remaining, ATHOC has a great deal of preparation and challenge ahead. The IPC is confident that the Paralympic Summer Games in Athens will be a tremendous success. We are enjoying an excellent relationship with the Organising Committee.

The closer relationship between the IOC and the IPC had led to the Athens 2004 Paralympic Games organisers scrapping the entry fee for Paralympic athletes for the first time. As with the Salt Lake 2002 Paralympic Winter Games, an integrated organising committee would plan and run both the Olympic and the Paralympic Games.

Split from WeMedia

When the IPC had signed the Memorandum of Understanding with WeMedia in October 2000, the hope was that all media delivery arrangements and secure income would accrue from this one relationship. But when Thomas Reinecke, Chief Operating Officer, reported to the IPC Executive Committee in Salt Lake City in March 2001, things were described as being at a critical stage. IPC had not received the first agreed instalment and began to take responsible action to protect future broadcasting arrangements. By the time the Executive met prior to the General Assembly in Athens in December 2001, the IPC had taken back control of all broadcasting rights from WeMedia, and appropriate correspondence was agreed in order to initiate dealings to recover lost revenue from the company. There was great disappointment that the very promising proposals of WeMedia were obviously not going to bear fruit – the timing overlapped with the decline in growth in Internet-reliant companies. Subsequently, in 2002, the IPC contracted out to International Sports Broadcasting (ISB) to become the host broadcaster for the Athens 2004 Paralympic Games. ISB's extensive experience included acting as host broadcaster for the Sydney 2000 Olympic Games. Its role was to distribute to national and international broadcasters comprehensive audio and video feeds of all main events, together with live feeds from certain venues and daily summaries.

Steadward to be Conferred with Title of Honorary President

As the elections for new officers of the IPC approached, attention turned to the best possible ways of continuing to benefit from the vast experience and relationships of Bob Steadward. At the completion of his period of office, Steadward would have held the highest office for twelve years, through thorny as well as exhilarating times. But the nature of such a position had generated a vast amount of goodwill and personal contacts that would be hard to replace immediately. François Terranova took a suggestion to the Management Committee that some sort of senior position should be created for Bob Steadward, particularly aimed at permitting him to represent the IPC as an IOC member. In order to allow discussion of this in detail at the March 2001 Executive Committee meeting in Salt Lake City, Steadward handed over the Chair to York Chow and left the meeting. The relationship with the International Olympic Committee was seen as the primary basis for IPC's future well being, and the IPC Executive Committee needed to ensure that it kept a presence in the IOC's 'inner circle'. It was feared that, as Steadward retired as IPC President, the incoming IPC President might not be elected to membership of the International Olympic Committee, even if nominated. Throughout the discussions about the appointment of Steadward to the role of Honorary President, only sparing mention was made of any wish to honour the long-serving President; this was much more a practical matter of the survival and prosperity of the International Paralympic Committee.

The Cooperation Agreement in place between the IOC and the IPC stated that the IPC President would be co-opted on to the IOC, but there was a lack of clarity over the actual meaning of this, as there was no facility for this within the IOC at present. There was soon also to be a new President of the International Olympic Committee, and any personal agenda of Juan Antonio Samaranch would not necessarily be continued with the same verve by his successor. In fact there was no cause for alarm as the IOC did later ensure that the representation was connected to the IPC President's position rather than being dependent upon election as an individual member of the IOC. But this would only be after the new IPC President had come to office, and required a change of procedures within the IOC itself. However, in the interim, York Chow worded a motion:

> That the Executive Committee propose the General Assembly of IPC to award Dr Robert Steadward the status of Honorary President of the IPC. He shall chair a new IOC Liaison Commission of the IPC and continue to represent IPC in future liaison with the IOC. The Chairman of the IOC Liaison Commission will be co-opted as a member of the Executive Committee of IPC and his role will be reviewed by the Executive Committee after a four year period.

This motion was carried. However, later in the same meeting the subject was revisited. There was a feeling of discomfort at how the IOC might react to a commission being set up without its consultation. An amended motion was carried unanimously, removing reference to any commission, but keeping Steadward in a position of Honorary President, as liaison with the IOC and in a 'senior Executive position within the IPC'. The General Assembly would need to decide this matter because it required a constitutional change. The Legal Committee would examine the most appropriate clarification to give to the General Assembly, including recommendations for voting rights and tenure.

During Bob Steadward's years in office he had proved himself to be an outstanding diplomat. As was natural, the President of the IPC was not able to keep everyone happy, however. There was a building concern that as the time came for a change of President, Bob Steadward's personality, so valued as the means by which some doors were opened in earlier days, could overshadow the truly professional outlook and proven teamwork that was now the driving force behind the IPC. Steadward had also held a consistent view that the International organisations of sport for people with a disability (IOSDs) should be moved to a more subsidiary role on the fringe of IPC's operation; this created understandable tensions. The disability sports organisations had brought the Paralympic Movement to life, and felt strongly that they should not be sidelined – they should be fundamental in decision making.

A number of alternative views had developed by the time the Executive Committee met in Kuala Lumpur, after the Strategic Planning Congress at the end of April 2001. The specific change to the constitution was put forward that would create a position of Honorary President. The personal nature of this position relating to Bob Steadward was replaced by a more general appointment for the immediate past President of IPC to become the Honorary President. The term was fixed at four years, with full voting rights on the Executive Committee.

Sport Science Committee Renamed

Michael Riding reported to the Executive Committee in March 2001 that the Sports Science and Medical Department of IPC recommended securing rights to the intellectual property of the VISTA Conference as the official property of the International Paralympic Committee, although there was agreement this would not be achieved until a later date. Details of the operational arrangements for the VISTA series were consolidated, with a bidding procedure formalised, a regular cycle established, and distribution of proceedings regularised. The Sport Science Committee was renamed the IPC Sport Science, Research and Education Committee at this meeting. Another important step for IPC was to apply to the International Council of Sport Science and Physical Education (ICSSPE) for membership of the 'Associations Board'. IPC had joined ICSSPE in 1996, when Bob Steadward had attended the ICSSPE meetings in Dallas in conjunction with the Pre-Olympic Scientific Congress. Gudrun Doll-Tepper, President of ICSSPE, had been involved in many aspects of IPC work, as well as having been President of the International Federation of Adapted Physical Activity (IFAPA). The link between the International Paralympic Committee and the International Council of Sport Science and Physical Education has proven to be a very fruitful one, and this relationship continues today.

Executive Committee Decide on INAS-FID

The report of the Investigation Commission was discussed in detail at the IPC Executive Committee meeting in March 2001. Owing to the sensitivity of the subject, no record was made for the minutes, and copies of the report were collected in at the end of the debate. Five motions were passed relating to the situation of athletes with intellectual disability. The first stressed that the investigation had 'proven beyond doubt that the process of assessment, verification and certification of intellectually disabled athletes was not carried out, supervised or audited'. Further, specific blame was apportioned to Fernando Martin Vicente and Felipe Gutiérrez Garcia, as President and Technical Officer of INAS-FID respectively. The motion also expelled them from the IPC immediately, as they were judged to be 'primarily responsible for this serious violation'.

The second motion demanded that INAS-FID review its eligibility criteria and process. It would have to prove, to the full satisfaction of the IPC, that it had put in place clear mechanisms for defining eligibility, for accrediting assessors and for accurately documenting the procedures. As for the previous motion, the IPC Executive Committee passed this unanimously. Next the IPC turned to the National Paralympic Committees. These were asked to review the status of all athletes who submitted inaccurate or invalid documentation to the Sydney 2000 Paralympic Games. The nations were to follow the

Spanish model of an independent investigation committee, and were to produce results for the IPC Investigation Commission within three months (not later than 31st May 2001). Medals won by these athletes had to be returned to IPC via their National Paralympic Committee.

INAS-FID was required to admit its 'responsibility and accountability' in these matters, and IPC insisted that it had to set right the policies and leadership at the first opportunity – the INAS-FID General Assembly in April 2001. In an unusual move, the IPC Executive Committee voted unanimously that INAS-FID had to expel those of its own Executive Committee members who had voted in support of Fernando Martin Vicente at the last INAS-FID Executive Committee meeting. There was to be some criticism that this standpoint of the IPC Executive Committee was heavy handed, and could be viewed as an intrusion in the internal operation of an autonomous international federation. But, in the view of the IPC, the credibility of the Paralympic Movement had been put at risk by the action or inaction of INAS-FID, and the IPC Executive believed this to be appropriate conduct.

The last motion of the IPC Executive Committee at the March meeting emphasised that INAS-FID was to remain suspended from IPC membership until it had resolved the policy and political issues. It could put its new policies and results of its investigations before the IPC at any time for consideration. As a show of respect to the athletes themselves, the IPC agreed to allow provisional recognition of suitably defined athletes, subject to verification by a new eligibility committee appointed jointly by IPC and INAS-FID. Events could also be planned for the future, including the 2002 Paralympic Winter Games in Salt Lake City.

Management of information was to be sensitively done; National Paralympic Committees would receive summaries of the investigation report and the Executive Committee's motions, but the Press was only to receive the resolutions themselves.

Kuala Lumpur IPC Strategic Planning Congress, April 2001

The future path of the International Paralympic Committee was under review in Malaysia when the Strategic Planning Congress opened on 26th April 2001. These meetings brought together more than 250 delegates from 77 countries, hosted by the Malaysian Paralympic Council, with support from the Ministry of National Unity and Social Development and the Ministry of Youth and Sports Malaysia. Bob Steadward spoke in a media release of the progress that had been gained as a result of the successes of the Sydney 2000 Paralympic Games, not only with regard to the numbers of athletes and the quality of the sport, but also with the intense media interest: 'The IPC has to ensure that this positive development will continue in the future. A lot of effort is needed to offer the top athletes of the world with a disability the opportunity to compete in first-class competitions under the same conditions as non-disabled elite athletes.'

At the Opening Ceremony of the Congress, Bob Steadward offered the assembled delegates three pieces of advice that he hoped might help them. Firstly, he advised them to preserve the 'unity of governance' that keeps everyone together. This was also a warning to put aside the overprotection of personal constituencies: 'Make no mistake, domination of one faction over another, sharpened by personal agendas, will gradually result in the absolute power of the individual. Sooner or later this will lead to total destruction.' Secondly Steadward asked the Congress to 'observe and cultivate good faith, peace and harmony towards all nations'. Steadward urged the International Paralympic Committee towards greater effort on developing nations: 'solidarity, support, and encouragement and opportunity'. Finally he urged them to 'maintain a vision and continue to look forward'.

Steadward pointed to the great progress of the Paralympic Movement in terms of milestones: the International Coordinating Committee; the Arnhem Seminar in 1987; the establishment of the International Paralympic Committee in Düsseldorf in September 1989; the 1995 Tokyo Congress and the Task Force's work. The most tangible achievements were to be seen in Paralympic Games in Tignes Albertville, Barcelona, Lillehammer, Atlanta, Nagano and Sydney. Steadward's important introductory comments highlighted the achievements of the past 12 years, but also pointed out the challenges the IPC had faced, and were still facing:

- drugs: powerlifting in particular, World Anti-Doping Agency relations;
- INAS-FID: ethics, values, principles, reputation, credibility;
- marketing and television: WeMedia;
- classification: reduction in events, functional;
- new sports and programme changes.

The IPC President posed questions that needed to be considered in Kuala Lumpur. Some of these had been raised in the context of the Task Force's investigations: should the IPC be responsible solely for the organisation of the Paralympic Winter and Summer Games, or also for regional and world championships? Should the roles and functions of the elected officers of the International Paralympic Committee be changed in the light of the establishment of a professional staff and a permanent headquarters? Should the nature and composition of the Executive Committee and other bodies within the IPC be reassessed? Steadward quoted Charles Du Bos' adage about determination and sacrifice: 'The important thing is: to be able at any moment to sacrifice what we are for what we could become'.

The Congress agreed certain essential 'guiding principles'. York Chow provided a thorough summary of the ideas on governance of the IPC: the General Assembly was described as 'having ownership'. This intended to affirm the General Assembly's primacy in all matters. Governance and management needed to ensure a working interface; the new, professional administration had to mesh seamlessly with the political strata of the International Paralympic Committee. It was seen as inevitable and desirable that the power and authority of the IPC was actually spread out in the organisation. There was a consistent call for transparency in management and effectiveness in communication, reflecting the democratic nature of the organisation. The Executive Board – that would eventually replace the Executive Committee – needed to have balance in its representation. In supporting the National Paralympic Committees, the IPC would have to ensure that all athletes were catered for, in both developed and developing countries. There was a repeat of the same discontent between the two factions in the Paralympic Movement: international federations wished to retain their direct involvement in all matters, while the National Paralympic Committees, and thereby the member nations, wished to have a single organisation to deal with – and subscribe to.

When the Task Force had gathered views in 1995 and 1996, the nations had expressed themselves forcefully and with passion. It is not surprising that many of the same issues and proposed solutions emerged from the Planning Congress. This time it was within a more reasonable timeframe, and the call for change would be confirmed without there being a correlating knee-jerk wish to change everything overnight. The discussion on governance led to significant statements of consensus:

- that eventually the IPC would be responsible solely for the Paralympic Games;
- that the future of the original disability sports organisations (IOSDs) was still a controversial subject, but that they should be focused on development;
- that the sports would be nurtured towards independence, but through close integration and partnership with the international federations for sports;
- that there should be a concept of partnership and synergy – the phrase 'no-one leaves the IPC' was endorsed;

- the organisation must serve the needs of all members, watchful of the widening gap between developed and developing countries;
- the IPC must cater for elite sports but also promote sports for people with disabilities more generally;
- the representation of the regions was emphasised, noting that there would be a tendency for increased numbers of athletes to come from developing countries as progress was made;
- that the IPC has a role and responsibility to assist the relationship between the National Paralympic Committees and the National Olympic Committees, as well as assisting the sports to cooperate with the international federations.

Above all the International Paralympic Committee must 'provide the united forum for the Paralympic Movement'.

While examining the roles and responsibilities of the different units within the IPC, the Congress provided clear direction for the future. Gudrun Doll-Tepper, ICSSPE President, chaired the group that made very practical suggestions for the future. The need for change arose from alterations in the fundamental nature of the Paralympic Movement and the needs of the membership, including: the rapid expansion of numbers of member nations and athletes; a greater number of disability groups and an increased number of sports; a closer connection between the IPC and the IOC; the establishment and development of National Paralympic Committees; and the existence of a professional headquarters-based administration. The recommendations of her panel would form an important part of the strategic planning (Box 8.1).

Box 8.1 Recommendations of the working group

Recommendations:

I. Athletes should play a greater role within the governance of the IPC and its members (in principle and practice).
  - Development of platforms and forums for athlete feedback and policy development (e.g. IPC Athletes' Congress).
  - That the IPC's policies should reflect athlete representation throughout the organisation (i.e. NPC, Regions, Sports, IPC, and new Commissions).
  - The IPC must adequately fund the IPC Athletes' Committee and related initiatives to ensure the achievement of an athlete centred organisation.
  - Development of a Paralympic Athlete Hall of Fame network to assist in the athlete retirement process and create athlete network structure.
  - Involve more retired athletes in the classification development and assessment process on national and international levels
  - The awareness, education, and participation of athletes on the governance of the IPC must be a fundamental principle and practice.
II. The IPC should draft a strategic plan to be endorsed by the General Assembly:
  - This plan should be based on a strategic review and on consultation with all constituencies with a sense of urgency and focus on results.
  - Two-way communication between the IPC and the NPCs and regions is vital for the future success of the movement.
  - The plan should take into consideration the different structures and stages of development that the NPCs are at.
III. There is a need for examination and redefinition of the roles and responsibilities of the IOSDs within the IPC.

IV. The IPC and the NPCs should increase their commitment to regional development:
   ▪ Focus shall be put on narrowing the gap among countries and regions in terms of athletes' participation, competition opportunities and input to governance.
   ▪ Knowledge transfer in terms of classification, coaching and general information to less developed countries shall be boosted.
V. The Sports shall have stronger representation in the IPC:
   ▪ Full membership of the sports in the IPC is considered necessary.
   ▪ Sports decision-making structures need to be reviewed and clarified.
   ▪ The Sports shall pursue individual paths towards their future structure according to their specific situation/IFs.
VI. Improvement of the financial situation of the IPC
   ▪ The Paralympic Solidarity programme needs to be expanded to meet the needs of the developing nations.
   ▪ Marketing strategy needs to be developed and implemented (urgent matter).
VII. The IPC should define its relationship to the IOC, the International Sports Federations and other external partners, including definition of roles and responsibilities.

Structural change was discussed in the section chaired by Garry Wheeler, host of the Congress. They looked at the rationale behind structural change (to improve communication, credibility and transparency, and to counteract a 'top heavy' organisational structure), and the necessary elements that contribute to successful change (consensus, commitment, unity, shared vision). In addition to the growth of sport opportunities for athletes with a disability, the International Paralympic Committee had to respond to significant shifts in sports governance more widely. The closing comments of the summary paper from Wheeler's group were very matter of fact: 'Change will be difficult. Change will take time. Change must be planned. Courage is required to make changes which contribute to the greater good of the organization.'

The productivity of the Strategic Planning Congress was prodigious. In the reporting process, the concise summations do not adequately echo the passion and enthusiasm of the discussions, although they are accurate in their communication of the process. York Chow, the Congress Chairman, reported his conclusions at the end of the discussions. He recorded the agreed vision and mission statements, as well as identifying the core values that the Congress had reviewed.

• The vision of the International Paralympic Committee (IPC) is to be indisputably recognised as one of the most successful and influential sports organisations in the world; to gain international respect and reputation as a major advocate for the promotion of the rights, recognition and equality of athletes with a disability throughout the world; and to meet the needs of those athletes as they pursue and achieve excellence in sport.
• The mission of the International Paralympic Committee (IPC) is to serve our worldwide community of athletes with a disability though the creation, development and promotion of sport opportunities. The Mission is to be served through participation at Paralympic Games, multi-disability world and regional championships, and through the provision of administrative support services including but not limited to marketing strategies, development, communication networks and the like.

Core values were agreed to be: sport for all; democratic, open and participative organisation; athletes-centred; teamwork and leadership integrity; respect and trust; quality of life. Chow also listed the major concerns of the delegates at the Planning Congress. Although the list could appear to be superficial in some ways, it reflected the caring nature of the gathered representatives. A new vocabulary was being employed that aligned itself with political correctness and modernity: open, direct communication; empathy; opportunity; optimism; unity – sharing and caring; extremes of development in NPCs; athletes' inclusion; regional structure and leadership; sports infrastructure; global positioning.

The IPC President wrote to the membership only a few days after the Strategic Planning Congress closed. He professed to want to convey his personal insights on the process they were engaged in. At some length – a ten page letter – Steadward outlined most of the recommendations of the Congress. A letter such as that sent by Steadward to members of the IPC marks how personal his leadership was – but it also suggests an eye to the legacy he knew he would be judged by. He emphasised how much of the Strategic Planning Congress actually mirrored the work of the Task Force some years earlier. But the Task Force had reached its conclusions within a more pressured time frame, and with the employment of less overtly democratic methods. In Steadward's letter, he stressed the changes that really needed to be made immediately, and those which could stand further consideration. He also laid strong emphasis on the relationship between the IPC and the IOC. The involvement of IPC representatives on 13 IOC Commissions was reinforced.

The IPC now had representation in a wide range of areas of the IOC:

- Carol Mushett   Commissions for Culture and Olympic Education
- Kjartan Haugen   Athletes' Commission
- Beatrice Hess   Women in Sport Commission
- Michael Riding   Medical Commission
- Nabil Salem   Press Commission
- York Chow   Radio and Television Commission
- Jens Bromann   Sport and Law Commission
- Bob Steadward   Sport and Environment Commission
- André Auberger   Sport for All Commission
- Thomas Reinecke   2002 Coordination Commission for Olympic Games
- Miguel Sagarra   2004 Coordination Commission for Olympic Games
- François Terranova   2006 Coordination Commission for Olympic Games
- Bob McCullough   Evaluation Commission for the Games of the XXIX Olympiad (2008)

Steadward had been invited to participate n the IOC Olympic Truce Foundation. The International Paralympic Committee had also created four of its own commissions: Women in Sport; Development; Athletes with Severe Disabilities; and Ethics.

Update on INAS-FID in Kuala Lumpur

Thomas Reinecke and José Luis Campo had represented the IPC at the General Assembly of INAS-FID in Mexico on 3rd April 2001. They reported back to the IPC Executive Committee on the meetings, and they also gave their impressions of the organisation more broadly. It was felt that there was a lack of structure to INAS-FID, and proven organisational competence was still absent. There was even some question over its lawful character because allegedly INAS-FID was not legally registered any-where. Unfortunately for IPC, the motion to suspend INAS-FID from membership and the motion to permit 'provisional recognition' of athletes to compete in sanctioned IPC events were judged to be contradictory. The IPC Legal Committee urged the establishment of consistency: either to suspend INAS-FID and prohibit its athletes from competing or to lift suspension altogether. The IPC constitution did not provide for the athletes of a suspended organisation to participate in any IPC events.

Although it was the National Paralympic Committees of the respective athletes that were entering them, it was INAS-FID that was supposed to be regulating eligibility – as its equivalent to the classification system of athletes with other disabilities. No eligibility committee had yet been set up, and the Salt Lake 2002 Paralympic Winter Games were very close at hand.

Jos Mulder had been elected as the new President of INAS-FID, and reports were stressing that he was making strenuous efforts to rebuild and take forward the structures of the organisation. Although Mulder was clearly moving along with as much vigour as he could possibly manage, Bob Steadward described INAS-FID as: 'a fragile and wounded organization which needed assistance from the (Paralympic) Movement'. An air of negativity was associated with the whole issue of eligibility for athletes with intellectual disability, and this was a problem that IPC had to deal with urgently. Even with Hans Lindström's urging of the IPC Executive Committee to hold fast with the resolutions passed at the previous meeting, they voted to remove the part that would have allowed athletes to be provisionally recognised for competition. Bob Steadward made it absolutely clear that provisional recognition was not appropriate at that moment, without greater assurances in place and a more secure organisational configuration. In saying this he also asserted that IPC wished to protect the interests of legitimate athletes with intellectual disability, while ensuring that the Paralympic Movement was not further discredited.

LOOKING FORWARD TO ATHENS

Agreement Signed with the International Olympic Committee, June 2001

On 19th June 2001 Bob Steadward and Juan Antonio Samaranch signed a groundbreaking Agreement on the Organization of the Paralympic Games. The purpose of the Agreement was to overtly bond the organisation of the Olympic Games and the Paralympic Games in the eyes of the organising committees and the public, for the 2008 and 2010 Games. The Agreement was a continuation of the progress made to apply similar principles to both the Olympic and Paralympic Games organisations. Samaranch made a statement emphasising the organisational and fiscal integrity offered by linking the IOC and IPC in the Games: 'Today is an important day for the Olympic Movement. This Agreement is the result of many years of close relationship between the IOC and the IPC. Its aim is to secure the organization of the Paralympic Games with full integration of both organising committees and financial guarantee.' This Agreement was complementary to the document signed by the same two parties in October 2000. There had been a growing range of cooperative activities since the Sydney agreement, including meetings and visits specifically relating to Paralympic Games organisation, but also extending to joint activities affecting various populations of the sporting world.

IPC and the World Anti-Doping Agency

In July 2001 IPC announced that the World Anti-Doping Agency (WADA) was to be present as an observer at the Salt Lake 2002 Paralympic Winter Games. This was to assist the IPC in the development of a versatile and meticulous doping control programme. The two organisations signed an accord that would bring them together to combat the illicit use of drugs. The agreement was more of a symbolic gesture at this stage, because the International Paralympic Committee could not have maintained credibility for long without publicly demonstrating that it was serious about the eradication of doping in sport. It needed to sign up to WADA's ethos in order to retain credibility. Dick Pound, now Chairman of WADA, strongly endorsed the participation of the Paralympic Movement, saying that WADA's focus had been in the Olympic sports arena until now: 'Unfortunately, the threat of doping exists throughout sport, and Paralympic athletes deserve the same protection from dope cheats as do all other athletes'. As part of its involvement, the IPC would be able to participate in the evolution of a 'WADA anti-doping code'. In addition to establishing doping control testing both in and out of competition, an education programme was to be launched, aimed at every level of sport for athletes with a disability. Bob Steadward pronounced the benefits to IPC of the formal relationship with the World Anti-Doping Agency: 'Our cooperation with WADA will be a great asset for the IPC's anti-doping efforts. It is our target to keep future Paralympic Games doping-free'.

Unity, Tolerance and Respect, Athens, December 2001

The last few meetings for Bob Steadward as President of the International Paralympic Committee were held in Athens in December 2001. When the Executive Committee met, the relationship with the International Olympic Committee was an early agenda item. A November meeting between IPC and IOC had concentrated on the implementation of the third part of the agreement on marketing and broadcasting. At that time the IOC was in the process of creating its own solution for host broadcasting that would eventually become Olympic Broadcasting Services (OBS). The 2001 IPC–IOC Agreement included the principle that the Olympic broadcaster would also be the Paralympic broadcaster.

The promising adventure with WeMedia had not worked out, as reported earlier. The company just did not have the robustness to warrant any legal recourse by IPC to recover lost revenue. The IPC President was able to reassure the members of the Executive Committee that the relationship between IPC and WeMedia was entirely over.

Thomas Reinecke informed the delegates that a Marketing Manager, Andreas Schönemann, had been recruited from 1st January 2001. Bob McCullough also suggested that the Marketing Task Force should be resurrected to help provide direction for the new member of staff.

When Bob Steadward delivered his final Presidential Address, he urged the members of the International Paralympic Committee to acknowledge three 'pillars' on which the success of the Paralympic Movement should be based: 'Unity, tolerance and respect'. He took the General Assembly through a brief history of the Paralympic Movement. Steadward had been active at every stage of the emergence of the International Paralympic Committee over the past 12 years, and had shared such a strong personal investment in the success of the organisation. He outlined the most urgent business of the IPC in the near future (Box 8.2).

Box 8.2 Future IPC business

- Protect the added value of the Paralympic Games
- Work towards universality
- Solidarity:
  - All nations
  - All sports
  - All disabilities
- Women – participation
- Severe disability – opportunities
- Development
- Preserve credibility of the Games:
  - Doping in sport
  - Ethics – cheating
  - Litigation – Court of Arbitration for Sport (CAS)

- Independence and autonomy of sport
- Classification
- Bridging the gap
  - IOSDs
  - Sport Committees
  - Nations
  - Regions
- Marketing
  - Benefiting the Games
  - Athletes
  - NPCs.

A Lively General Assembly in Athens, December 2001

The IPC General Assembly met on 7th December 2001, with representatives of 75 nations; 5 IOSDs and 22 sports were in attendance. The new members were welcomed: Andorra, Central African Republic, Chad, Gabon, Gambia, Laos, Lesotho, Mauritania, Mongolia, Rwanda and Uzbekistan.

When York Chow reported back to the membership on the follow-up to the Strategic Planning Congress earlier in 2001, he was able to tell them that he had received responses from 56 countries to the questionnaire on specific questions arising. Detailed analysis could now take place, leading to the development of significant proposals for the future direction of IPC.

Marketing came under fire again in the General Assembly. There was a broadly expressed discontent with the ineffective direction of the IPC's marketing policies. When Nabil Salem gave his report on marketing and communication, focusing on host broadcasting and television rights, along with the negotiations for a marketing agreement, the delegate from the Netherlands read out a strongly worded statement:

> It turns out that within the Executive Committee no coordinated approach to the marketing and sponsorship problem has taken place. We don't approve of this. It is according to our opinion of the highest importance and necessity that the new Management and Executive Committee approach this kind of problem in a coordinated and structured way.

The statement went on to be critical of the move towards total reliance on the International Olympic Committee, believing that the IPC was in a 'weak negotiating position'. These were not unreasonable concerns. The International Paralympic Committee had so far found it difficult to translate the success of the Sydney 2000 Paralympic Games into long-term marketing strategies and relationships. The IPC had to begin to succeed in this essential sphere in order to guarantee its security.

Thomas Reinecke added to his written report, describing the negotiations with the IOC on marketing and media rights. He explained that the Paralympic Games were to be 'covered by the Olympic Broadcasting Corporation from 2008 or 2010 on, whereby the Olympic broadcaster would provide a live feed and signal similar to the services provided in Sydney. There would be a share of revenue from the rights sale.' Reinecke added that the marketing negotiations were more complex and they were in the initial stages of discussions.

When André Auberger presented his report on the finances of the International Paralympic Committee, there was another critical pronouncement from the Netherlands. This emphasised that the IPC was entering a difficult phase in its budget; the projections did not give confidence in the financial security of the organisation. Until the benefits from agreements with the IOC kicked in, IPC would need to be watchful in its housekeeping.

The relationship with the International Olympic Committee also gave impetus to the strategic initiatives reported by Carol Mushett, IPC Technical Officer. She listed the areas under review:

- re-evaluation of the IPC Handbook criteria for programme evaluation (due to limitations in number of sports, disciplines and events);
- reduction in the number of events for the Summer Paralympic Games;
- review of the number of disability classes for each sport;
- review of current structuring of sports, including relationships with international federations recognised by IOC;
- development of formal agreements between IPC and each sport;
- development of National Technical Officials;
- limitation of 4000 Summer Paralympic athletes and 800 Winter Paralympic athletes, resulting from firm sport-specific quotas;
- review of the team delegation quota formula;
- review of the Paralympic programme, including events, sport allocations and qualification processes, in order to balance the programme. 'That balance must reflect our athletes' diversity, which includes gender, disability and region.'

Voting on INAS-FID Suspension at Athens General Assembly

The General Assembly needed to vote on the ratification of the suspension of INAS-FID. The Executive Committee had amended the wording slightly since the motion had been sent out, and agreed:

> The suspension of INAS-FID by IPC will be lifted provided that INAS-FID specifically acknowledge and accept the following:
>
> 1. That the IPC Protest Procedures for Classification and Eligibility that are applied universally at the Paralympic Games and IPC Championships shall include athletes with intellectual disability.
> 2. The IPC Handbook including:
>   – Item 2.1, Chapter 5, Section II. A competitor who cannot participate on reasonably equal terms in a sport for 'able-bodied' because of a functional disadvantage due to a permanent disability is eligible for that sport within the IPC Programme
>   – Item 2.2, Chapter 5, Section II. The minimum handicap is determined in and by each sport depending on functional factors
>   – Item 1.1, Chapter 5, Section II. Sport specific functional classes and classification rules are described under the specific rules respectively. Amendments of the classification rules by the Sports Assemblies.
>
> In the cases of the forthcoming Salt Lake 2002 Paralympic Winter Games and 2002 World Championships in which the event programmes, schedules and standards have been established and distributed, the inclusion of ID athletes will not be possible.

This motion was carried with 79 voting in favour, 12 against, and five abstentions. Bob Steadward took time to thank Jos Mulder for his efforts in helping to resolve the difficulties, and during a subsequent break in the proceedings, the President of INAS-FID signed an agreement accepting the motion as passed by the IPC General Assembly.

In reality INAS-FID had little choice: refusal to sign would have excluded it from any meeting table in the future. The benefits to INAS-FID were imperceptible for the time being.

New President: a 'Team Player'

When the General Assembly discussed and voted on the appointment of the outgoing President as Honorary President of IPC, Bob Steadward handed over the Chair to York Chow. There was clearly not universal acceptance of the concept, but the vote went in favour of Steadward being 'conferred the title of Honorary President of the IPC, his roles and responsibilities will be determined by the IPC President and Executive Committee'. The General Assembly voted with 58 in favour, 37 opposed and two abstentions.

The General Assembly pushed the more mundane business to one side in order to carry out the elections that would bring a new regime into being. Bob Steadward had completed three terms in office, acting as midwife at the birth of IPC and nurturing the infancy of the organisation. A new President would be in his seat before delegates left Athens. A true appraisal of the impact of Steadward on the progress of the Paralympic Movement is always going to be emotive and unscientific. Without doubt, the first President of IPC did foster the organisation through growing pains, maintaining a diplomatic stance in the presence of the factionalism that still caused tensions. Dedication and sacrifice would be associated with Bob Steadward's ambition, but also a focus on the International Olympic Committee that some saw as narrow. Steadward's strong drive had upset people along the way, and his principles served to make the IOSDs feel marginalised. It is likely that he would have welcomed the opportunity to take the Presidency through for another term. His own elevation to IOC member was a diverting honour, until the benefits of this formal recognition could be returned to become an advantage for the International Paralympic Committee as a result. Without the cultivation of a personal affiliation between Bob Steadward and Juan Antonio Samaranch, who was a sincere promoter of the Paralympic Movement, it is possible that the IPC would still be struggling to see clearly into the future.

The nominees for the IPC Presidency were Phil Craven, Bob McCullough, Hans Lindström and François Terranova. All these individuals had strong backgrounds within the Paralympic Movement, and their expertise and passion were unquestioned. The outright winner of the ballot for the Presidency was Phil Craven, President of the International Wheelchair Basketball Federation. As a five times Paralympic competitor and as a high-level sports administrator, Craven also impressed the voting members with his fervour and energy.

In November 2001 the Presidential candidates had been asked to submit a statement that indicated their outlook and the issues they identified as most vital. Phil Craven identified several important characteristics about himself: an ability to listen and to act; a determination to fight injustice. Craven considered that there were untapped resources within the Paralympic Movement. He signalled that he would help to 'unlock skills' by encouraging athletes to help themselves as well as the Movement. 'Management of change' would be achieved by encouragement of forthrightness and sincerity: 'Committee members must be encouraged to actively contribute to, and work hard between, meetings'. Importantly for the members, Craven was aware of the need to build personal relationships – he pointed to his confidence in being able to engage with the new President of the International Olympic Committee, Jacques Rogge. Overall, the most important message that emanated from Phil Craven's candidacy was that of 'teamwork'. There was no solo crusade in Craven's manifesto; this was all about sharing in a valuable quest for the very greatest opportunities for athletes with a disability. Phil Craven had shown himself to be unyielding and resolute in his efforts on behalf of the International Wheelchair Basketball Federation. His uncompromising attitude had sometimes put him at loggerheads with other authorities. He was now in a position to turn his hand to the bigger picture of the Paralympic Movement: perhaps a case of the poacher turning gamekeeper.

The new Officers of the International Paralympic Committee for the term 2001 to 2005 were (including those elected at this time and those elected later or *ex officio*):

President	Philip Craven (UK)
Vice President Policy and Planning	York Chow (Hong Kong)
Vice President Games Liaison	François Terranova (France)
Vice President Marketing	Nabil Salem (Egypt)
Technical Officer	Carol Mushett (USA)
Medical Officer	Björn Hedman (Sweden)
Treasurer	John Teunissen (Netherlands)
Secretary General	Miguel Sagarra (Spain)
Chief Operating Officer	Thomas Reinecke (Germany)
Athletes Representative	Kjartan Haugen (Norway)

Regional Representatives:

Americas	Jose Luis Campo (Argentina)
East Asia	Yasuhiro Hatsuyama (Japan)
Europe	Bob Price (UK)
Middle East	Abdulhakim Al-Matar (Saudi Arabia)
South Pacific	Greg Hartung (Australia)
Summer Sports Representative	Fred Jansen (Netherlands)
Winter Sports Representative	Jack Benedick (USA)
CP-ISRA Representative	Colin Rains (Great Britain)
IBSA Representative	Enrique Pérez (Spain)
INAS-FID Representative	Jos Mulder (Netherlands)
ISMWSF Representative	Bob McCullough (Australia)
ISOD Representative	Juan Palau Francas (Spain).

The day following the General Assembly brought the newly composed Executive Committee together for the first time. The intention was to introduce the new members to the rest of the Committee, but also to cover some particularly important subjects. Key topics included: taking forward the strategic review of the IPC; the establishment of a Paralympic Foundation; the participation of athletes with a severe disability; the role and responsibilities of elected officers and staff; and the position of Honorary President. This last subject is worth mentioning because there was such a considerable change of direction in this matter from the earlier discussions. The General Assembly had passed the motion: 'Dr Steadward is conferred the title of Honorary President of IPC, and his roles and responsibilities will be determined by the IPC President and Executive Committee'. Although this was a flexible final position, the original idea had been to use Steadward's personal placement within the IOC to ensure the security of the International Paralympic Committee's influence in the IOC. Through this honour Bob Steadward was also going to be rewarded for his longstanding service to the IPC. Phil Craven immediately drew attention to the IPC constitution's clarity in stating that liaison with the IOC was the responsibility of the Executive Committee, through the President. The meeting 'agreed to reconfirm the principle that the liaison with the IOC will go through the IPC President'. It was then logical that the debate should lead to a questioning of how appropriate it was for an Honorary President to have a position on the Executive Committee, and the Executive Committee then formally agreed that Steadward should 'have tasks that were not directly associated to the work of the Executive Committee'. Constructive suggestions included involvement of the Honorary President in the museum, the Foundation, or the awards committee – but obviously not an involvement of a political nature.

Redefining the Impossible: Salt Lake City, USA, March 2002

Opening the Eighth Paralympic Winter Games, Phil Craven certainly had a different style from his predecessor. Raw enthusiasm and much less formality were projected in the IPC President's first welcome speech at a Paralympic Games. Craven had attended the Olympic Games prior to the Opening Ceremony of the Paralympics, and he was clearly fired up by the experience. On 6th March, Craven spoke mainly to the athletes in welcoming all those gathered in the Rice-Eccles Olympic Stadium. He congratulated the Paralympic athletes as a whole:

> You redefine the impossible. You succeed by focusing your minds, driving your bodies and achieving what many would consider the impossible . . . This synergy of mind and body creates the Paralympic Spirit, which is pounding in the hearts of Salt Lake's incredible team of 4000 volunteers. I hope that all of you will breathe in this spirit over the next nine days. It will last you a lifetime.

Craven then invited the President of the United States, George W. Bush, to declare the Salt Lake 2002 Paralympic Winter Games open. Festivities had been prepared on a glorious scale. The entertainment included Donny Osmond, Stevie Wonder, Vanessa-Mae and Billy Gilman. Eric Weihenmayer, the first climber with visual impairment to reach the summit of Mount Everest, handed over the Paralympic Flame to US Paralympians Muffy Davis and Chris Waddell.

The Games saw a total of 416 athletes from 36 countries competing over the period from 7th to 16th March. Newcomers to the Paralympic Winter Games included Andorra, Chile, the People's Republic of China, Croatia, Greece and Hungary. It was notable that the minimum eligibility rules were being applied, and that qualifying standards for each sport meant that there was a diminution in the number of athletes compared with Nagano in 1998. Ice events took place in the E Center, while Alpine competition was held at the Snowbasin Ski Area. Nordic events were located in Soldier Hollow. Spectators crammed in to the most popular ice sledge hockey events, and a total of more than 200 000 tickets were sold during the competition period. Income from ticket sales exceeded

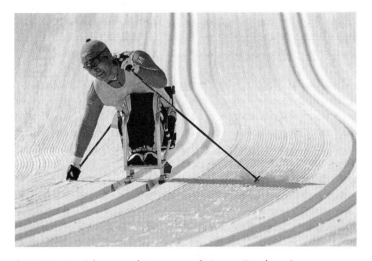

Figure 8.1   Salt Lake City 2002 (photograph courtesy of Lieven Coudenys).

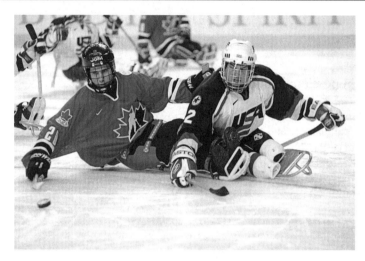

Figure 8.2   Salt Lake City 2002 (photograph courtesy of Lieven Coudenys).

US$2.5 million, pleasingly beyond the projected amount. A Norwegian called Ragnhild Myklebust made everyone pay attention when she was again victorious in the sit-skiing competition – retiring as a Paralympian at the ripe age of 58 years, but having collected 17 gold medals in her time (and one bronze as well). Another indefatigable lady was 36-year-old Sarah Will (USA). Her Alpine successes in the mono-ski category included gold in the downhill, the slalom, the Super-G and the giant slalom.

During the Paralympic Winter Games, the IPC held a reception on 13th March 2002 to present four people who had served the Movement exceptionally with the Paralympic Order. The citation declared that the Paralympic Order: 'is awarded to persons who have illustrated the Paralympic ideal through their actions, who have achieved remarkable merit in the sporting world of the disabled, or who have rendered outstanding services to the Paralympic cause, either through their personal achievement or their contribution to the development of sport for the disabled'. IPC President Phil Craven presented Gudrun Doll-Tepper, Gertrude Krombholz, Hans Lindström and Bob McCullough with the silver medal. Following a decision taken by the IPC Executive Committee at Salt Lake City, the gold, silver and bronze medals of the Paralympic Order would be amalgamated in future to a single award.

State Governor Mike Leavitt, interviewed for the *Deseret Morning News* in Utah on 17th March 2002, was struck by the commitment of the Paralympic athletes he met during the Games. He visited the ice sledge hockey athletes after a game: 'It was a serious locker room,' he said, 'with all the scents and intensity of a world-class competition ... Frankly, I have a hard time relating to their disabilities sometimes, but the fact that I can be an athlete that does my best, I do understand. This is about the human spirit. The Paralympians' motto is "No excuses, no limits." I find that inspiring.'

The 2002 Olympic Winter Games had taken the phrase 'Light the Fire Within' as its theme. This was certainly also applicable to the Paralympic Winter Games in 2002. In an interview by the *Salt Lake Tribune*, the new President of the International Paralympic Committee had to respond to his reputation as a rebel. The interviewer, Mike Gorrell, pointed to Craven's dismissal from the British wheelchair basketball team in 1976, after confrontations about the competence of the coaching staff. Eventually reinstated, Craven went on to have a lengthy and successful competitive career. He claimed to have learned that change is best effected by positively working from the inside.

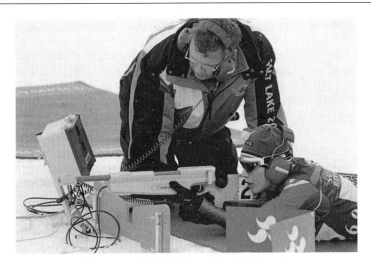

Figure 8.3   Salt Lake City 2002 (photograph courtesy of Lieven Coudenys).

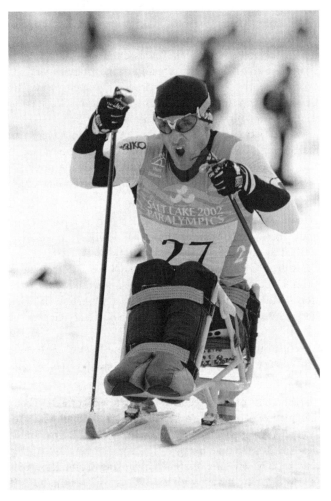

Figure 8.4   Salt Lake City 2002 (photograph courtesy of Lieven Coudenys).

The Executive Committee Does Business at Salt Lake City

The International Paralympic Committee had brought the Executive Committee together on the eve of the 2002 Paralympic Winter Games. The first key subject was that of relations with the International Olympic Committee. In accordance with the IOC Charter, a letter was received saying that the IOC had withdrawn the membership of Bob Steadward with the end of his occupation of the position of President of IPC. Phil Craven told the Executive Committee that further communication had led to an indication that the IOC was likely to offer membership again to the new IPC President, on the basis of his position rather than as an individual. The next opportunity for this to happen would be the IOC Session in November 2002. In fact, Phil Craven would make his way on to this important stage, but not until the 115th Session of the International Olympic Committee (IOC) in Prague, in July 2003 – due to changes being made in the Olympic Charter to clarify the membership process. But the recent Olympic Winter Games had offered extensive opportunities for the promotion of the Paralympic Movement, particularly through formal and informal meetings with Jacques Rogge, IOC President, and Gerhard Heiberg, Chairman of the IOC Marketing Commission. It was at this time that news was given that Visa had obtained the marketing rights for the Paralympic Winter Games in Salt Lake City, as well as the 2004 Paralympics. The implications of this favourable support for these Games had yet to be assessed, but it was a big step.

The IPC's Marketing Working Group was accorded more formal status at the meeting, on the recommendation of the Management Committee. They would become a Marketing Standing Committee, with the members Nabil Salem, John Teunissen, Tony Sainsbury, Thomas Reinecke and Andreas Schönemann. Broadcasting was also discussed at the March meeting, and it was felt less important that broadcasting was driven as a revenue-producing mechanism. The benefits were more likely to be from greater positive exposure – an investment primarily. Some thought that broadcasting was likely to be an advantage when pursuing sponsorship in future.

Returning to the relationship between the IPC and the IOC, decisions were needed as to who would represent the IPC on the Beijing 2008 Coordination Commission. The Management Committee had wanted particular care to be taken over this matter because it was the point at which the IOC–IPC Agreement would come into effect. The Management Committee recommended the following.

- The position (on the Coordination Commission) must be filled by a person with executive authority and Dr Steadward should therefore be removed from that position immediately.
- The position must be filled by an elected officer not by paid staff.
- Negotiation is needed with IOC to change the present IOC–IPC agreement and ensure a broader representation of IPC on the commission as this commission would replace the present IPC Games Liaison Committee for the 2008 Games and beyond. A combination of elected officers and staff members was needed to ensure operational continuity. The Secretary General was instructed to write to the IOC on this.
- The IOC should be informed that IPC was going through a review of its structures and that in an interim measure the President was appointed to the Coordination Commission.

Colin Rains reminded the members of the Executive Committee that the IPC had relied heavily on the former President over the last 12 years, and he asked that they should all 'observe the sensitivity of the issue'. Steadward and André Auberger would remain on the Sport and Environment and the Sport For All Commissions respectively, for the time being.

The contract between the IOC and the Beijing Organising Committee of the Olympic Games (BOCOG) precluded the need for a contract with the IPC as well, as the IOC–IPC agreement meant that the one contract served both Games. But a separate agreement would settle the specific arrangements and conditions for the success of the Paralympic Games.

At this meeting there was also acceptance of the Management Committee's recommendation that there should only be one Paralympic Order, rather than subsections of bronze, silver and gold. This would apply to any other awards of the International Paralympic Committee.

Manchester Hosts Commonwealth Games

Her Majesty Queen Elizabeth II opened the XVII Commonwealth Games in Manchester on 25th July 2002. This sporting celebration was a master showpiece of sport for athletes with a disability, as ten full medal events were offered. The sports available to elite athletes with a disability were athletics, lawn bowls, powerlifting, swimming and table tennis. The Commonwealth Games Organization had been among the first to embrace inclusive opportunities for athletes with a disability, many years before. A particularly successful aspect of the Commonwealth Games was the huge television viewing figures, producing a very positive reflection of the Paralympic Movement. It was estimated that almost half of the UK television audience watched the Opening Ceremony, for example. The IPC President was obviously impressed with the whole phenomenon: 'The Commonwealth Games Organising Committee has done a wonderful job of making these games truly inclusive. The atmosphere in Manchester is marvellous.' At the next meeting of the IPC Executive Committee in Bonn in October, formal congratulations were extended to the 'leadership of the 2002 Commonwealth Games in Manchester, and especially to Tony Sainsbury, for hosting successful fully inclusive events for athletes with disabilities'. The Commonwealth Games had consistently provided important opportunities for leaps forward in sport for athletes with a disability.

Paralympic Games Preparation Discussed in Bonn, October 2002

The Bonn meetings, on 11th and 12th October 2002, received reports from the Athens 2004 organisers, as well as the Torino 2006 and Beijing 2008 organisers. The Athens Managing Director, Mr Ioannis Spanudakis, and Ms Karyofylli, Paralympic Games General Manager, supplied detailed papers relating to progress on the Games. Two particular issues were covered during the presentation: approval of the location of venues, and the appointment of a host broadcaster. In addition, members of the Executive Committee wished to have clarification of the provision of horses for the equestrian events – a review was underway to decide whether the hosts would provide horses or the competitors should arrange for their own. Discussion moved to the broadest sense of accessibility. There was some concern about the extent of services and security of participants who were visually impaired. As expected, IBSA suggested that it should assist and advise in this particular area. The host broadcaster would be ISB, as had been expected, which would undertake provision of all broadcasting services as well as managing the sale of TV rights. In return it would collect an administration fee and a percentage of sales proceeds. After examining some specific aspects of this relationship, it was agreed that Xavier Gonzalez should have authority to proceed according to the adopted principles. Gonzalez, who had been appointed interim Chief Operating Officer in July following the resignation of Thomas Reinecke, was the Paralympic Games Liaison Director. Gonzalez had brought to his work in the IPC a wealth of experience and expertise from his lengthy involvement in Paralympic organising committees. He had held senior posts of responsibility at the Barcelona 1992 Olympic Games and Atlanta 1996 Paralympic Games before being appointed General Manager of Sport and Games Operation for the Sydney 2000 Paralympic Games, and then Managing Director of Salt Lake 2002.

The Torino 2006 contract was still being negotiated, but the IPC Executive Committee pressed the organising committee to ensure that the General Assembly of the IPC could be held in Torino in 2003, consistent with the normal procedure. The technical concerns rested with the intention to utilise the same slopes as for the Winter Olympic Games – some gradients might need to be looked at closely for suitability. There was a consensus that all disciplines should take place in Sestrière. Confidence was evident in the presentation of the Torino officials. Tiziana Nasi, President of the Paralympic Section of the Torino 2006 Organising Committee (TOROC) pronounced: 'The Torino Paralympics will be a historical event, as it was in Rome in 1960 that the Olympic and Paralympic Games were held in the same place for the first time'. The Executive Committee strongly urged the Torino organisers to do all that they could to ensure that there was identical handling of the Olympic and Paralympic athletes – in particular that there should be no requirement for entry fees. The TOROC team verified that this was a feature of the contract.

Zhang Quiping, Deputy Director of the Sports Department of the Beijing Organising Committee for the Olympic Games (BOCOG), gave a brief initial presentation, together with Yang Yang, BOCOG Programme Manager. Because these were to be the first Games under the IPC–IOC contract system, discussions had already taken place together with Gilbert Felli. All events would take place in Beijing, except the sailing competitions, which had to be located in Qingdao. One acknowledged shortfall was in the number of well-trained technical experts and classifiers. The BOCOG representatives stressed that they were actively engaged in the development of strategies to build up numbers of officials in time for the Paralympic Games, and that they would salute the IPC's input and assistance in this process. Carol Mushett suggested that a number of members and organisations should be encouraged to become involved in what was a time-consuming process. Sports, regional organisations and individuals would be called upon to generate a 'systematic mentoring programme'. This should lead to a responsible and appropriate level of provision for the Beijing 2008 Paralympic Games.

The International Olympic Committee announced that it had accepted the candidature of Vancouver (Canada), Salzburg (Austria), Pyongchang (Korea) and Bern (Switzerland) to host the Olympic and Paralympic Winter Games in 2010. Not every city that makes a submission goes through to the decisive round. In total there had been eight applicants by the May deadline. The cities that did not receive the IOC Executive Committee's blessing were: Sarajevo (Bosnia-Herzegovina), Jaca (Spain), Harbin (China) and Andorra La Vella (Andorra). The Prague Session of the IOC in July 2003 would determine which city should be awarded the Olympic and Paralympic Games for 2010.

INAS-FID Still Not Up to the Mark, According to IPC

There was a need to deliver an account of the eligibility and protest procedures for athletes with an intellectual disability. Jos Mulder had suggested that the two eligibility advisors for INAS-FID, Trevor Parmenter and Jennifer McTavish, should attend the IPC Executive Committee meeting. They had all met with Bjorn Hedman and Carol Mushett, IPC Medical and Technical Officers respectively, on 9th October. What was described as a 'major breakthrough' was recounted to the IPC Executive Committee a few days later. The officials of INAS-FID had accepted that proof of fulfilment of certain imperative conditions would make readmission possible. The conditions were:

- More stringent verification procedures whereby primary documentation must be provided on the assessment of intellectual disability
- Development of a sports related component to eligibility, i.e. linking the impact of the impairment to the sports specific function
- Piloting a protest procedure which is in line with the IPC Policy.

While this was a very satisfactory situation, the full rigour of the conditions laid down by the IPC General Assembly had not been met. The connection to functional classification was a much more complex process for athletes with intellectual disability, and Jos Mulder considered that INAS-FID would require more time to fine-tune. They felt they could meet the terms of the demands, but it was not possible to accurately place a timetable on compliance. But there was a real need to finalise the event programme for the Athens Summer Paralympic Games of 2004, and the entries for the IPC Swimming World Championships in Mar Del Plata were about to close. When the IPC Executive Committee reconvened on 12th October 2002, a statement from INAS-FID was read out. In it the INAS-FID officials acknowledged that there had been a loss of confidence and that questions relating to integrity were associated with the eligibility, verification and registration of INAS-FID athletes. They asked for 'more time to help rebuild the confidence between itself and IPC, and achieve the required clarity. Accordingly, it is determined to work toward these aims in the spirit of cooperation with IPC.' INAS-FID would not compete in the Mar Del Plata Swimming Championships, and acknowledged that it might not be able to enter athletes in the Athens 2004 Paralympic Games unless it resolved the issues satisfactorily.

For its part, the International Paralympic Committee formally congratulated INAS-FID for its efforts and progress so far, but emphasised that there was still a way to go. At the present time athletes with an intellectual disability could not be included in the Athens 2004 Paralympic Games programme: 'Full medal events for athletes with an intellectual disability will be reinstated to IPC sanctioned competitions one month after the IPC Management Committee and the relevant Sport Assembly Executive Committee are satisfied that all conditions, as contained within the General Assembly motion 1, are met by INAS-FID'. A deadline for a final decision on inclusion of events for Athens would be 31st January 2003, at the Management Committee meeting.

The IPC had ruled against the involvement of athletes with an intellectual disability at the Athens 2004 Paralympic Games. The deadline of 31st January 2003 did not bring evidence that the organisation had satisfactorily resolved the difficulties of eligibility and verification. INAS-FID was given leave to appeal to the IPC Executive Committee at the 34th meeting that took place between 4th and 6th April, in Athens. As expert witnesses, Bernard Atha and Hans Lindström worked together with Jos Mulder in their one-hour presentation. The evidence that Lindström set out was based on the question of how appropriate it was for athletes with intellectual disability to submit to a sport-specific functional classification mechanism, when their disability was cognitive rather than physiological. Bernard Atha took the Executive Committee back to the original context of the suspension, to Sydney 2000. The response of the INAS-FID authorities to each IPC requirement was examined, and Atha stressed that INAS-FID could not be faulted on its willingness to comply. He had suggested to the IPC Executive Committee that athletes with an intellectual disability were only just embarking on the long struggle against ignorance and prejudice that people with physical disabilities and visual impairment had largely come through in the second half of the twentieth century. Some athletes with other disabilities had shown an active reluctance to welcome those with intellectual disabilities into the Paralympic Games. Atha generously put this attitude down to 'misunderstanding and lack of knowledge rather than ill will'.

It was agreed that some delays had come about because INAS-FID appeared not to fully comprehend some of the requirements, and clarification had helped accelerate the cause more recently. In particular there was some concern about whether INAS-FID could actually comply fully with the original General Assembly motion, in view of Hans Lindström's emphasis on the proposed classification procedure being inappropriate for athletes with an intellectual difficulty. Jos Mulder submitted a detailed motion to the IPC Executive Committee. It gave rise to extended discussion, and eventually led to agreement by Mulder to amendments that would be more acceptable to all parties. The motion asked:

The IPC Executive Committee to approve that:

- Athletes with intellectual disability will be included in the Athens 2004 Paralympic Games, in a limited number of exhibition events
- The establishment of a joint IPC/INAS-FID Eligibility Verification Committee as proposed in IPC's letter of 28th March 2001 and agreed by INAS-FID
- The appointment as members of that Committee of two individuals by IPC, two individuals by INAS-FID, and a Chairman to be appointed by those four
- That IPC and INAS-FID shall review the position immediately after Athens.

The motion was passed with 16 votes in favour and one abstention. Jos Mulder asked that he should be able to have the information about which events could be demonstration events in Athens in time for the INAS-FID General Assembly the following week. He felt that he could ensure that there was little danger of the INAS-FID membership turning this offer down on receipt of the details. In a press release, Phil Craven indicated the great support that IPC would still give to all athletes with an intellectual disability. He said that the decision to include exhibition events in the Athens 2004 Paralympic Games was evidence of this support: 'With this move, the IPC can provide INAS-FID athletes with sporting opportunities at a high level, whilst safeguarding the Paralympic Games'.

Strategic Review Gains Momentum, and the Medical Committee Restructures Itself

The Strategic Review of IPC was approaching its next stage: the appointment of a consultancy to conduct a review. The Executive Committee ratified the decision of the Management Committee to place the contract with the McKinsey Sports Practice Group. Six representatives from this firm informed the IPC Executive Committee of their proposed methodologies and schedule for what they called the 'diagnostic phase'. It was important for the IPC to appoint a Steering Group to meet regularly with the McKinsey people every four to six weeks. Phil Craven, Bob Price, Greg Hartung, Paul De Pace, Ljiljana Lubisic, the newly elected athletes' representative, and Xavier Gonzalez made up the group. A cautionary observation was made at the Executive Committee: that all stakeholders must remain fully informed of the debate in order to secure satisfactory acceptance of eventual proposals in the General Assembly. McKinsey and the Steering Committee would need to ensure that adequate information was presented to the Management and Executive Committees, so that the very best suggestions for the future reached the General Assembly – and in a way that they were likely to receive greatest acclamation in that forum.

The meetings in Athens in April 2003 were also arranged so that a total of seven hours could be devoted to workshops and discussions about the Strategic Review. The plenary sessions worked towards consensus on recommendations under four main headings: development, fundraising, sports independence, and governance and structure. The Steering Committee concluded that the demands of the Paralympic Movement in the modern context called for a wider range of 'value-adding activities', some of which would need additional financial resources. The Steering Committee recognised three key concerns that the IPC would need to tackle: 'improving the organisation's marginal income base, enhancing the service portfolio to the IPC's members and clarifying roles and responsibilities within the organisation'.

IPC medical matters and sport science matters needed a different structure, as a result of a period of independent development. Björn Hedman, IPC Medical Officer, described the changes that would foster closer relations between the experts concerned with different aspects of science. The IPC Medical Committee would comprise the IPC Medical Officer and the Chairpersons of the Sport Science and Education Sub-Committee, the Classification Sub-Committee and the Anti-Doping Sub-Committee.

This would mean the Medical Committee would be made up of Björn Hedman, Yves Vanlandewijck, Conrado Rodriguez Jaubert and José Antonio Pascual. Hedman also proposed that two other Ad Hoc committees should be created to improve the flow of information and expertise: one to collect together the Medical Officers of the International Organisations of Sport for the Disabled (IOSD), and the other formed of representatives from the IPC regions.

Public Relations

It was time, once again, to update the image of the International Paralympic Committee to the outside world. To this end the IPC commissioned the public relations firm, Scholz & Friends, to bring a suitably modern symbol and meaning to the IPC's public presence. The Executive Committee agreed the recommendation of the Management Committee to adopt the new logo and motto: 'Spirit in Motion'. The logo was a clever adaptation of the well-known shapes and colours of the IPC over the past years; the three modified *Tae-Geuks*, in blue, red and green, were now arranged in a more circular style. The public relations company handed the International Paralympic Committee a statement to explain the 'new image'.

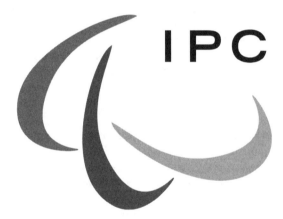

The shape of the new logo was chosen to complement the rephrased vision of the IPC: 'To enable Paralympic athletes to achieve sporting excellence and to inspire and excite the world'. 'Spirit in Motion' was explained by the IPC in *The Paralympian* (no. 2, 2003) as

> expressing the inspirational character of the Paralympic Movement as well as elite performance of Paralympic athletes. It also stands for the strong will of every Paralympian. The word 'Spirit' is derived from the notion that the IPC, like the athletes it represents, has a drive to compete and to succeed. But the IPC not only stages high performance sporting events, the strong message of the Movement accompanies it: the Paralympic Spirit. 'Motion' relates to the idea that the IPC is truly moving forward – an organisation that realises its potential and is now striving to achieve it. Motion is ever present in the Movement, be it through athletes setting new records or the never-ending enthusiasm of volunteers and staff.

SportAccord Convention in Madrid

From 12th to 16th May 2002 the International Paralympic Committee participated in an international convention aimed at discussing several common issues in modern sports. The meetings were organised so that a different theme was taken to lead the day's meetings: designing for sport, hosting and managing sports events, sport business, sport broadcast and sponsorship, law and sport, and technology. Phil Craven presented a paper with the title: *Sport and Education: A Blueprint for the Future*, as well as the IPC maintaining a display booth with information about the Paralympic Movement. This conference for leaders of international sports also gave the opportunity for the IPC Management Committee to meet, and to receive the news that the IPC President, Phil Craven, had been nominated for election as an IOC member.

Commission for Athletes with a Severe Disability

The first meeting of the Commission for Athletes with a Severe Disability took place in March 2003. During this important gathering a number of priorities were laid down as foundations for future work. James Thompson, four-times Paralympian in the sport of boccia, chaired the meetings. The initial hub needed to be an assessment of the present situation, and to develop strategies for enhancing the opportunities for athletes with a severe disability. Thompson identified the specific concerns of education to reduce prejudice, and the raising of awareness of the contribution of athletes with a severe disability. Some research would be needed before concrete proposals could be drawn up. In particular there was a very low response rate to a questionnaire that had been sent out to member nations asking for views on what they considered to be the definition of 'severe disability'. Only 16 of the 160 National Paralympic Committees had responded at all. The Commission put together some guidelines for identifying those athletes with a severe disability. It suggested that an athlete with a severe disability was:

- an athlete who requires assistance from a person during competition based on the rules of the sport; and/or
- an athlete who requires support staff for daily living functions based on the Paralympic Games environment (including for travel/transportation, personal support, transfers).

The Commission wished to look forward to the future rather than to get stuck analysing the past. There was agreement of the merit of encouraging athletes and former athletes with a severe disability to move into the ranks of senior organisational positions. But education would be a significant portion of the Commission's drive: the National Paralympic Committees, IOSDs and the wider sporting world needed to understand the context in which these athletes operated. Promotion of sport opportunities at grass-roots level would need the support of several agencies, and the IPC needed to help facilitate this secure base for individuals with a severe disability to experience the values of competitive sport. Having identified the mission as the promotion of an athlete-centred inclusive participation by all athletes, the Commission reported that this would be achieved by upholding certain principles:

- becoming an integral part of the new strategic plan;
- ensuring that existing systems effectively support the involvement of individuals with severe disabilities, including participation in the process of governance;
- exploring possible changes to rules and regulations;
- becoming an important component of development programmes for athletes and leaders;
- exploring issues related to event (class) combination guidelines;
- maintaining ongoing communication and feedback;

- examining practices regarding sport staff quotas;
- enhancing promotion and awareness activities and materials.

The Commission for Athletes with a Severe Disability recognised that the tasks of the future would include: 'continuing data analysis; consideration and implementation of new operational ideas; providing input to ongoing policy and programme development; and seeking a balanced Paralympic programme'.

Phil Craven Elected as IOC Member

The 115th Session of the International Olympic Committee, on 2 July 2003, voted to elect Phil Craven, IPC President, as a member of the International Olympic Committee. Craven acknowledged the tribute of this recognition, in a typically low-key manner: 'I am honoured and excited about the opportunity to represent the Paralympic Movement in the IOC. In the last 18 months, the partnership between the IPC and the IOC has gone from strength to strength. My election today confirms it.'

At the same IOC Session, the host city for the 2010 Winter Olympic and Paralympic Games was announced. Vancouver was awarded the Games, and it was stressed that a contract would be drawn up that would continue the requirement of the organising committee to host both Olympic and Paralympic events in the same venue in sequence.

On 25th August 2003 in Lausanne, Jacques Rogge and Phil Craven signed an amendment to the 2001 IOC–IPC Agreement. This was a logical step following the formal links that had begun with the October 2000 Cooperation Agreement. The thrust of the 2003 amendment was that guaranteed income would be forthcoming from the organising committees of the Paralympic Games for 2008, 2010 and 2012, from broadcasting rights and marketing. The rights and responsibilities for broadcasting and marketing were to be transferred directly to the organising committee of these Games. The amounts contained within the amendment should mean almost complete financial security for the International Paralympic Committee in future – even if this was not due to arrive until 2008. The income was to be: US$9 million for the 2008 Paralympic Games, US$4 million for the Winter Paralympic Games of 2010 and US$10 million for the Summer Paralympic Games of 2012. In a press release, Jacques Rogge stressed the willingness of the IOC to continue its support: 'This is a big day for the Olympic Movement. The IOC is happy to be able to support the IPC for these forthcoming editions of the Paralympic Games and, in doing so, to strengthen its relations with the Paralympic Movement.' From Phil Craven's point of view the position for the IPC could not be better: 'The amendment lays an excellent foundation for the IPC's quest to fully develop the Paralympic Movement – a huge task, which we can now begin to explore. It also emphasises the close partnership which continues between the IOC and the IPC.' Although the 2001 agreement specifically related to Beijing 2008 and Vancouver 2010, the organising committees of Salt Lake 2002, Athens 2004 and Torino 2006 chose to employ the model of having one organising committee for both Olympic and Paralympic Games. The amendment served also to emphasise the success of the relationship between the IPC and the IOC in the years since Phil Craven and Jacques Rogge had each come to office.

VISTA Conference 2003, Bollnäs, Sweden

The Swedish Sports Organization for the Disabled hosted the 2003 VISTA Conference at Bollnäs from 11th to 14th September 2003. Kari Marklund, President of the Swedish Sports Organization for the Disabled, along with Ingemar Wedman, President of the Swedish Development Centre for Disability

Sport, welcomed the 200 delegates from almost 50 countries. At the Opening Ceremony, Kennet Fröjd, Director of the Swedish Development Centre for Disability Sport said: 'It is a great recognition and honour for SUH to host the most important development conference during a Paralympic cycle within the Paralympic Movement'.

A very strong line-up of presentations was assembled, with keynote papers from Gudrun Doll-Tepper (*Participation in Paralympic Games*), Yves Vanlandewijck (*Science for Success*), Björn Hedman (*Classification in Paralympic Sports*) and Chris Nunn (*Coaching for Paralympic Gold: Experiences and Future Implications*). The conference was organised into eight rewarding topic areas: gender equity; youth in Paralympic sport; organisation of the sports counselling service; performance enhancement through sport science: what do we know?; classification; education; intellectual disabilities; and severe disabilities.

Andy Parkinson, IPC Anti-Doping and Classification Manager, chaired a fascinating and constructive panel discussion at the close of the VISTA 2003 Conference. The panel included Phil Craven, Tim Johansson, Yves Vanlandewijck, Chris Nunn, Gudrun Doll-Tepper and Ljiljana Ljubisic. The well-established VISTA cycle has proven to be a formative source of inspiration and sharing of ideas on Paralympic issues.

Evolution, not Revolution

Phil Craven approached his first General Assembly, in November 2003, by compiling a biennial report. This lengthy document recorded and characterised the work of the International Paralympic Committee over the past two years. The report was both documentary and personal. Craven's editorial style consisted of giving credit to the stakeholders and demanding more from them for the future. He endorsed the steering done within the Kuala Lumpur Strategic Review, leading to the Strategic Review that had only just been concluded.

The self-assessment began with the IPC President showing his colours as a team player by characteristically spreading his praise around: 'First and foremost it is our athletes who inspire me. It is to serve them, by promoting their best interests and increasing their visibility that guides my official duties and gives me motivation and great pleasure.' Craven insisted that the proposals from the Strategic Review were for evolution, not revolution. He was concerned to work to give the athletes 'visibility and protection'. The paternalistic overtones were apt for this occasion: the IPC was embarking on a surge of public growth, fostered by a secure partnership with the International Olympic Committee. The economic realisation had been achieved through an attractive partnership with Visa that affected financial services until December 2004, and other high-impact proposals were under discussion that would have very significant benefits if they were realised.

Engineering the Future, Torino General Assembly, November 2003

The 2003 General Assembly of the International Paralympic Committee began on 21st November in Torino, Italy. The Organising Committee of the Torino 2006 Paralympic Winter Games (TOROC) played host to the IPC family at the Fiat Storico, a museum in a former factory of the car manufacturer. The National Paralympic Committees of Botswana, Congo, Ghana, Malta, Mauritius, Tanzania, Togo and Turkey were admitted as members of IPC. As expected, progress reports were presented by the Organising Committees of the Paralympic Games of Athens 2004, Torino 2006, Beijing 2008 and Vancouver 2010. Prior to the General Assembly there had been an IPC Conference on 20th and 21st November, with discussions on four major topics: development, fundraising, inclusion of athletes with an intellectual disability and sport independence.

A new procedure was adopted for reckoning the IPC membership fee, making it more comfortable for some NPCs. Countries with a Gross National Product of less than US$500 would be exempt from paying the membership fee.

The Paralympic Order was presented to seven first-rate servants of the Paralympic Movement: Yasuhiro Hatsuyama (Japan), Colin Rains (UK), Hector Ramirez (Argentina), Donald Royer (Canada), Jean Stone (UK), Carl Wang (Norway) and Xavier Gonzalez (Spain).

The 2001 Strategic Planning Congress in Kuala Lumpur had proposed a review of the organisational structures of the IPC. The external appraisal of the IPC, undertaken by the McKinsey Group, served to direct the Management and Executive Committees to put forward proposals that would take the IPC into its next phase. The report, *The IPC in Five Years*, was presented to the Strategic Review Steering Committee in December 2002. The extensive debate led to the IPC President contacting every IPC member by letter on 18th June 2003 to solicit reactions. The responses were extensive, and two major motions were devised to reflect the opinions of the membership: one on governance and organisational structure and another on governance of multi-disability competitions.

Central principles for the future were agreed for a new governance and organisational structure along the following lines: 'Adherence to the democratic values of IPC; separation of governance and management; ownership and joint responsibility of the IPC; simplification of the decision making process; and ensuring universality'.

The motion proposed a restructuring of the main organs of the IPC. The detail is recorded here for accuracy (Box 8.3).

The intention was to elect the President, Vice President and Board Members without specific portfolios in mind. Built in was the wish to elect the broadest representation of the IPC stakeholders, but to retain the cohesively democratic nature of the IPC. The committees of the IPC were to be established as advisory satellites to the Governing Board, which would appoint chairperson and members. Distinct from the IPC Committees were to be the four IPC Councils. These would continue to bring together specific members of the Paralympic Movement in proven groupings: Sports, IOSDs, Regions and Athletes. A management team was to be formed, composed of the management staff of IPC, and directed by the Chief Executive Officer. The principle aim would be to implement the Strategic Plan and the 'delivery of the goals'. The two key positions within IPC's proposed structure were to be the President and the Chief Executive Officer. The President's role was defined as the 'Keeper of the Vision and the Mission ... the Chief Governance Officer' and the Chairperson of the Governing Board.

When this motion on governance and organisational structure was put forward in the 2003 General Assembly, it was passed with 79 votes in favour and seven votes against. With no abstentions, the necessary two-thirds majority was easily reached. The second major strategic change was impelled by the motion on governance of multi-disability sports. The wording of the motion was such that the IPC constitution relating to the objects of the Association required changes so as to read:

Article 2.1 c. For the Championships Sports: award, sanction and where appropriate assist in the coordination and supervising of world and regional multi-disability games and championships as the governing body for that sport recognized by IPC.

To facilitate the process of independence of any IPC Championship Sport when democratically agreed by the respective Sports Assembly and in accordance with the IPC regulations as agreed by the Executive Committee.

In describing the rationale for the motion, the Executive Committee explained that the overwhelming consensus of the Strategic Review process was that the IPC should concentrate on the Paralympic

---

Box 8.3 Motion for restructuring the IPC

The General Assembly (GA):

- The General Assembly is the ultimate governing body of the IPC
- The General Assembly is responsible for defining the Vision and the general directions of the organization
- The different stakeholders of the Paralympic Movement will have representation at the General Assembly with full membership
- The following autonomous organizations will become full members of the IPC General Assembly: the NPCs, the IOSDs, the Regions and the Sports

Note: In the transition period each Sport and Region will be granted speaking and voting rights until they choose to obtain independence from IPC.

The IPC Governing Board (GB). The Governing Board's main responsibilities are:

- To interpret the Vision set by the General Assembly
- To ensure that the directions set by the General Assembly are implemented
- To set the broad goals of the Strategic Plan
- To monitor the performance of the delivery of the goals

The composition of the Governing Board is the following:

- One President, elected by the General Assembly
- One Vice-President, elected by the General Assembly
- Ten Board members, elected by the General Assembly
- One Athletes' Representative, ex-officio member with vote, elected by the Athletes' Council
- The Chief Executive Officer, ex-officio member without vote.

Games. This had also been the upshot of the Task Force Report before it. Most crucially the motion was not intended to oblige any move on the part of the sports towards independence: it was to smooth the progress of such ambition, if desired, and yet the IPC would oversee the steps towards independence so as to ensure that the end product was a 'democratic, viable and self-sustainable organisation that enhances the opportunities for the athletes and respects the principles of the Paralympic Movement'. The IPC was acknowledging the prerogative of any IPC championship sport (a sport not included on the Paralympic programme) to become autonomous, 'without prejudging which organizational model it adopts (whether it be the inclusion within an Olympic International Federation or the creation of an independent federation for a Paralympic Sport, etc)'. As for the motion on governance and organisational structure, fundamental principles were also laid down in achieving the results:

- A clear mandate from the respective sports membership as outlined in the IPC Handbook
- An implementation plan and timetable that takes into consideration and addresses the needs of all parties
- Agreements, outlining responsibilities for each party, will be signed with the Sports.

Appropriate time was given for clarification of this motion, particularly to reassure members that not all sports would be expected to press forward with independence, and to reassure National Paralympic

Committees that they would be central to the process. When it came to a vote the required majority of two-thirds to effect a constitutional change was achieved: 65 votes for, 18 against and 3 abstentions. Many could see the sense of movement in this direction.

The General Assembly accepted that the Commission for Women in Sport should be the responsible body to address relevant Paralympic issues, but some details of the motion relating to its mandate and specific work did not receive such full backing. The recommendations were:

- That the Commission for Women in Sport supervises gender equity in Paralympic sport with advisory and consultative responsibilities to the IPC Executive Committee, IPC Headquarters, Sports, NPCs and IOSDs.
- That the General Assembly confirms the continuation of the Commission for Women in Sport to work with other stakeholders to ensure that standards and policies are established and that equitable participation in Paralympic sport and representation of women in all decision-making structures is achieved.
- That the General Assembly further endorses the recommendation made by the Commission for Women in Sport that the IPC, NPCs, Sports, IOSDs and IFs belonging to the Paralympic Movement shall immediately establish a goal to be achieved by December 2005 that at least 15% of all officers in all their decision making structures be held by women with the intent of achieving 30%representation by 2009.

There was some concern that the imposition of quotas was undesirable, and against the grain of the IPC's past identity. Ann Cody, a former US Paralympian, reassured the members of the General Assembly that compliance with these percentages should only be on the basis of positioning the most qualified and very best people to do the jobs – inevitably there would be discomfort at this sort of positive discrimination. It was also pointed out that these recommendations were in line with the International Olympic Committee's policies on representation by women. Thirty votes went against the motion, 52 in favour, and seven abstentions: the motion was carried. The opponents included some who were sceptical about the means of ensuring that quotas could be fulfilled without positive discrimination; this could not guarantee that the best-qualified person would be offered the job. The concerns voiced at the General Assembly were somewhat eased by the explanation that the quotas being referred to were targets only; they could not be imposed on the National Paralympic Committees. There was no suggestion that meeting the target was more than a recommendation – it was not to become a condition for membership.

The inclusion of athletes with an intellectual disability had received extensive airing at the conference session prior to the General Assembly. There had been some progress made already through the establishment of a Joint Eligibility Verification Committee. The South African representative proposed a motion, seconded by the Netherlands, which restated the IPC position with regard to INAS-FID:

That the General Assembly decide, in principle, whether INAS-FID should be a member of the Paralympic Movement through a process whereby the future of athletes with an intellectual disability within IPC should be based on a report to be developed by the IPC Executive Committee. This report should be presented to the Special General Assembly to be held in 2004 provided that INAS-FID has proved that it has developed a watertight, reliable, valid and proven system for the inclusion of ID athletes in all IPC competitions in terms of the IPC Constitution, rules and regulations and motion number 1 of the 2001 General Assembly. In the alternate, a proposal to exclude ID athletes from all IPC events should be presented.

Because the motion did not have any bearing on the IPC constitution, it required only a simple majority to get through. The onus was placed firmly on INAS-FID to establish acceptable eligibility testing; in particular, INAS-FID had to research sport-specific eligibility testing. With strong support, the motion was accepted by the General Assembly (69 for, 13 against, four abstentions). The next item on the agenda was a motion from the USA to immediately replace INAS-FID with Special Olympics International as the sole representative of athletes with an intellectual disability. This was a hasty move to plug a gap that had not quite opened up yet! As a result of the success of the previous motion in keeping INAS-FID in the primary position, the USA withdrew the motion.

Athens Prepares to Welcome the World

The Olympic Games had seen Athens pull out all the stops to ensure that practical difficulties were overcome – there had been massive provision of security, and the facilities were completed and judged to be excellent. The peculiar scandal of Konstandinos Kenteris and Ekaterina Thanu – allegedly evading drug testing by far-fetched sight-seeing, traffic accident and hospitalisation, puzzled commentators of the Olympic Games more than anything seen in many years. But the overall message to the host nation was expressed in a headline from Owen Slot, Chief Sports Reporter for *The Times*, London: 'Thanks Athens, sorry we doubted you' (Tuesday 31st August 2004). Indeed, Phil Craven later also instructed the world to apologise to Athens for having doubts about its ability to deliver Olympic and Paralympic Games of global quality. The highlights of the Olympic Games were too numerous to capture, but they included the performances of Kelly Holmes (UK), Guo Jingjing (China), Ian Thorpe (Australia), Michael Phelps (USA), Carolina Klüft (Sweden) and Hicham El Guerrouj (Morocco).

As the Athens 2004 Paralympic Games drew closer, attention turned to the detailed arrangements of the venues and competition events themselves. Athens would see the celebration of a Paralympic Games to benefit from the IOC–IPC Cooperation Agreement for the first time. A single organising committee had been responsible for all arrangements leading up to the Games. Paralympic athletes were not required to pay for their participation, for the first time.

The Paralympic Games were staged from 17th to 28th September, using the same venues as the Olympic Games. The Paralympic Village was located in the Municipality of Acharnes at Lekanes, 11 kilometres from the Athens Olympic Stadium. A total of 3806 athletes competed in the Paralympic Games in Athens, the gender split being 2646 men and 1160 women. As ever, the Athens 2004 Paralympic Games relied on an army of volunteers – some 8863 were engaged to help make the phenomenon a success. Over 850 000 tickets were sold to spectators for the Paralympic Games, twice the estimate of the organisers. The time zones allowed live television coverage to be significantly greater worldwide than it had been in Sydney in 2000. In the United Kingdom it was calculated that more than 10 million viewers tuned in during the Games. Congestion and transport chaos had been predicted. Venues may not all have been completely ready for pre-competition access, but athletes would care less about this than the specific preparation and acclimatisation for their events.

However, the more recent past had produced immediate concerns about security. The Athens 2004 Paralympic Games would be the first summer Games since the 9/11 terrorist attacks on New York and Washington. Although it may be argued that the preceding Olympic Games might have provided a more attractive stage for terrorist attention, any such targeting would have an inevitable knock-on effect for the Paralympic Games. The precedents of terrorism at the 1972 Munich Olympic Games and the pipe bomb in Atlanta in 1996 were realistic evidence of the possibility. Both the United States and the United Kingdom expressed concern about the effectiveness of the security proposed for Athens. An unprecedented US$750 million had been allocated to security for the Olympic Games, with the Paralympic Games benefiting from the same arrangements, and numerous countries as well as NATO were providing advice. Perhaps as a result of all this, both Olympic and Paralympic Games proceeded without incident.

New events for Athens included five-a-side football, handcycling, women's judo and women's sitting volleyball. Handcycling had its successful debut at the 2002 World Cycling Championships in Altenstadt, Germany, and entered the Paralympic cycling programme as a full medal status event. The complete programme of sports was: archery, athletics, boccia, cycling, equestrianism, wheelchair fencing, football five-a-side, football seven-a-side, goalball, judo, powerlifting, sailing, shooting, swimming, table tennis, wheelchair basketball, wheelchair rugby, wheelchair tennis, volleyball.

The Athens 2004 Paralympic Games were declared open at the Opening Ceremony on Friday 17th September 2004 by the President of the Greek Republic, Costis Stephanopoulos. A Greek long jumper, Georgios Toptsis, lit the Cauldron to symbolically reawaken the phenomenon of the Paralympics. Phil Craven, in his speech at the Opening Ceremony, declared:

> The real heroes of the evening are the athletes. We are here to celebrate you and your sport, but there is more to it than that. You are a beacon of inspiration for millions of people around the world: for those who cannot be in the stadium tonight; for young athletes, who, watching you, will set their sights higher; for the families, friends and organizations that support those young athletes.

Craven went on to stress the inextricable connections between the sporting endeavour at the highest levels and the philosophy that must accompany it: 'The essence of the Paralympic spirit is a Greek heritage, expressed in just two words: "Kalos" and "Kagathos": harmony and excellence paired with nobility and ability'. The Opening Ceremony was beamed to millions in Europe and North America,

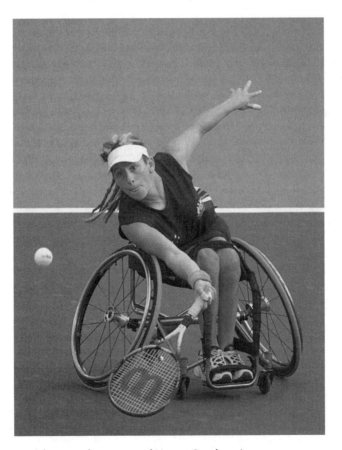

Figure 8.5   Athens 2004 (photograph courtesy of Lieven Coudenys).

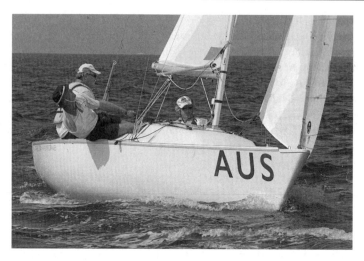

Figure 8.6   Athens 2004 (photograph courtesy of Lieven Coudenys).

but reportedly there were also audiences of 10 million in China and 8 million in Japan – where the time was 3.00 am!

A Japanese swimmer was the most successful at sweeping up the medals: Mayumi Narita won seven individual golds, one relay gold and one bronze medal. China won 141 medals (63 gold, 46 silver and 32 bronze) coming out at the top of the table, with Great Britain and Spain bringing in the second and third places respectively. This was the Paralympics of Chantal Petitclerc of Canada, who had not managed to bring her power and consistency along in her previous Paralympic Games. Petitclerc won five gold medals on the track, taking the titles in 100 m, 200 m, 400 m, 800 m and 1500 m. Along the way she managed to lodge three world records. In cycling, Australia ruled the roost, claiming 14 of the available Paralympic medals. Spain and Portugal rose to prominence in the boccia competitions, sweeping up six and five medals for their respective countries. In equestrian events, Great Britain managed to show particularly well. Deborah Criddle and Lee Pearson were awarded three golds each. The venue for goalball was the scene of a remarkable repeat: the gold medals went to Denmark in the men's competition and to Canada in the women's competition – exactly as they had in Sydney four years before. The appreciative crowd soon became used to the uncanny silence necessary for the game to be played properly.[1] As each goal was scored there was a release of pure delight as everyone gasped and roared their support, only to return to silence for play to resume.

Dominance was total from the Hong Kong wheelchair fencing team, winning eight gold medals. The women's team won gold in every event except one – in which they only managed silver! In athletics, the most remarkable new name was Oscar Pistorius, the 17-year-old sprinter from South Africa. He took gold in 200 m and bronze in 100 m (T44), breaking world records in the 200 m. Pistorius was a big success due to his youthful approach to athletics, his drive and passion, and his obvious potential. There will be plenty more to come from Pistorius.

Provision in the Olympic Village was caring and thorough. In the Library there was great interest in a Braille embosser, enlarging monitor and audio aids for visually impaired participants to be able to surf the Internet and use the computer facilities. The enlarging monitor could make ordinary text from books and magazines more manageable for those in need of larger print. There was quite a queue at times for

---

[1] Goalball is a game for athletes with visual disabilities, and is played with a large ball with a bell inside.

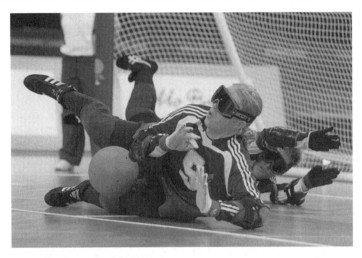

Figure 8.7   Athens 2004 (photograph courtesy of Lieven Coudenys).

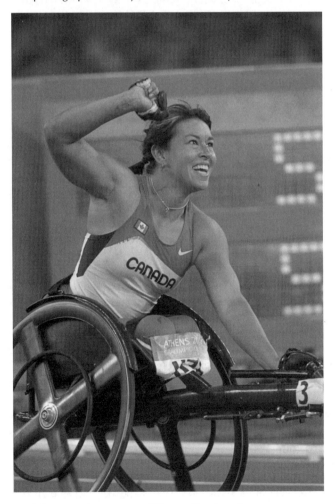

Figure 8.8   Athens 2004 (photograph courtesy of Lieven Coudenys).

the use of these facilities once the word had spread about their availability. The main dining hall, 'Philoxenos' was the setting for endless rumination over detailed sporting discussion, but also for budding friendships among people from all of the 136 nations represented at the Paralympic Games. One way that the Organising Committee ensured that there were shorter lines inside the dining facility was by the provision of street entertainers located just outside 'Philoxenos'. The crowds were often huge. The list of films shown at the open air cinema seems to reflect the thrill-seeking nature of the elite athletes: S.W.A.T., Panic Room, Trapped, I-Spy, Spiderman and more.

A tragic road traffic accident that claimed the lives of seven schoolchildren marred the euphoria of the closing of the Paralympic Games, when a bus carrying them crashed while travelling to the Games. There had been tremendous support from the children of Greece, with more than 70 000 schoolchildren being taken to watch the Games. As a mark of respect the Closing Ceremony took on a more sombre tenor, and ended in under an hour. Phil Craven said: 'Tonight should have been a night only for celebration. The children of Greece, especially, have learnt first hand the meaning of the 'Paralympic Spirit'. They are the messengers of a better world. This simple truth magnifies the tragedy that has befallen their families and friends.' The integrity with which the whole gathering shared the sense of loss was heart-wrenching. In conclusion, Phil Craven again congratulated the people of Greece on their 'passion', 'friendliness and hospitality', saying that it would have a long-lasting impact beyond the closing of the Games. Craven exhorted the athletes and the many spectators in the more subdued Olympic Stadium to: 'Continue to carry that sparkle in your eyes and keep the flame burning in your hearts'.

CONCLUSION: PARALYMPIC MOVEMENT: HOW FAR HAVE WE COME?

Any appraisal of the development of the Paralympic Movement would have to include an appreciation of the immensely strong influence of a few individuals. Ludwig Guttmann must rank as the most important figure in the emergence of a new impetus for people with disabilities. Although Guttmann's energies were aimed at a relatively small portion of what is now the broader Paralympic Family, his actions and his philosophy broke down barriers and paved the way for the worldwide phenomenon of Paralympism. At times those who worked with him were frustrated by the immovable determination of Guttmann's convictions. But due credit must be accorded him for his crusading activities from the late-1940s onwards. His doggedness and his resolve certainly stirred support in people of crusading zeal. But the dominance of Guttmann's influence also provided its own barrier to progress in some areas. Pieter Joon, during the Barcelona 1992 Paralympic Games, reflected on the development of the Paralympic Movement under the influence of Ludwig Guttmann. He gave an account of the tensions and restrictions associated with developing an international umbrella organisation. Joon suggested that the death of Guttmann in 1980 may have 'freed' international federations of their binding to a dominant paternalistic influence. But Joon correctly pointed out that there was no motivation at the time for the disparate international federations to cooperate – so the International Coordinating Committee had a tougher time moving forward. Funding was also greatly constrained: the altruistic International Fund Sport Disabled eventually proved awkward and demanding. When the International Paralympic Committee was founded, it appeared at first to be structured along the same lines as the international disability sport organisations – favouring administration rather than sports. The clear cry of the participants in the Paralympic Movement was for a democratically established, athlete-centred organisation that would move towards being more sport based.

With the gradual acceptance of functional classification, the international federations that had exerted so much influence in the earlier period of the Paralympic Movement had a much less indispensable significance. Concentration on a more sports-specific rather than disability-specific ethos made the IOSDs tangential to the main purpose of the IPC. In a tactful attempt to provide purpose for the IOSDs, the Task Force recommended (and the Strategic Review endorsed) that the international federations should become more involved in grass-roots development. This has proved to be very fruitful.

Advancement in the Paralympic Movement was greatly enhanced by sustained affirmative assistance from the International Olympic Committee, particularly through the personal inspiration of the President, Juan Antonio Samaranch. The basis of the present valuable rapport between the IPC and the IOC can be attributed to the cultivation of Samaranch's eagerness for a positive rapport between the two organisations. The fruitful relationship between corresponding Presidents has certainly continued with Phil Craven and Jacques Rogge; a more businesslike and less personal interaction that reflects the scale of the organisations they each head. The exchange of ideas is almost continuous: regular visits for members of commissions and office staff of headquarters. This relationship should continue to fortify the Paralympic Movement in the future, not least by securing the financial future of IPC. As the International Paralympic Committee became more sophisticated, and as the direction of development became more identifiable, there was a clear modelling of the IPC's administrative structures on those of the International Olympic Committee. Some participants and stakeholders criticised this, concerned about a loss of integrity and even a threat to independence. But the administrative model was a proven one, and the IPC would do well to manage its administration as effectively as the IOC. In matters of governance and politics, the two organisations have remained very different; this is entirely appropriate for IPC, and provides much of its strength. The other benefit was that of allowing the two organisations to intermesh rather more easily when there were initiatives that could overlap and thereby benefit one or both parties. This was to be borne out in the IPC's approach to bidding procedures, medical and doping policies, marketing and media rights distribution. More recently, the regular placement of IPC nominees on IOC commissions has aided the identity of athletes with a disability as full members of the sporting fraternity, while also reflecting the need for the IOC to broaden its representation in the 21st century.

There were examples of outstanding service to the Paralympic Movement by individuals – often volunteers – wherever one looked. In terms of staffing appointments, a very significant advantage was gained when Xavier Gonzalez was appointed Chief Executive Officer in January 2005. Gonzalez had been Paralympic Games Director, and then stepped into Thomas Reinecke's shoes as Interim Chief Operating Officer, until his permanent position was ratified as CEO. With his arrival in such a vital position, the International Paralympic Committee gained within its headquarters operation the benefit of his extensive and varied work with Paralympic Organising Committees.

Following in the footsteps of Guttmann, there has been a multitude of people with remarkable influence in their own particular areas. The presidents and committee members of the respective international federations, the officers of the International Coordinating Committee and the International Paralympic Committee, each have contributed to the wealth of the Paralympic Movement. The worth of Bob Steadward, as first President of the International Paralympic Committee, should not be underestimated. He exerted a pastoral influence over the growing organisation, bringing a sense of unity and steadfastness to a potentially fractious group of individuals. Steadward's persistent countering of Guttmann's 'medical model' of disability with the 'social model' proved to be essential to a modern outlook on disability. But, as with Juan Antonio Samaranch towards the end of his period of office, there began to be an awe-inspiring narrowness of identity of the Paralympic Movement with one person – the President. This was to be anticipated given the personal influence Steadward had come to exert on the Paralympic Movement. He was a confident leader: firm but diplomatic, always present and visible. As is also often the case, powerful individuals can have their 'hobby-horses' or particular views – these would come to the surface more frequently the longer one person is in office.

Having done an unparalleled job of bringing the International Paralympic Committee to the shoulder of the International Olympic Committee, and thus to a guaranteed future, it was appropriate that Steadward could not stand for re-election in 2001. Phil Craven, elected President of the International Paralympic Committee to succeed Steadward, has embarked on steering the organisation to realise strategic modifications in areas of governance and administration, as well as in Paralympic Games organisation – proposals that were initially recommended by the Task Force to which he had been appointed in 1995. The needs of the Paralympic Movement have changed in many respects from the early days of the International Paralympic Committee; the size of the phenomenon is huge, including servicing a massively complex organisation, and globally spectacular sporting celebrations every two years. Craven, a distinguished Paralympic athlete over many years and a respected sports administrator, has been known as a tough opponent both on court and around a meeting table. At times, Craven had rocked the boat in his years as President of the International Wheelchair Basketball Association, but no one has doubted his motivation or his resolve. He is poised to use his gritty, uncompromising character to secure the future for athletes with a disability.

Of particular significance has been the role of the sports in the success story of the IPC. The international federations and the sports structures have been the corner stone of the IPC. Volunteers have always been the mainstay of sporting development, and this has been even more obvious as sport for individuals with a disability has progressed. Moving away from disability-based sports organisations towards self-governing sports organisations and federations has allowed a more democratic participation of the athletes in the material decisions about their own sport. The International Paralympic Committee has been true to this objective and relies heavily on its sports structures.

Problems for the future will include rationalisation of marketing strategies so as to generate realistic operational income to be able to fulfil the objectives of the International Paralympic Committee. There are signs of great progress in this regard.

Greater clarity is being achieved in the relationship that the IPC is forging with the International Olympic Committee. There will be a constant debate about the proximity of the Paralympic Movement to the International Olympic Committee, as neutral coexistence is never straightforward. But there is a more harmonious employment of effort as a result of the accords between the two organisations. The more recent relationship has demonstrated a practical delivery of services and operational integration. Far from being beneficial in only one direction, both partners confidently function side by side with mutual respect. This is now much more of a partnership than the IOC supporting a needy junior. It has become clear that the IPC members of IOC commissions are wanted for their contributions to the Olympic Movement. With the steady and strong advancement of the recent few years, particularly through its organisational development, the IPC has located itself alongside the IOC as a player in the global political arena for sport more broadly.

Beyond financial survival and beyond the Paralympic Games spectaculars, the IPC must enhance its services to athletes. To do this it must help the National Paralympic Committees and Regions to achieve more in training and support outside Paralympic competition, as well as continuing to enrich the lives of so many people through the highest quality Paralympic Games.

To find a reasonable answer to the complex position of athletes with an intellectual disability is easier said than done. It is desirable to see the return of INAS-FID athletes to the Paralympic competition cycle, but this should not be without first ensuring that there are practicable and sustainable processes by which to ensure fair competition.

Among its other ongoing roles, the International Paralympic Committee has accepted the mission of addressing the issues of athletes with a severe disability and the issues of women in sport. These are truly meaningful challenges, but for a Movement that has already broken down so many societal barriers there can be no doubt of the positive outcomes the future will bring. A refreshing and revealing sign of the modern outlook on the concept of disability can be seen in an interview with

Tanni Grey-Thompson published in the *Daily Telegraph* (29th September 2004). The British wheel-chair athlete with 11 Paralympic gold medals to her name was responding to the notion that she had 'suffered' from spina bifida: 'I've never, ever *suffered* from being born with spina bifida ... I saw a Chinese athlete missing both arms tapping out a text message on his mobile using his toes. When he saw us looking he came over with a huge grin to show us how it was done.'

Sport is a powerful instrument for social change, and for the realization of individual goals. The Paralympic Movement has come of age; now a mature adult accepting responsibility for those in need of support and their own empowerment. The International Paralympic Committee has carved out a worthy mission, and the work of the future will be precious in its service to individuals with a disability. But there will be challenges offered through difficulties and controversies. As Theodore Roosevelt said: 'Far and away the best prize that life offers is the chance to work hard at work worth doing'.

Bibliography and Resources

I am grateful to the International Olympic Committee and the International Paralympic Committee for their help in obtaining the research material for this publication. Their confidence has been necessary in order for me to have the restrictions lifted on access to normally confidential papers. Unless otherwise stated, the detailed analysis of this book is based on personal interviews and material made available by the International Olympic Committee at the Olympic Museum and Research Centre in Lausanne, and the International Paralympic Committee Headquarters in Bonn.

BIBLIOGRAPHY

Albrecht, Gary (1976) *The Sociology of Physical Disability and Rehabilitation*. Pittsburgh: University of Pittsburgh Press.

Amako, T. (1967). Workshops for Paraplegics in Japan. *Paraplegia*, 5: 131–132.

Ammons, D. (1986). World Games for the Deaf. In Sherrill, C. (Ed.). *Sport and Disabled Athletes: The 1984 Olympic Scientific Congress Proceedings Volume 9*. Champaign, IL: Human Kinetics.

Anderson, J. (2003). Turned into Taxpayers: Paraplegia, Rehabilitation and Sport at Stoke Mandeville, 1944–1956. *Journal of Contemporary History*, 38 (3): 461–475.

Atha, B.P. (1994). Issues in Classification in Sport for the Mentally Handicapped. In R. Steadward, E. Nelson and G. Wheeler (Eds), *VISTA '93: The Outlook: Proceedings of the International Conference on High Performance Sport for Athletes With Disabilities* (pp. 304–309). Edmonton, AB, Canada: Rick Hansen Centre.

Atlanta Paralympic Organizing Committee. (n.d.). *The Triumph of the Human Spirit*. Atlanta, GA: ATOC.

Bailey, S.J. (1996). *Science in the Service of Physical Education and Sport*. Chichester: John Wiley and Sons Ltd.

Bailey, S.J. and Vamplew, W. (1999). *100 Years of Physical Education 1899–1999*. Warwick: Warwick Printing Co.

Bedbrook, G.M. (1987). The Development and Care of Spinal Cord Paralysis (1918 to 1986). *Paraplegia*. 25: 172–184.

Berridge, M.E. and Ward, G.R. (1987). *International Perspectives on Adapted Physical Activity*. Champaign, IL: Human Kinetics.

Berthe, P. (1964). 18th Olympic Games, 2nd Paralympic Games. In *The 1964 International Stoke Mandeville Games for the Paralysed in Tokyo*. Aylesbury, UK: Hunt Barnard.

Bourke, J. (1991, July). Athletics Functional Classification Paper. In *Proceedings of Kevin Betts Sports Science Symposium on Functional Classification*. Aylesbury, England: ISMGF.

Brandmeyer, G.A. and McBee, G.F. (1986) Social Status and Athletic Competition for the Disabled Athlete, In Sherrill, C.

Brasile, F.M. (1990). Wheelchair Sports: a New Perspective on Integration. *Adapted Physical Activity Quarterly*, 4 (7): 3–11.

Brasile, F.M. (1992). Inclusion: a Developmental Perspective–a Rejoinder to Examining the Concept of Reverse Integration. *Adapted Physical Activity Quarterly*, 9: 293–304.

Burns, S.R. (1955). *Committee Report*. Amateur Athletic Association for the Deaf International Games.

Caton, M. (2003). [Question on Learning-Disabled Athletes] House of Commons Hansard, 31 March, Column 766–780.

Chappel, R. (1994). Classification in Cerebral Palsy Athletes. In *Proceedings of the Second Paralympic Congress* (pp. 93–99). Lillehammer, Norway: Royal Norwegian Ministry of Cultural Affairs.

Comité International des Sports des Sourds (1961). *Bulletin* No. 25, April 1961.

Comité International des Sports des Sourds (1962). *Bulletin* No. 30, July 1962.

Comité International des Sports des Sourds (1985). XV World Games for the Deaf. *The Silent News*, Commemorative Edition.

COOB '92 (1993). *Paralympics '92: Barcelona 1992, IX Paralympic Games Official Report*. Barcelona: Enciclopedia Catalonia, S.A.

Damanski, M. (1964). The Paraplegic Patient as a Social Problem. *Paraplegia*. 2: 169–177.

DePauw, K.P. (1985). History of Sports for Individuals with Disabilities. *Able Bodies*, 4: 1, 3.

DePauw, K.P. (1986a). Research on Sport for Athletes with Disabilities. *Adapted Physical Activity Quarterly*. 3: 292–299.

DePauw, K.P. (1986b). Toward Progressive Inclusion and Acceptance: Implications for Physical Education. *Adapted Physical Activity Quarterly*. 3: 1–5.

DePauw, K.P. and Gavron, S. J. (1995). *Disability and Sport*. Champaign, IL: Human Kinetics.

DePauw, K.P. and Rich, S. (1993). Paralympics for the Mentally Handicapped. *Palaestra*. 9: 59–64.

Doll-Tepper, G., IPCSSC and IFAPA (1994). *The Future of Sport Science in the Paralympic Movement*. Berlin: German Olympic Institute.

Doll-Tepper, G., IPCSSC and IFAPA (1995). *The Paralympic Movement: New Directions and Issues in Sport Science*. Berlin: German Olympic Institute.

Doll-Tepper, G. *et al.* (Eds) (1990). *Adapted Physical Activity: An Interdisciplinary Approach*. Berlin: Springer-Verlag.

Eason, R, Smith, T. and Caron, F. (Eds) (1983). *Adapted Physical Activity: From Theory to Application*. Champaign, IL: Human Kinetics.

Eisenberg, M., Griggins, C. and Duval, R. (Eds) (1982) *Disabled People as Second-Class Citizens*. New York: Springer Publishing Co.

Fundacion ONCE (1993). I Paralympic Congress (Barcelona 1992). Madrid: ONCE.

Goffman, E. (1963). *Stigma: Notes on the Management of Spoiled Identity*. Englewood Cliffs, NJ: Prentice-Hall, Inc.

Goldman, S. (1997). Athlete First. *Olympian*, May/June, pp 10–15.

Goldstein, T., Simonds, T. and Sanders, C. (1994) *Succeeding Together: People with Disabilities in the Workplace*. Northridge, CA: California State University.

Goodman, S. (1986). *The Spirit of Stoke Mandeville: The Story of Sir Ludwig Guttmann*. London: William Collins Sons and Co. Ltd.

Gregory, S. and Hartley, G. (1991). *Constructing Deafness*. London: Pinter Publishers.

Guttmann, L. (1945). New Hope for Spinal Cord Sufferers. *New York Medical Times*. 73: 318.

Guttmann, L. (1949a). Readjustment to a New Life. *The Cord*. 2: 21.

Guttmann, L. (1949b). The Annual Stoke Mandeville Games. *The Cord*. 3: 24.

Guttmann, L. (1952). On the Way to an International Sports Movement for the Paralysed. *The Cord*. 5.

Guttmann, L. (1953a). *British Medical History of World War II: Surgery*. London: HMSO.

Guttmann, L. (1953b). The Treatment and Rehabilitation of Patients with Injuries of the Spinal Cord. In Guttman, L. *British Medical History of World War II: Surgery* (pp. 431–516) London: HMSO.

Guttmann, L. (1954a). Looking Back on a Decade. *The Cord*. 6 (4): 9–23.

Guttmann, L. (1954b). Statistical Survey of One Thousand Paraplegics and Initial Treatment of Traumatic Paraplegia. *Proceedings of the Royal Society of Medicine*, 47: 1099–1109.

Guttmann, L. (1958). *Modern Trends in Diseases of the Spinal Column*. London: Butterworth.

Guttmann, L. (1960). The International Stoke Mandeville Games in Rome. *The Cord*.

Guttmann, L. (1962a). Sport and the Disabled. *Sport Medicine* 367–391. London: Arnold.

Guttmann, L. (1962b). The First 10 Years of the International Stoke Mandeville Games for the Paralysed. *The Cord*. 14: 30–39.

Guttmann, L. (1964). The International Stoke Mandeville Games for the Paralysed in Tokyo. *Physiotherapy*. 51: 252–3.

Guttmann, L. (1965). Reflections in Sport for the Physically Handicapped. *Physiotherapy*.

Guttmann, L. (1967a). History of the National Spinal Injuries Centre, Stoke Mandeville Hospital, Aylesbury, *Paraplegia*. 5: 115–126.

Guttmann, L. (1967b). Sport for the Disabled as a World Problem: *Proceedings of the International Seminar, British Council for Rehabilitation*. Brighton. Rehabilitation.

Guttmann, L. (1971). Sport for the Disabled. *Times Educational Supplement*. July 16, pp. 31–32.

Guttmann, L. (1973a). Sport and Recreation for the Mentally and Physically Handicapped. Conference on Sport for All. Royal Society of Health, 1–6.

Guttmann, L. (1973b). *Spinal Cord Injuries: Comprehensive Management and Research*. Oxford: Blackwell Scientific Publications.

Guttmann, L. (1976). *Sport for the Disabled*. Oxford: Alden Press.

Hansen, R. and Taylor, J. (1987). *Rick Hansen: Man in Motion*. Vancouver BC: Douglas and McIntyre.

Huber, C.A. (1984). An Overview and Perspective on International Disabled Sport: Past, Present Future. *Rehabilitation World*. 8: 8–11.

Hunt, P. (Ed.) (1966). *Stigma: The Experience of Disability*. London: Chapman.

IBSA. and Fundacion ONCE (1994). *Sport and Disability Meeting: Summer Course of the Madrid Complutense University Foundation*, San Lorenzo de El Escorial, 19th August 1994.

Jackson, P. (1990). *Britain's Deaf Heritage*. Edinburgh: Pentland.

Jennings, A. (1996). *The New Lords of the Rings*. New York: Simon and Schuster.

Jernigan, K. (1993). Resolution 93/01. *National Federation of the Blind Convention*, Dallas, Texas, 9th July 1993.

Jochheim, K. and Strohkendl, J. (1973). The Value of Particular Sports of the Wheelchair-Disabled in Maintaining Health of the Paraplegic. *Paraplegia*. 11: 173–178.

Kasai, Y. (1964). Hosts to the Games in Tokyo. In *The 1964 International Stoke Mandeville Games for the Paralysed in Tokyo*. Aylesbury, UK: Hunt Barnard.

Labanowich, S. (1988). A Case for the Integration of the Disabled into the Olympic Games. *Adapted Physical Activity Quarterly*. 5: 264–272.

Landry, F. (1992). Olympism, Olympics, Paralympism, Paralympics: Converging or diverging notions and courses on the eve of the third millennium? Paper presented at the *First Paralympic Congress*, 31st August 1992, Barcelona.

Legg, D., Emes, C., Stewart, D. and Steadward, R. (2004). Historical Overview of the Paralympics, Special Olympics and Deaflympics. *Palaestra*. 20 (1): 30–38.

Leonard, G. (1974). *The Ultimate Athlete*. New York: Viking Press, Inc.

Lieberman, L.J. and Houston-Wilson, C. (2002). *Strategies for Inclusion: A Handbook for Physical Educators*. Champaign, IL: Human Kinetics.

Lindström, H. (1990). The Dramatic Birth of a New International Body for the Disabled. *Palaestra*. 6: 12–15.

Lindström, H. (1994a). Integration in Sports for Persons with Disabilities: An Overview. In Steadward, E. Nelson and G. Wheeler (Eds), *Vista '93: The Outlook: Proceedings of the International Conference on High Performance Sport for Athletes With Disabilities* (pp. 333–344). Edmonton and Jesper, Alberta: R. Hansen Center.

Lindström, H. (1994b). Integration of Sports for Athletes with Disabilities on International Level: Perspectives for the Future. In *Proceedings of the Second Paralympic Congress* (pp. 273–284). Lillehammer, Norway: Royal Norwegian Ministry of Cultural Affairs.

Lockwood, R. (1987). *Physical Education and Disability*. Parkside, Australia: ACHPER.

Masham S. in the Cord (Anniversary Issue)

Massingale J.D. and Swanson, R.A. (Eds) (1997). *The History of Exercise and Sport Science*. Champaign, IL: Human Kinetics.

McKenzie, R. Tait (1909). *Exercise in Education and Medicine*. Philadelphia: W.B. Saunders Company.

Mester, J. (1994). *Sport Sciences in Europe 1993: Current and Future Perspectives*. Aachen: Meyer and Meyer.

Miller, J.O. (1984). Sport for Disabled Australians. In Sherrill, C. (Ed.) *Sport and Disabled Athletes: The 1984 Olympic Scientific Congress Proceedings Volume 9*. Champaign, IL: Human Kinetics.

Morgan, W. (2007). *Ethics in Sport*. Champaign, IL: Human Kinetics.

Munro, D. (1945). Treatment of Patients with Injuries of the Spinal Cord and Cauda Equina Preliminary to Making Them Ambulatory. *Clinics*. 4: 448–474.

Munro, D. (1950). Two Year End Results in the Total Rehabilitation of Veterans with Spinal Cord and Cauda Equina Injuries. *New England Medical Journal*. 242: 223–235.

Paciorek, M.A. and Jones, J.A. (1989). Sports and Recreation for the Disabled. Masters Press.

Padden, C. and Humphries, T. (1988). *Deaf in America: Voices from a Culture*. London: Harvard University Press.

Peterson, R.W. (1990). *Cages to Jump Shots*. New York: Oxford University Press.

Price, B. (1998). Paralympic Compatibility with the Olympic Movement. *International Olympic Academy Proceedings*. 38, 15–30 July.

Reinecke, T. and Reiff, S. (2002). Paralympics: celebrating sporting excellence of athletes with a disability. *ICSSPE Bulletin*. 35, May.

Riddoch, G. (1941). Phantom limbs and body shape. *Brain*. 64: 197–222.

Roaf, R. (1972). International Classification of Spinal Injuries. *Paraplegia*. 10: 78.

Rosenberg, Janet and Phillips, William R. F. (Eds) (1980) *The Origins of Modern Treatment and Education of Physically Handicapped Children*. New York: Arno Press.

Ruckert, H. (1980) *Olympics for the Disabled, Holland 1980, Commemorative Book*. Netherlands: Stichting Olympische Spelen voor Gehandicapten.

Salt Lake Organizing Committee (2000). Salt Lake 2002. *Paralympic Media Update*. Fall/Winter.

Samaranch, J.A. (1994). *Sport and Disability Meeting, 19th August 1994*. Madrid: ONCE Foundation.

Scruton, J. (1960). The 1960 International Stoke Mandeville Games. *The Cord*. Special Edition, 14–21.

Scruton, J. (1964). *The 1964 International Stoke Mandeville Games for the Paralysed in Tokyo*. Aylesbury, UK: Hunt Barnard.

Scruton, J. (1998). *Stoke Mandeville: Road to the Paralympics*. Aylesbury: The Peterhouse Press.

Seaman, J. and DePauw, K. (1989). *The New Adapted Physical Education: A Developmental Approach*. Palo Alto, CA: Mayfield.

Shephard, R.J. (1990). *Fitness in Special Populations*. Champaign: Human Kinetics.

Sherrill, C. (Ed.) (1984). *Sport and Disabled Athletes: The 1984 Olympic Scientific Congress Proceedings Volume 9*. Champaign, IL. Human Kinetics.

Sherrill, C. (Ed.) (1986). *Sport and Disabled Athletes*. Champaign: Human Kinetics.

Sherrill, C. (1989). Yang and Yin of the 1988 Paralympics. *Palaestra*. 5(4), 53–59, 76.

Sherrill, C. (1993). *Adapted Physical Activity, Recreation and Sport: Crossdisciplinary and Lifespan* (4th ed.). Dubuque, IA: Brown and Benchmark.

Songster, T.B. (1984). The Special Olympics Sport Program: An international sport program for mentally retarded athletes. In Sherrill, C. (Ed.) *Sport and Disabled Athletes: The 1984 Olympic Scientific Congress Proceedings Volume 9*. Champaign, IL: Human Kinetics.

Steadward, R.D. (1992). Excellence: The future of Sports for Athletes with Disabilities. In Williams, T., Almond, L. and Sparkes, A. (Eds) *Sport and Physical Activity: Moving Towards Excellence* (pp. 293–299). London, UK: E and FN Spon.

Steadward, R.D., Nelson E.R. and Wheeler G.D. (1994). *The Outlook*. Edmonton, AB: Rick Hansen Center.

Stewart, D. (1993). *Deaf Sports: The Impact of Sports within the Deaf Community*. Washington DC: Gallaudet University Press.

Strohkendl, H. (1991, July). The Relevance of Understanding Sport-Specific Functional Classification in Wheelchair Sports and its Future Development. In *Proceedings of Kevin Betts Sports Science Symposium on Functional Classification*. Aylesbury, England: ISMGF.

Strohkendl, H. (1996). The 50th Anniversary of Wheelchair Basketball: A History, New York, Waxman Publishing Company.

Taylor, G. and Bishop, J. (Eds) (1991). *Being Deaf: The Experience of Deafness*. London: Pinter Publishers.

Thiboutot, A., Smith, R.W. and Labanowich, S. (1992). Examining the concept of Reverse Integration: A Response to Brasile's "New Perspective" on Integration. *Adapted Physical Activity Quarterly*. 9: 283–292.

Whitteridge, D. (1983). Ludgwig Guttmann. 3 July 1899–18 March 1980. *Biographical Memoirs of Fellows of the Royal Society*. 29 (Nov.): 226–244.

Wilcox, S. (Ed.) (1989). *American Deaf Culture*. Burtonsville, Maryland: Linstock.

Williams, T., Almond, L. and Sparkes, A. (Eds) (1992). *Sport and Physical Activity*. Spon Press.

Winnick, J. (1990). *Adapted Physical Education and Sport*. Champaign, IL: Human Kinetics.

Yabe, K., Kusano, K. and Nakata, H. (1994). *Adapted Physical Activity: Health and Fitness*. Springer Verlag.

JOURNALS

Active Living Magazine
Disability Today Publishing Group
P.O. Box 2659
Niagara Falls, NY 14302-9945

Adapted Physical Activity Quarterly
International Federation of Adapted Physical Activity

Disability Today
Disability Today Publishing Group
P.O. 2659
Niagara Falls, NY 14302-9945

International Paralympic Committee Newsletter

Sports N' Spokes
Paralyzed Veterans of America
801 Eighteenth Street, NW
Washington, DC 20006-3517

Palaestra
Circulation Dept., Challenge Publication
P.O. Box 508
Macomb, IL 61455

CORRESPONDENCE

Archer, Stephen M. to Otto Mayer, 23rd April 1963
Brundage, Avery to Armand Massard, David Lord Burghley, H.R.H. Prince Axel of Denmark, Mr. Mohammed Taher, Dr Miguel A. Moenck, Count Paolo de Revel, Mr. Otto Mayer, 14th September 1954
Brundage, Avery to Cesare Magarotto and Vittorio Ieralla, 20th December 1954.
Brundage, Avery to S. Robey Burns, 6th August 1955.
Brundage, Avery to S. Robey Burns, 22nd August 1955.
Brundage, Avery to V. Tschernishev, Editor, Sovietskaja Russia, 8th August 1956.
Brundage, Avery to Antoine Dresse, 7th August 1958.
Brundage, Avery to J.P. Nielsen, 18th June 1961.
Brundage, Avery to S. Robey Burns, 15th July 1961.
Brundage, Avery to John H. Norton, 11th May 1956.
Brundage, Avery to David Peikoff, 13th January 1965.
Brundage, Avery to Jerald Jordan, 15th March 1965.
Burns, S. Robey to Avery Brundage, February 1955.
Burns, S. Robey to Otto Mayer, 29th March 1955
Burns, S. Robey to Avery Brundage, 15th August 1955
Burns, S. Robey to Otto Mayer, 26th September 1955
Burns, S. Robey to Otto Mayer, 14th June 1961
Burns, S. Robey to Avery Brundage, 11th July 1961
Burns, S. Robey to Avery Brundage, 26th July 1961
Burns, S. Robey to Otto Mayer, 26th July 1961
Dresse, Antoine to Otto Mayer, 10th October 1953
Dresse, Antoine and Ryden, Oscar to Members of the International Olympic Committee, 22nd October 1954
Dresse, Antoine to Otto Mayer, 25th July 1955
Dresse, Antoine to Otto Mayer, 28th May 1958
Dresse, Antoine to Avery Brundage, 8th September 1958
Dresse, Antoine to Otto Mayer, 6th May 1961
Dresse, Antoine and J.P. Nielsen to Otto Mayer, 3rd June 1961
Ferris, Daniel J. to Avery Brundage, 7th April 1961.

Hillegers, Marjolijn to Hans Lindström, 27th November 1986.
Jordan, Jerald M. to Avery Brundage, 9th October 1962.
Jordan, Jerald M. to Avery Brundage, 1st March 1965.
Labanowich, Stan to Juan Antonio Samaranch, 5th March 1984.
Lindström, Hans to M. Hillegers, 10th November 1986.
Magarotto, Cesare and Ieralla, Vittorio to Avery Brundage, 20th December 1954
Magarotto, Cesare to Otto Mayer, 2nd July 1955
Magarotto, Cesare to Otto Mayer, 7th August 1955
Mayer, Otto to E Conti, 13th March 1951
Mayer, Otto to Antoine Dresse, 14th October 1953
Mayer, Otto to Cesare Magarotto, 11th July 1955
Mayer, Otto to CISS, 19th August 1961
Mayer, Otto to CISS, 24th June 1955
Mayer, Otto to IOC Executive Committee Members, 6th August 1954
Mayer, Otto to S. Robey Burns, 24th June 1955
Mayer, Otto to Federazione Sport Silenziosi d'Italia, 3rd October 1955
Mayer, Otto to S. Robey Burns, 3rd October 1955
Mayer, Otto to Avery Brundage, 3rd June 1958
Mayer, Otto to S. Robey Burns, 3rd August 1961
Mayer, Otto to Stephen M. Archer, 29th April 1963
Miller, F. Don to Dale Wiley, 28th April 1981
Neumann to Samaranch, 3 February 1983
Peikoff, David to Avery Brundage, 25th November 1964
Peikoff, David to Avery Brundage, 11th January 1965
Samaranch, Juan Antonio to Stan Labanowich, 16th March 1984
Westerhoff J.W. to A. Lentz, 18th November 1966

PAPERS RELATING TO THE INTERNATIONAL COORDINATING COMMITTEE

Paper on the position of the ICC towards the United Nations, Arnhem, 14th January 1986
The structure and future of ICC, Observations ICC minutes August 1986, page 2
The structure and future of ICC
ICC Administration
Concept agreement International Coordinating Committee (ICC) of World Sports Organisations for the Disabled, Agenda 1st Session ICC Meeting 30th January–1st February 1987
Paralympics Administration, Enclosure 15, Agenda 1st Session ICC Meeting 30th January–1st February 1987
To the Presidents and Secretary Generals of: CP-ISRA, IBSA, ISMGF and ISOD re: ICC Seminar, December 24th 1986, from Marjolijn Hillegers
Report of Ad Hoc Committee

IPC EXECUTIVE COMMITTEE MINUTES

Minutes of 1st IPC Executive Committee Meeting, Duisberg, Germany, 23rd September 1989
Minutes of 2nd IPC Executive Committee Meeting, Brugge, Belgium, 30th November – 1st December
Minutes of 3rd IPC Executive Committee Meeting, Groningen, The Netherlands, 15th – 17th July 1990
Minutes of 4th IPC Executive Committee Meeting, Brugge, Belgium, 16th and 17th November 1990
Minutes of 5th IPC Executive Committee Meeting, Lillehammer, Norway, 9th and 10th May 1991
Minutes of 6th IPC Executive Committee Meeting, Budapest, Hungary, 1st and 3rd November 1991
Minutes of 7th IPC Executive Committee Meeting, Tignes, France, 29th – 31st March 1991
Minutes of Business Meetings of IPC Executive Committee, Barcelona, Spain, 7th and 10th September 1992
Minutes of 8th IPC Executive Committee Meeting, Manchester, England, 5th and 6th December 1992

Minutes of 9th IPC Executive Committee Meeting, Lillehammer, Norway, 18th – 21st March 1993
Minutes of 10th IPC Executive Committee Meeting, Berlin, Germany, 9th, 12th and 13th September, 1993
Minutes of 11th IPC Executive Committee Meeting, Lillehammer, Norway, 7th – 10th March 1994
Minutes of 12th IPC Executive Committee Meeting, Paris, France, 18th – 20th November 1994
Minutes of 13th IPC Executive Committee Meeting, Atlanta, USA, 28th – 30th April 1995
Minutes of 14th IPC Executive Committee Meeting, Tokyo and Nagano, Japan, 5th and 11th November 1995
Minutes of 15th IPC Executive Committee Meeting, Cairo, Egypt, 3rd – 5th March 1996
Minutes of 16th IPC Executive Committee Meeting, Atlanta, USA, 12th – 14th August 1996
Minutes of 17th IPC Executive Committee Meeting, Lisle, France, 24th – 26th January 1997
Minutes of 18th IPC Executive Committee Meeting, Nagano, Japan, 22nd – 23rd May 1997
Minutes of 19th IPC Executive Committee Meeting, Sydney, Australia, 4th, 5th and 9th November 1997
Minutes of 20th IPC Executive Committee Meeting, Nagano, Japan, 4th March 1998
Minutes of 21st IPC Executive Committee Meeting, Lausanne, Switzerland, 19th – 20th May 1998
All remaining committee minutes published on-line

Index